Handbook
Orthopaed

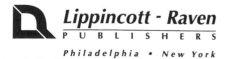

Edited by

Raymond G. Hart, M.D., M.P.H.
Assistant Clinical Professor
Department of Emergency Medicine
University of Louisville
Louisville, Kentucky;
University of Illinois at Chicago
Chicago, Illinois

Timothy James Rittenberry, M.D.
Associate Professor of Clinical Emergency Medicine
Department of Emergency Medicine
University of Illinois at Chicago
Chicago, Illinois;
Director of Emergency Medical Education
Department of Emergency Medicine
Illinois Masonic Medical Center
Chicago, Illinois

Dennis T. Uehara, M.D., F.A.C.E.P.
Clinical Assistant Professor
Department of Surgery
University of Illinois at Rockford;
Chairman
Department of Emergency Medicine
Rockford Health System
Rockford, Illinois

Illustrations by Quinn Heath

Lippincott - Raven
P U B L I S H E R S
Philadelphia • New York

Acquisitions Editor: Elizabeth Greenspan
Developmental Editor: Rebecca Irwin Diehl
Manufacturing Manager: Kevin Watt
Production Manager: Robert Pancotti
Production Editor: Christina Zingone
Cover Designer: J.E. Norton
Indexer: Nanette Cardon
Compositor: Compset
Printer: R. R. Donnelley–Crawfordsville

Printed in the United States of America

9 8 7 6 5 4 3 2 1

Library of Congress Cataloging-in-Publication Data
Handbook of orthopaedic emergencies / editors, Raymond G. Hart,
  Timothy James Rittenberry, Dennis T. Uehara; illustrated by Quinn
  Heath.
       p.   cm.
    Includes bibliographical references and index.
    ISBN 0-7817-1610-1
    1. Orthopaedic emergencies—Handbooks, manuals, etc.   I. Hart,
  Raymond G.   II. Rittenberry, Timothy J.   III. Uehara, Dennis T.
    [DNLM: 1. Orthopaedics–methods handbooks. 2. Emergency Medicine–
  methods handbooks.   3. Wounds and Injuries–therapy handbooks.
  4. Extremities–injuries handbooks.   WE 39 H2358 1999]
  RD750.H36   1999
  617.4´7026–DC21
  DNLM/DLC
  for Library of Congress   98-4109
                                                                  CIP

To Raymond F. and Mary Lenihan Hart
for their love, guidance, and support.

R.G.H.

To family, friends, and all my teachers
who took the time to care.

T.J.R.

In memory of Ronnie Lee, colleague, co-conspirator,
and good friend.

D.T.U.

Handbook of
Orthopaedic Emergencies

Contents

I. Orthopaedics

II. Upper Extremity Orthopaedics

III. Lower Extremity Orthopaedics

IV. Spine

V. Pediatric Orthopaedics

VI. Special Topics in Emergency Medicine

Contributing Authors

Brian N. Aldred, M.D., F.A.C.E.P. *Clinical Assistant Professor, Department of Surgery, University of Illinois at Rockford; Staff Physician, Emergency Department, Rockford Memorial Hospital, 2400 North Rockton Avenue, Rockford, Illinois 61103*

Felix Ankel, M.D. *Assistant Professor of Clinical Emergency Medicine, Emergency Medicine Program, University of Minnesota Medical School, 420 Delaware Street Southeast, Minneapolis, Minnesota 55455; Assistant Residency Director, Department of Emergency Medicine, Regions Hospital, 640 Jackson Street, St. Paul, Minnesota 55101–2595*

Jefferson D. Bracey, D.O., F.A.C.E.P. *Assistant Professor, Department of Surgery, University of Nevada School of Medicine, Reno, Nevada 89501; Director of Cost Containment and Utilization Management, Departments of Emergency Medicine and Trauma, University Medical Center, 1800 West Charleston, Las Vegas, Nevada 89102*

Todd H. Chaffin, M.D., F.A.C.E.P. *Rockford Memorial Hospital, 2400 North Rockton Avenue, Rockford, Illinois 61103*

Harold W. Chin, M.D. *Clinical Assistant Professor, Department of Medicine, University of Chicago, 5841 South Maryland Avenue, Chicago, Illinois 60637; Attending Physician, Department of Emergency Medicine, Lutheran General Hospital, 1775 West Dempster Street, Park Ridge, Illinois 60068*

Paul J. Donovan, D.O., F.A.C.E.P. *Medical Director, U.S. Ski Team Physician, Northern Berkshire Sports Medicine, The Sports Medicine Institute; Staff Physician, Emergency Department, North Adams Regional Hospital, Hospital Avenue, Suite 307–Doctors Building, North Adams, Massachusetts 01247*

Wesley P. Eilbert, M.D., F.A.C.E.P. *Clinical Assistant Professor, Department of Emergency Medicine, University of Illinois at Chicago, 1740 West Taylor Street, Chicago, Illinois 60612; Director of Undergraduate Education, Department of Emergency Medicine, Mercy Hospital and Medical Center, 2525 South Michigan Avenue, Chicago, Illinois 60616*

Wendy S. Filener, M.D. *Clinical Fellow, Department of Emergency Medicine, Tufts University School of Medicine, 136 Harrison Avenue, Boston, Massachusetts 02111; Resident, Department of Emergency Medicine, Baystate Medical Center, 759 Chestnut Street, Springfield, Massachusetts 01199*

Angelo Grillo, M.D. *Instructor, Department of Surgery, Thomas Jefferson Medical College, 1025 Walnut Street, Philadelphia, Pennsylvania 19107; Attending Physician, Department of Emergency Medicine, Christiana Care Health System, 4755 Ogletown-Stanton Road, Newark, Delaware 19718*

Raymond G. Hart, M.D., M.P.H. *Assistant Clinical Professor, Department of Emergency Medicine, University of Louisville, 706 Colonel Anderson Parkway, Louisville, Kentucky 40222; University of Illinois at Chicago, 1740 West Taylor Street, Suite 1600, Chicago, Illinois 60614*

Teresita M. Hogan, M.D. *Associate Professor, Department of Emergency Medicine, University of Illinois at Chicago, 1740 West Taylor Street, Chicago, Illinois 60612; Residency Director, Department of Emergency Medicine, Resurrection Medical Center, 7435 West Talcott Avenue, Chicago, Illinois 60631*

Melinda S. Jasani, M.D., F.A.A.P. *Department of Emergency Medicine, St. Christopher's Hospital for Children, Erie Avenue at Front Street, Philadelphia, Pennsylvania 19134*

Neil B. Jasani, M.D. F.A.C.E.P. *Clinical Instructor, Department of Emergency Medicine, Thomas Jefferson University, 1025 Walnut Street, Philadelphia, Pennsylvania 19107; Associate Residency Director, Department of Emergency Medicine, Medical Center of Delaware, 4755 Ogletown-Stanton Road, Newark, Delaware 19718*

Patricia Lee, M.D., F.A.C.E.P. *Clinical Assistant Professor, Department of Emergency Medicine, University of Illinois at Chicago, 1819 West Polk Street, Suite, 618 (M/C 724), College of Medicine, West Chicago, Illinois 60612; Attending Physician, Department of Emergency Medicine, Illinois Masonic Medical Center, 836 West Wellington Avenue, Chicago, Illinois 60657*

Brian A. Macaulay, M.D., F.A.C.E.P. *Assistant Clinical Professor, Department of Emergency Medicine, University of Illinois at Chicago, 1819 West Polk Street, Suite 618 (M/C 724), College of Medicine West, Chicago, Illinois 60612; Director, Department of Emergency Medicine, Norwegian American Hospital, 1044 North Francisco Avenue, Chicago, Illinois 60622*

Valerie Neylan, M.D., F.A.C.E.P. *Assistant Professor and Associate Residency Director, Department of Emergency Medicine, University of Illinois at Chicago, 1740 West Taylor Street, Suite 1600 (M/C 722), Chicago, Illinois 60612*

Robert E. O'Connor, M.D., M.P.H. *Clinical Associate Professor, Department of Emergency Medicine, Thomas Jefferson University, 1025 Walnut Street, Philadelphia, Pennsylvania 19107; Director of Education and Research, Department of Emergency Medicine, Christiana Care Health System, 4755 Ogletown-Stanton Road, Newark, Delaware 19718*

Kenji Oyasu, M.D. *Assistant Clinical Professor, Department of Emergency Medicine, University of Illinois at Chicago, 1740 West Taylor Street, Chicago, Illinois 60612; Staff Physician, Department of Emergency Medicine, Lutheran General Hospital, 1775 West Dempster Street, Park Ridge, Illinois 60068*

Thomas S. Pannke, M.D., F.A.C.E.P. *Assistant Professor, Department of Surgery, University of Illinois at Rockford; Attending Physician, Emergency Department, Rockford Memorial Hospital, 2400 Rockton Avenue, Rockford, Illinois 61103*

Charles F. Pattavina, M.D., F.A.C.E.P. *Assistant Professor, Department of Medicine, Brown University, Thayer Street, Providence, Rhode Island 02906; Chief, Department of Emergency Medicine, The Miriam Hospital, 164 Summit Avenue, Providence, Rhode Island 02906*

John T. Piotrowski, M.D. *Associate, Department of Emergency Medicine, University of Illinois at Chicago, 1740 West Taylor Street, Chicago, Illinois 60612; Attending Physician, Department of Emergency Medicine, Illinois Masonic Medical Center, 836 West Wellington Avenue, Chicago, Illinois 60657*

Stephen J. Playe, M.D. *Assistant Professor, Department of Emergency Medicine, Tufts University School of Medicine, 136 Harrison Avenue, Boston, Massachusetts 02111; Residency Program Director, Department of Emergency Medicine, Baystate Medical Center, 759 Chestnut Street, Springfield, Massachusetts 01199*

Arthur F. Proust, M.D., F.A.C.E.P. *Clinical Assistant Professor, Department of Surgery, University of Illinois at Rockford; Assistant Director, Emergency Department, Rockford Memorial Hospital, 2400 North Rockton Avenue, Rockford, Illinois 61103*

Timothy James Rittenberry, M.D. *Associate Professor of Clinical Emergency Medicine, Department of Emergency Medicine, University of Illinois at Chicago, 1740 West Taylor Street, Suite 1600, Chicago, Illinois 60614; Director of Emergency Medical Education, Department of Emergency Medicine, Illinois Masonic Medical Center, 836 West Wellington Street, Chicago, Illinois 60657*

Alok C. Saxena, M.D., F.A.C.E.P *Associate Professor of Clinical Medicine, Departments of Surgery, Internal Medicine, and Trauma, University of Nevada School of Medicine; Director of Education, Department of Emergency Medicine, University Medical Center, 1800 West Charleston Boulevard, Las Vegas, Nevada 89102*

Joseph L. Tasto, M.D., M.S. *Director of Medical Research and Technology, HT Medical, Inc., 6001 Montrose Road, Suite 902, Rockville, Maryland 20852*

David A. Townes, M.D., M.P.H. *International Emergency Medicine and Public Health Fellow, Attending Physician, Department of Emergency Medicine, University of Illinois at Chicago, 1740 West Taylor Street, Chicago, Illinois 60612*

Mary Jo Wagner, M.D. *Assistant Professor, Program in Emergency Medicine, Michigan State University College of Human Medicine; Associate Director, Department of Emergency Medicine, Saginaw Cooperative Hospitals, Inc., 1000 Houghton Avenue, Saginaw, Michigan 48602*

Diana Rae Williams, M.D., M.H.P.E. *Director of Education, Department of Emergency Medicine, MacNeal Memorial Hospital, 3249 South Oak Park Avenue, Berwyn, Illinois 60402*

Robert W. Wolford, M.D. *Associate Professor and Vice Chair, Program in Emergency Medicine, Michigan State University College of Human Medicine; Director, Department of Emergency Medicine, Saginaw Cooperative Hospitals, Inc., 1000 Houghton Avenue, Saginaw, Michigan 48602*

Matthew W. Wols, M.D. *Attending Physician, Department of Emergency Medicine, Norwegian American Hospital, 1044 North Francisco Avenue, Chicago, Illinois 60622*

John L. Zautcke, M.D. *Assistant Professor, Medical Director, UIC O'Hare Clinic, Department of Emergency Medicine, University of Illinois at Chicago, 1740 West Taylor Street, Suite 1600, Chicago, Illinois 60614*

Preface

This text is for the emergency medicine community. The Editors conceived and developed it as a concise, reliable text for education and easy reference in the emergency department setting. Chapter topics were chosen to cover the vast spectrum of emergency medicine orthopaedics. Authors were selected for their expertise, experience, and geographic diversity. We hope the text proves valuable and insightful to all those who practice and care deeply about emergency medicine.

R.G.H.
T.J.R.
D.T.U

Acknowledgments

The Editors thank all those who assisted in the compilation of this text. Thanks in particular to Jackie Strange, Rose Bradford, and Angel Farris for manuscript organization and assistance. We also express our deep appreciation to Elizabeth Greenspan and Rebecca Irwin Diehl of Lippincott—Raven Publishers for their editorial assistance and guidance. Next, many thanks to our illustrator, Quinn Heath, for his excellent work. Finally, and most especially, thanks to all the authors who committed countless hours to complete the project.

R.G.H.
T.J.R.
D.T.U.

Permissions for Figures

Chapter 9

Figure 1: Adapted from Uerhara D, Rudzinski JP. Injuries to the shoulder complex and humerus. In: Tintinalli JE, Ruiz E, Krome RI, eds. *Emergency Medicine: a Comprehensive Study Guide/American College of Emergency Physicians,* 4th ed. New York: McGraw-Hill, 1996; 1236.
Figure 4: Adapted with permission from Herscovici D, Sanders R, DiPasquale T, Gregory P. *Clinical Orthopaedics and Related Research,* 1995; 318:54.

Chapter 11

Figure 4: Adapted from Neer CS. Displaced Proximal humeral fractures: Part I. Classification and evaluation. *J Bone Joint Surg* 1970; 52A: 1077–1089.

Chapter 13

Figure 4: Reprinted with permission from Chin HW, Vitotsky J. Ligamentous wrist injuries. *Emergency Medicine Clinics of North America* 11:3, 1993.
Figure 7: From Chin HW, Vitotsky J. Ligamentous wrist injuries. *Emergency Clinics of North America.* 11:3, 1993: 730. Figure 10.

Chapter 19

Figure 2: Rittenberry TJ, Sloan EP. *Emergency Medicine: A Problem Solving Approach,* ed. Hamilton et al. 1991; 752. Figure 43-2.

Chapter 20

Figure 9: Rittenberry T, Sloan EP. *Emergency Medicine: An Approach to Clinical Problem Solving,* ed. Hamilton et al. 1991; 780. Figure 43-14.
Figure 10: Rittenberry T, Sloan EP. *Emergency Medicine: A Problem Solving Approach,* ed. Hamilton et al. 1991.
Figure 13: Rittenberry T, Sloan EP. *Emergency Medicine: A Problem Solving Approach,* ed. Hamilton et al. 1991; 756. Figure 43-14.

Chapter 25

Figure 3: Rittenberry T, Hassfeld G. *Emergency Medicine: A Problem Solving Approach,* ed. Hamilton et al. 1991; 752. Figure 41-8.

Chapter 26

Figure 8: Ogeden JA. *Skeletal injury in the child,* 2nd ed. Philadelphia: WB Saunders; 400. Figure 10-100.

Orthopaedics

1

General Orthopaedic Principles

Raymond G. Hart and Brian A. Macauley

I. **Principles and classification of fractures.** A fracture is a break in the continuity of a bone. The term covers all types of disruptions, from microscopic to severely comminuted injuries. Fracture description should be concise and accurate. Certain facts must be communicated to the referring physician regarding the mechanism of injury, the type of fracture present, and associated soft tissue injuries. A system for describing fractures using orthopaedic terminology is outlined below.

  A. **Exact anatomic location.** The name of the bone and the location within the bone is first described. Long bones are typically divided into thirds, with a fracture being in the proximal, middle, or distal third. If a fracture is through a specific anatomic part of a bone, that terminology is preferred (e.g., a fracture through the neck of the femur).

  B. **Fracture line or pattern.** The fracture line is its direction through the bone relative to the bone's long axis.

    1. **Transverse.** The fracture line is perpendicular to the long axis of the bone (Fig. 1). This injury is usually due to direct trauma and is typically stable.

    2. **Oblique.** The fracture line runs at an oblique angle to the long axis of the bone (Fig. 2). This injury results from indirect trauma and is normally associated with less soft tissue damage and faster healing than a transverse fracture.

    3. **Spiral.** The fracture line curves in a spiral fashion around the bone (Fig. 3). It is caused by a torsional or rotational force.

    4. **Comminuted.** Fractures in which more than two fragments are present are termed comminuted (Fig. 4). Such fractures are often associated with significant soft tissue injury and are unstable.

      a. **Butterfly.** This is a type of comminuted fracture with a characteristic butterfly-shaped fragment.

      b. **Segmental.** The bone is fractured at two distinct levels. Reduction of this fracture is difficult and nonunion common.

    5. **Impacted.** This is a fracture in which the ends are driven into each other. Cancellous bone is typically involved, and union often occurs rapidly. A **torus** fracture is a pediatric impaction fracture in which the cortex of a long bone buckles, with no loss of cortical continuity.

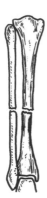

Fig. 1.   Transverse fractures.

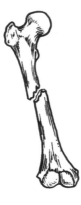

Fig. 2.   Oblique fracture.

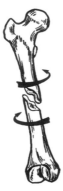

Fig. 3.   Spiral fracture.

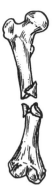

Fig. 4. Comminuted fracture.

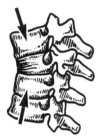

Fig. 5. Compression fracture.

6. **Compression.** This occurs in cancellous bone, when an excessive axial load compresses the bone beyond its limits. It typically occurs in the vertebral bodies (Fig. 5).

7. **Depressed.** This is a fracture of the cortical bone caused by a localized force that breaks and depresses one segment below the level of surrounding bone.

C. **Displacement.** Bone fragments that have shifted relative to each other are displaced. In describing the abnormality, the position of the distal fragment is noted relative to the proximal one. The degree of shifting should be estimated by determining the percentage of fracture surfaces in contact. Fractures with total displacement are unstable and may lead to progressive shortening. This interferes with reduction, and union is difficult.

1. **Bayonette deformity.** The fracture fragments are 100% displaced, shortened, and overlapping.

2. **Distraction deformity.** Fracture fragments are displaced along the long axis of the bone. Dis-

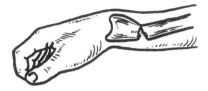

Fig. 6.   Fracture of distal radius with dorsal angulation.

tracted segments with gaps greater than 0.5 cm may require a lengthy healing time.

D. **Angulation.** The angle between the longitudinal axes of the main fracture fragments must be measured. Fractures that demonstrate significant angulation must be reduced or function will be compromised. In weight-bearing areas, abnormal stress to joints due to angulation may lead to osteoarthritis. Angulation is described in several ways:

   1. The relationship of the bone distal to the fracture site with respect to the proximal is described (e.g., a Colles fracture is a distal radial fracture with dorsal angulation of the distal fragment) (Fig. 6).

   2. An alternative description is the direction in which the apex of the fracture fragments points (e.g., a Colles' fracture is a distal radial fracture with the apex angled volarly). The terms **ulnar, radial, volar,** and **dorsal** are used if the fracture is in the forearm and hand. In the foot, **plantar** and **dorsal** are used.

   3. The terms **valgus** and **varus** describe the angular relationship of the distal part to the proximal part around a known axis. *Valgus* means that the distal part is angled laterally relative to the proximal part, and *varus* means that the distal part is angled medially.

E. **Axial rotation.** Fragments that are rotated with respect to each other must be recognized. To avoid overlooking rotation, radiographs should include the joints above and below the injury. Differences in the measured diameters of the bone fragments can also be used to detect rotation.

F. **Additional modifiers**

   1. **Incomplete versus complete fractures.** A fracture is complete if both cortices of the bone are interrupted and incomplete if only one is involved. A **greenstick fracture** is an incomplete fracture in children in which the cortex and periosteum are broken on one side only. It occurs in young bones that are porous, less brittle, and more apt to bend than to break completely (Fig. 7).

   2. **Stable versus unstable fractures.** Unstable fractures are those that tend to displace after re-

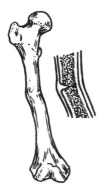

Fig. 7.   Greenstick fracture.

duction, whereas stable fractures remain in place after reduction.

3. **Complicated versus uncomplicated fractures.** Complicated fractures are those in which there is significant soft tissue damage to major nearby structures (nerves, vessels, ligaments, and muscles). Uncomplicated fractures involve only minimal soft tissue damage.

4. **Extraarticular versus intraarticular fractures.** Intraarticular fractures are those in which the fracture line extends into the joint space. Extraarticular fractures are those in which the fracture line does not enter the joint space.

5. **Open (compound) fracture versus closed (simple) fracture.** A closed fracture is one in which the skin overlying the fracture site is intact. An open fracture is one in which the skin over the fracture site is broken. Open fractures may occur when a bone fragment from within breaks out through the skin or when some outside force penetrates both the skin and bone. The latter scenario has a poorer prognosis, as there is often greater soft tissue damage and a greater risk of contamination. Open fractures are surgical emergencies, and most require operative treatment. Initial management involves application of sterile gauze soaked in povidone-iodine (Betadine), intravenous broad-spectrum (e.g., cephalosporin) antibiotics, and preparation for operative debridement. Neurovascular status must be carefully assessed. Open fractures vary in severity according to the bone damage, the nature and size of the wound, the contamination potential, and the mechanism of injury.

   a. **Grade I** injuries are minor. The wound length is less than 1.0 cm, bone and soft tissue

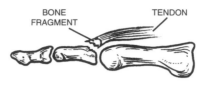

Fig. 8.   Avulsion fracture.

      damage is small, and contamination is minimal.

    b. **Grade II** injuries involve larger wounds but without extensive loss or devitalization of soft tissue. There is no vascular injury and only moderate contamination.

    c. **Grade III** injuries involve extensive wounds with significant soft tissue damage, vascular injury, and heavy contamination.

  G. **Specific fractures**

    1. **Stress fractures.** Stress fractures are caused by repetitive loading beyond the tolerance of a bone. Each individual stress causes minute fractures that, over time, develop into a complete fracture. Patients present with pain but without a definite history of trauma. The classic example is the second metatarsal fracture in army recruits ("march" fracture).

    2. **Pathological fractures.** These occur in bones weakened by preexisting disease. The strength of the bone is compromised and often only minor trauma precipitates a fracture. Osteoporosis, infection, and tumors are common causes of pathological fractures.

    3. **Avulsion fractures.** Traction on a ligamentous attachment to bone or a forcible muscular contraction that pulls attached bone away causes an avulsion fracture (Fig. 8).

    4. **Named fractures.** A list of fracture eponyms is given in Table 1.

II. **Fracture biomechanics and mechanism of injury**

  A. **Biomechanics.** Bone is composed of minerals, which provide rigidity, and collagen, which provides tensile strength. The compressive strength of bone is greater than its tensile strength, so that when bone is subjected to an excessive stress, it will fail first with tension. Extrinsic factors important in bone fractures are the magnitude, duration, and direction of the force acting on the bone and the rate at which this force is applied.

  B. **Directly applied forces**

    1. **Tapping fracture.** An application of a small force to a localized area of bone produces a transverse fracture. Most of the energy is absorbed by the bone, and minimal soft tissue damage occurs.

Table 1. Fracture eponyms

Aviator's astragalus. Implies a variety of fractures of the talus; described after World War I as rudder bar is driven into foot during plane crash.

Barton's fracture. Displaced articular lip fracture of the distal radius; may be associated with carpal subluxation. Fracture configuration may be in a dorsal or volar direction.

Bennett's fracture. Oblique fracture of the first metacarpal base separating a small triangular fragment of the volar lip from the proximally displaced metacarpal shaft.

Bosworth fracture. Fracture of the distal fibula with fixed displacement of the proximal fragment posteriorly behind the posterolateral tibial ridge.

Boxer's fracture. Fracture of the fifth metacarpal neck with volar displacement of the metacarpal head.

Burst fracture. Fracture of the vertebral body from axial load, usually with outward displacement of the fragments. May occur in the cervical, thoracic, or lumbar spine.

Chance fracture. Distraction fracture of the thoracolumbar vertebral body with horizontal disruption of the spinous process, neural arch, and vertebral body.

Chauffeur's fracture (Hutchinson's fracture). Oblique fracture of the radial styloid, initially attributed to the starting crank of an engine being forcibly reversed by a backfire.

Chopart's fracture and dislocation. Fracture and/or dislocation involving Chopart's joints (talonavicular and calcaneocuboid) of the foot.

Clay-shoveler's (coal-shoveler's) fracture. Spinous process fracture of the lower cervical or upper thoracic vertebrae. Injury initially attributed to workers attempting to throw upward a full shovel of clay, but the clay, adhering to the shovel, would cause a sudden flexion force opposite to the neck musculature.

Colles' fracture. General term for fractures of the distal radius with dorsal displacement, with or without an ulnar styloid fracture.

Cotton's fractures. Trimalleolar ankle fracture with fractures of both malleoli and the posterior lip of the tibia.

Die-punch fracture. Intraarticular fracture of the distal radius with impaction of the dorsal aspect of the lunate fossa.

Dupuytren's fracture. Fracture of the distal fibula with rupture of the distal tibiofibular ligaments and lateral displacement of the talus.

Duverney's fracture. Fracture of the iliac wing without disruption of the pelvic ring.

Essex-Lopresti's fracture. Fracture of the radial head with associated dislocation of the distal radioulnar joint.

Galeazzi's fracture. Fracture of the radius in the distal third associated with subluxation of the distal ulna.

Continued.

Table 1. *Continued.*

Greenstick fracture.   Incompletely fractured bone in a child, with a portion of the cortex and periosteum remaining intact on the compression side of the fracture.

Hangman's fracture.   Fracture through the neural arch of the second cervical vertebra (axis).

Hill-Sachs fracture.   Posterolateral humeral head compression fracture caused by anterior glenohumeral dislocation and impaction of the humeral head against the anterior glenoid rim.

Holstein-Lewis fracture.   Fracture of the distal third of the humerus with entrapment of the radial nerve.

Hutchinson's fracture.   See *Chauffeur's fracture.*

Jefferson's fracture.   Comminuted fracture of the ring of the atlas due to axial compressive forces. Fractures usually occur anterior and posterior to the lateral facet joints.

Jones fracture.   Diaphyseal fracture of the base of the fifth metatarsal.

Lisfranc's fracture dislocation.   Fracture and/or dislocation involving Lisfranc's (tarsometatarsal) joint of the foot. Lisfranc was one of Napoleon's surgeons and described traumatic foot amputation through the level of the tarsometatarsal joint.

Maisonneuve's fracture.   Fracture of the proximal fibula with syndesmosis rupture and associated fracture of the medial malleolus or rupture of the deltoid ligament.

Malgaigne's fracture.   Unstable pelvic fracture with vertical fractures anterior and posterior to the hip joint.

Mallet finger.   Flexion deformity of the distal interphalangeal joint caused by separation of the extensor tendon from the distal phalanx. The deformity may be secondary to direct injury of the extensor tendon or an avulsion fracture from the dorsum of the distal phalanx, where the tendon inserts.

Monteggia's fracture.   Fracture of the proximal third of the ulna with associated dislocation of the radial head.

Nightstick fracture.   Isolated fracture of the ulna secondary to direct trauma.

Posadas' fracture.   Transcondylar humeral fracture with displacement of the distal fragment anteriorly and dislocation of the radius and ulna from the bicondylar fragment.

Pott's fracture.   Fracture of the fibula 2 to 3 in. above the lateral malleolus with rupture of the deltoid ligament and lateral subluxation of the talus.

Rolando's fracture.   Y-shaped intraarticular fracture of the thumb metacarpal.

Segond's fracture.   Avulsion fracture of the lateral tibial condyle from the bony insertion of the iliotibial band.

Shepherd's fracture.   Fracture of the lateral tubercle of the posterior talar process.

Smith's fracture.   Fracture of the distal radius with palmar displacement of the distal fragment. Also referred to as a reverse Colles' fracture.

Table 1. *Continued.*

Stieda's fracture.   Avulsion fracture of the medial femoral condyle at the origin of the medial collateral ligament.

Straddle fracture.   Bilateral fractures of the superior and inferior public rami.

Teardrop fracture.   Flexion fracture/dislocation of the cervical spine with associated triangular anterior fragment of the involved vertebrae. Injury complex in unstable, with posterior ligamentous disruption.

Tillaux's fracture.   Fracture of the lateral half of the distal tibial physis during differential closure of the physis. The medial part of the tibial physis has already fused.

Torus fracture.   Impaction fracture of childhood as the bone buckles instead of fracturing completely.

Walther's fracture.   Ischioacetabular fracture that passes through the pubic rami and extends toward the sacroiliac joint. The medial wall of the acetabulum is displaced inward.

  2. **Crush injury.** A larger force applied to a larger area of bone will cause comminution or a transverse fracture, with extensive soft tissue damage.
  3. **Penetrating injury.** A large force—as via a gunshot wound—will cause extensive comminution and soft tissue damage in high-velocity impacts (>2000 ft/s) and moderate damage in low-velocity impacts.
 C. **Indirectly applied forces.** Indirect trauma is produced by a force that acts at a distance from the fracture site.
  1. **Traction or tension fracture.** A muscle that forcibly contracts and pulls away a piece of bone attached to its musculotendinous unit (i.e., avulsion fracture) will produce a transverse fracture.
  2. **Angulation fracture.** A force causing bending of the bone such that one side is under compression and the other under tension will cause a transverse fracture. The side under tension fractures first.
  3. **Rotational fracture.** A combination of horizontal and vertical stresses will cause fracture lines at 45 degrees to the long axis of the bone.
  4. **Compression fracture.** Excessive axial loads will cause either impaction fractures of cancellous bone or longitudinal fractures of cortical bone.
III. **Fracture healing**
 A. **Stages of fracture healing**
  1. **Inflammatory stage.** A fracture causes injury to the periosteum, bone marrow, and soft tissue.

Bleeding from these areas causes immediate formation of a fracture hematoma. Fracture ends within the clot are deprived of their blood flow, causing local necrosis and an intense inflammatory reaction. An influx of macrophages, chemoattractive substances, and fibroblasts occurs that activates cellular mechanisms. Blood vessels and granulation tissue grow in rapidly from surrounding tissues. A primary external callus forms and collagen tissue is laid down, replacing clot.

2. **Reparative stage.** Early bone formation begins in the subperiosteal regions of the external callus. A less developed endosteal callus produces cartilage that later becomes ossified. The critical step in fracture union is the formation of an intact bony bridge from the external calluses. Osteoclasts then tunnel across fracture lines and osteoblasts form new haversian systems. Gradually, collagenous tissue is replaced by new cortical bone.

3. **Remodeling stage.** After clinical union, osteoblasts and osteoclasts continue remodeling the bone until healing is complete. Haversian systems are laid down along lines of stress.

B. **Variables in fracture healing.** Both local and systemic variables influence the rate and degree of fracture healing. When normal healing occurs, but at a slower rate than usual, it is termed **delayed union**. A complete cessation of the healing process, in which fibrous tissue is never replaced by bony matrix, is termed **nonunion**.

1. **Systemic variables**

   a. **Age.** Young patients heal rapidly and have a remarkable ability to remodel and correct angulation deformities. These abilities cease once skeletal maturity is reached.

   b. **Nutrition.** A substantial amount of energy is needed for fracture healing to occur. An adequate metabolic state with sufficient carbohydrates and protein is necessary.

   c. **Systemic diseases and genetic abnormalities.** Diseases like osteoporosis, diabetes, and those causing an immunocompromised state will likely delay healing. Illnesses like Marfan's syndrome and Ehlers-Danlos syndrome cause abnormal musculoskeletal healing.

   d. **Hormones.** Thyroid hormone, growth hormone, calcitonin, and others play significant roles in bone healing. Corticosteroids impede healing through many mechanisms.

2. **Local variables**

   a. **Type of bone.** Cancellous (spongy) bone fractures are usually more stable, involve greater surface areas, and have a better blood supply than do cortical (compact) bone fractures. Cancellous bone heals faster than cortical bone.

b. **Degree of local trauma.** The more extensive the injury to bone and surrounding soft tissue, the poorer the outcome. Mild contusions with local bone trauma will heal easily, whereas severely comminuted injuries with extensive soft tissue damage heal poorly.

c. **Vascular injury.** Inadequate blood supply impairs healing. Especially vulnerable areas are the femoral head, talus, and scaphoid bones.

d. **Degree of immobilization.** The fracture site must be immobilized for vascular ingrowth and bone healing to occur. Repeated disruptions of repair tissue, especially to areas with marginal blood supply or heavy soft tissue damage, will impair healing.

e. **Intraarticular fractures.** These fractures communicate with synovial fluid, which contains collagenases that retard bone healing. Joint movement will cause the fracture fragments to move, further impairing union. When intraarticular fractures are comminuted, the fragments tend to float apart owing to loss of soft tissue support.

f. **Separation of bone ends.** Normal apposition of fracture fragments is needed for union to occur. Inadequate reduction, excessive traction, or interposition of soft tissue will prevent healing.

g. **Infection.** Infections cause necrosis and edema, take energy away from the healing process, and may increase the mobility of the fracture site.

h. **Local pathological conditions.** Any disease process that weakens the musculoskeletal tissue, like osteoporosis or osteomalacia, may impair union.

IV. **Recognition and treatment of fractures**

A. **Clinical features of fractures.** Fractures are suspected from the history and physical examination. On exam, pain and tenderness are consistent findings and may be the only evidence of a fracture. Deformity of the limb or angulation are both highly suggestive of a fracture. If the fracture is mobile, moving the involved part may create angulation or crepitus from the bone ends rubbing together. Loss of function is often noted but may be minimal in incomplete fractures. Finally, any neurovascular injury distal to the area should suggest an injury.

B. **Radiographic evaluation** (see Chapter 3). Radiographic examination is necessary to confirm any suspicion of fracture. Normal radiographs suggest but do not determine an absolute absence of injury. Many fractures will not be apparent, and soft tissue damage to ligaments and neurovascular structures may be overlooked (Table 2). Additional rules to remember regarding radiographs are as follows:

1. A fracture or dislocation may require two x-rays to be seen (anteroposterior and lateral); a single view should never be relied upon.

2. In angulated fractures of the forearm and lower leg, the joints above and below the fracture must be included on the radiographs. This is to exclude the possibility that the other bone is broken or dislocated.

3. In pediatric x-rays, "comparison" views are helpful, as normal epiphyses and centers of ossification may confuse the diagnosis of fracture.

4. Radiographs of all dislocations should be taken before and after reduction unless a delay would cause neurovascular compromise.

C. **Initial stabilization.** Patients require stabilization of life-threatening injuries before any orthopaedic assessment occurs. A systematic approach to the airway, breathing, and circulation (the "ABCs") is imperative. Blood loss from orthopaedic injuries can be extensive

Table 2.   Commonly associated injuries of fractures and dislocations

Fracture/dislocation	Associated injury
Clavicular shaft fracture	Subclavian vessels, brachial plexus, acromioclavicular joint
Shoulder dislocation	Brachial plexus, axillary nerve, subclavian vessels
First rib fracture	Subclavian vessels
Midshaft humeral fracture	Radial nerve
Supracondylar humeral fracture	Median nerve, brachial artery
Avulsion fracture of medial epicondyle	Ulnar nerve
Radial head dislocation	Posterior interosseus nerve
Distal radius/ulnar fracture	Median nerve, ulnar nerve
Proximal ulnar shaft fracture	Radial head dislocation
Radial shaft fracture	Distal radioulnar joint dislocation
Posterior hip dislocation	Sciatic nerve, acetabular fracture
Knee dislocation	Popliteal artery, tibial and common peroneal nerves
Upper fibular fracture	Peroneal nerve
Ankle dislocation	Anterior and posterior tibial artery
Calcaneual fracture	Lumbar compression fracture

and should be appreciated. Closed injuries of the femur, for example, may involve more than 1 L of blood loss, and pelvic fracture may involve several liters. Open fractures with bleeding are best treated with direct pressure on the site with a sterile gauze packet.

D. Fracture immobilization (See Chapter 6). Once a fracture is diagnosed or suspected, the extremity should be immobilized with a splint. No manipulation or reduction should occur unless significant vascular compromise exists. The advantages of splinting are as follows:

  1. It protects against further soft tissue injury, especially to nerves and vessels.
  2. It prevents fracture displacement and conversion of a closed to an open fracture.
  3. Pain is relieved.
  4. It allows for more efficient reabsorption of edema and blood.
  5. The incidence of fat embolism is decreased.
  6. It allows for easier transportation and radiographic examinations.

E. Types of splinting. Almost any splinting material can be used to stabilize a fracture temporarily. Cardboard, wood with padding, wire frames, metal strips, inflatable splints, pillows, or sandbags are effective initial materials. Plaster and casting material are commonly used in the emergency department setting. Neurovascular assessment should follow any manipulation or application of splinting material.

F. Definitive fracture treatment. Nonrigid support methods such as arm slings, bandages, and strapping may be used in certain types of fractures. Treatments that require increased fracture stabilization include internal and external fixation, cast immobilization, and continuous traction.

V. Joint and soft tissue injuries
  A. Joint injuries
    1. **Dislocation.** A dislocation is a total disruption of a joint such that there is complete loss of congruity between the articulating surfaces. It is described by naming the joint involved and modifying it by indicating the position of the distal bone.
    2. **Subluxation.** A subluxation is a partial dislocation. Partial articular contact remains between the bone surfaces.
    3. **Fracture/dislocation.** This is a dislocation complicated by a fracture through one of the bony parts of the joint. Stiffness and avascular necrosis are two common complications of this injury.
  B. Soft tissue injuries
    1. **Sprain.** A sprain is a tear in the ligamentous fibers that stabilize a joint. The grading system is as follows:
      a. **Grade I** sprains are those in which a small number of fibers are torn. No ligamentous in-

stability exists but tenderness and swelling are present.

b. **Grade II** injuries are those in which a moderate number of fibers are torn. Some degree of instability is noted on exam, but the instability is limited to a definite endpoint.

c. **Grade III** injuries are those with complete disruption of fibers and gross instability. There is no detectable endpoint on exam.

2. **Strain.** A strain is an injury to the musculotendinous unit that results from stretching or contraction of the muscles. It is graded from minor to severe, with severe strains involving complete disruption of the muscular unit.

3. **Tendinitis.** This is a painful inflammatory condition of the tendon, most often due to overuse.

4. **Bursitis.** Bursitis is a painful inflammation of the bursa due to an infectious or traumatic cause.

C. **Therapeutic use of heat and cold**

1. **Cold treatment.** Minor acute soft tissue injuries can be effectively treated with application of ice. Cold substances decrease blood flow, swelling, and inflammation; they also relieve pain and muscle spasm. Treatment is most effective during the first 72 hours after an injury. Cold packs should be applied for 20 minutes at a time, four times a day.

2. **Warm treatment.** Application of moist heat will increase blood flow and edema and produce an inflammatory response. Its effects are to increase muscle flexibility, improve joint mobility, and overcome chronic muscle tightness. Heat should never be used in acute injuries. Warm packs should be applied for 20 minutes at a time, about four times a day.

BIBLIOGRAPHY

Birnbuam JS. *The musculoskeletal manual,* 2nd ed. Orlando, FL: Grune & Stratton, 1986.

Callahan ML. *Current practice of emergency medicine,* 2nd ed. Philadelphia: BC Decker, 1991.

Chipman C. *Emergency department orthopaedics.* Rockville, MD: Aspen Systems, 1982.

Green DP, Bucholz RW. *Fractures in adults,* 3rd ed. Philadelphia: JB Lippincott, 1991.

Kozin SH, Berlet AC. *Handbook of common orthopaedic fractures,* 2nd ed. West Chester, PA: Medical Surveillance, 1992.

Kravis TC et al. *Emergency medicine,* 3rd ed. New York: Raven Press, 1993.

Leung PC. *Current practice of fracture management.* Hong Kong: Springer-Verlag, 1994.

Mallon WJ et al. *Orthopaedics for the house officer.* Baltimore: Williams & Wilkins, 1990.

McRae R. *Practical fracture management,* 2nd ed. Edinburgh: Churchill Livingstone, 1989.

Mercier LR. *Practical orthopaedics,* 4th ed. St. Louis: Mosby, 1995.

Rosen P et al. *Emergency medicine,* 2nd ed. St. Louis: CV Mosby, 1988.

Segelov PM. *Manual of emergency orthopaedics.* Edinburgh: Churchill Livingstone, 1986.

Simon RR, Koenigsknecht SJ. *Emergency orthopaedics,* 2nd ed. Norwalk, CT: Appleton & Lange, 1987.

The Orthopaedic History and Physical Exam

Raymond G. Hart and Joseph L. Tasto

I. **History.** A careful history is an important part of caring for orthopaedic injuries. The emergency physician should strive to be complete yet concise. The extent and nature of the injuries will determine the focus of the history.

  A. **Demographic data**

  1. **Age.** The same mechanism of injury can result in different injuries, depending on age. The classic example is a forward fall on an outstretched hand. This can produce a greenstick fracture in a child, a scaphoid fracture in a young adult, or a Colles' fracture in an elderly adult. At different ages, patients can present with various complications. For example, pediatric patients can sustain injuries to their growth plates and older patients may present with osteoporosis. In addition, treatment may vary depending on the age of the patient.

  2. **Sex.** Bone mass can differ between men and women, occasionally resulting in different injuries. For example, osteoporosis is more common in older women.

  3. **Dominant hand.** Whether the patient's dominant hand is injured may influence the management of the injury.

  B. **History of present illness**

  1. **Mechanism of injury.** Obtain a detailed account of the cause of the injury, including when it happened. Determine the amount of force that caused the injury. When injuries are more extensive than expected from the force, suspect underlying pathological conditions such as tumors. When injuries seem minor relative to the force, repeat exams and observation may be warranted. More soft tissue damage is expected when the force is direct rather than indirect. Determine all sites where the force was applied, being careful not to focus only on the most obvious site of injury.

  2. **Results of injury.** Ask whether the pain and/or swelling began immediately after the injury or was delayed. A "snap," "pop," or tearing sound heard or felt by the patient during the injury will increase the likelihood that a fracture or rupture of a ligament or tendon occurred. Inquire about any loss or changes in sensation, range of motion, or strength. Ask if the patient was able to use the affected limb after the injury. Determine if any

other injuries besides the presenting orthopaedic injury occurred.

3. **Previous treatment.** Inquire about treatments given before presentation to the emergency department.

C. **Past medical/surgical history.** Determine if there have been previous problems with the affected limb. Ask about previous orthopaedic injuries and past surgeries. Obtain information about possible systemic disorders that may affect diagnosis, treatment, or prognosis, such as bleeding tendencies, rheumatic diseases, immune deficiencies, cancer, diabetes, peripheral vascular disease, renal disorders, or metabolic diseases. Determine the patient's tetanus immune status.

D. **Medications.** Nonsteroidal anti-inflammatory drugs (NSAIDs), other pain medications, and muscle relaxants can mask symptoms or influence the exam. In addition, be aware of possible drug interactions between the patients' current medications and those that may be given in the emergency department for sedation or treatment.

E. **Allergies.** History of allergy must be taken into account, particularly because antibiotics and muscle relaxants are commonly used in the emergency department to treat orthopaedic injuries.

F. **Social history.** The patient's occupation may increase the significance of the injury, as may the use of alcohol and/or illicit drugs and when the patient last ate or drank.

G. **Family history.** A family history of rheumatic disease can be pertinent for a patient who presents with decreased range of motion (ROM) in several joints. In the case of a suspected pathological fracture, a history of cancer is important.

H. **Review of systems.** Fever and chills can be indicative of infection. Nausea and vomiting can preclude the administration of oral medications. Dizziness and syncope may indicate internal bleeding from the injuries.

II. **Physical exam.** A complete physical exam should be conducted before treatment or manipulation of the injury is performed. The injured body part should be fully exposed. Therefore, clothing covering the area should be removed, as well as any constricting jewelry. The orthopaedic physical exam will consist of inspection, palpation, and assessment of ROM, strength, reflexes, sensation, and vascular integrity. Assess the joints above and below the injury to ensure that they are intact.

A. **Inspection.** Inspect the entire injured area. Compare the injured limb with that of the unaffected side, looking for asymmetries. Look for deformities such as angulation, rotation, or shortening. Check for skin injuries such as abrasion, ecchymoses, or lacerations, which may suggest possible underlying pathology. Be sure to look for the classic signs of fracture: erythema, swelling, and deformity.

B. Palpation. Begin palpating the extremity contralateral to the injury to gain the patient's confidence and obtain comparative information. When the patient has a grossly obvious deformity, delay palpation, ROM, and strength testing until radiographs have been taken and pain has been controlled. Palpate for the point of maximal tenderness, crepitus, discontinuity, instability, and temperature.

C. Range of Motion. Both active and passive ROM testing should be performed. Do active ROM testing (patient initiates movement) before passive testing (examiner moves the joints) to assess the amount of pain and loss of function in the injured joint prior to manipulation. Compare the ROM of the injured extremity with that of the unaffected side. Tables 1 and 2 list the normal values of ROM for each of the joints. Zero degrees is defined to be the joint in extended anatomic position. A goniometer is useful for these measurements.

D. Strength. Strength testing allows for the assessment of the integrity of the motor pathways from the cerebral cortex through the spinal cord, out the peripheral nerves, and to the muscle. Compare the injured limb with the unaffected contralateral limb to ascertain the patient's baseline strength. Be aware that this part of the exam can be influenced a great deal by the patient's experience of pain. Table 3 lists the grading scale for muscle strength. Tables 4 and 5 list the primary muscles involved in the basic joint movements and the innervation of each.

E. Reflexes. Evaluate the deep tendon reflexes. The reflexes tested along with the respective nerve roots are listed in Table 6. The reflexes are graded as follows: 0 for no response; 1+ for diminished response; 2+ for normal response; 3+ for increased response; 4+ for hyperactive response. Diminished responses are indicative of lower motor neuron disturbances or myopathies, while increased responses are indicative of upper motor neuron disturbances.

F. Sensation. This is especially important in order to assess distal to the injury. Light touch and pinprick should always be tested. Two-point discrimination is helpful for assessing digital nerve function in hand injuries. Normal adults should be able to distinguish two points more than 5 mm apart on their fingers.

G. Vascular integrity. The vascular status is assessed by looking at skin color, feeling skin temperature, palpating peripheral pulses, and testing capillary refill. This is particularly important distal to the site of injury. Compare the pulses of the injured extremity with those of the unaffected side. If no pulse can be felt, use Doppler ultrasound to confirm its presence.

**Table 1. Range of motion: normal
values for the upper extremity**

Joint	Motion in degrees
Neck	
Flexion	45
Extension	45
Lateral bending	40
Rotation	70
Shoulder	
Flexion	150
Extension	45
Abduction	180
Adduction	45
Internal rotation	70
External rotation	80
Elbow	
Flexion	150
Extension	−5
Supination	90
Pronation	90
Wrist	
Flexion	80
Extension	70
Ulnar deviation	30
Radial deviation	20
Fingers	
Abduction	20
Adduction	0
MCP flexion	90
MCP extension	30
PIP flexion	100
PIP extension	0
DIP flexion	90
DIP extension	10
Thumb	
Abduction	70
Adduction	0
MCP flexion	50
MCP extension	0
IP flexion	90
IP extension	20

Key: MCP, metacarpophalangeal; PIP, proximal interphalangeal;
DIP, distal interphalangeal; IP, interphalangeal.

Table 2. Range of motion: normal values for the lower extremity

Joint	Motion in degrees
Lumbar supine	
Flexion	75
Extension	30
Lateral bending	30
Rotation	30
Hip	
Flexion	120
Extension	30
Abduction	45
Adduction	30
Internal rotation	35
External rotation	45
Knee	
Flexion	135
Extension	−10
Internal rotation	10
External rotation	10
Ankle/Foot	
Dorsiflexion	20
Plantarflexion	50
Subtalar inversion	5
Subtalar eversion	5
Forefoot abduction	10
Forefoot adduction	20
First MTP* flexion	45
First MTP extension	70

*Metatarsophalangeal.

Table 3. Grading scale for muscle strength

5	Movement against gravity with full resistance
4	Movement against gravity with some resistance
3	Movement against gravity
2	Movement with gravity eliminated
1	Slight muscle contraction, no movement
0	No contraction detected

Table 4. Innervation of the primary muscles of movement for the upper extremity

Joint movement	Primary muscles	Peripheral nerves	Nerve root
Shoulder			
Flexion	Deltoid (anterior portion)	Axillary	C5
	Coracobrachialis	Musculocutaneous	C5-6
Extension	Latissimus dorsi	Thoracodorsal	C6-8
	Teres major	Lower subscapular	C5-6
	Deltoid (posterior portion)	Axillary	C5-6
Abduction	Deltoid (midportion)	Axillary	C5-6
	Supraspinatus	Suprascapular	C5-6
Adduction	Pectoralis major	Medial and lateral pectoral	C5-T1
	Latissimus dorsi	Thoracodorsal	C6-8
External rotation	Infraspinatus	Suprascapular	C5-6
	Teres minor	Axillary	C5
Internal rotation	Subscapular	Subscapular	C5-6
	Pectoralis major	Medial and lateral pectoral	C5-T1
	Latissimus dorsi	Thoracodorsal	C6-8
	Teres major	Lower subscapular	C5-6
Scapular elevation	Trapezius	Spinal accessory	CN XI
	Levator scapulae	C3,C4	C3-4
Scapular retraction	Rhomboid major	Dorsal scapular	C5
	Rhomboid minor	Dorsal scapular	C5
Scapular protraction	Serratus anterior	Long thoracic	C5-7

Continued.

Table 4. *Continued.*

Joint movement	Primary muscles	Peripheral nerves	Nerve root
Elbow			
Flexion	Brachialis	Musculocutaneous	C5-6
	Biceps (in supination)	Musculocutaneous	C5-6
Extension	Triceps	Radial	C7
Supination	Biceps	Musculocutaneous	C5-6
	Supinator	Radial (deep branch)	C6
Pronation	Pronator teres	Median	C6
	Pronator quadratus	Median (anterior interosseous)	C8-T1
Wrist			
Flexion	Flexor carpi radialis	Median	C7
	Flexor carpi ulnaris	Ulnar	C8
Extension	Extensor carpi radialis longus	Radial	C6
	Extensor carpi radialis brevis	Radial	C6
	Extensor carpi ulnaris	Radial (posterior interosseous)	C7

Fingers			
Abduction	Dorsal interossei	Ulnar	C8-T1
	Abductor digiti minimi	Ulnar	C8-T1
Adduction	Palmar interossei	Ulnar	C8-T1
MCP flexion	Lumbricals: medial 2	Ulnar	C8
	lateral 2	Median	C7
PIP flexion	Flexor digitorum superficialis	Median	C7-T1
DIP flexion	Flexor digitorum profundus	Ulnar, Median (anterior interosseous)	C8-T1
Finger extension	Extensor digitorum communis	Radial (posterior interosseous)	C7
	Extensor indicis	Radial (posterior interosseous)	C7
	Extensor digiti minimi	Radial (posterior interosseous)	C7
Thumb			
Abduction	Abductor pollicis longus	Radial (posterior interosseous)	C7
	Abductor pollicis brevis	Median	C6-7
Adduction	Adductor pollicis	Ulnar	C8
MCP flexion	Flexor pollicis brevis, medial portion	Ulnar	C8
	lateral portion	Median	C6-7
IP flexion	Flexor pollicis longus	Median (anterior interosseous)	C8-T1
MCP extension	Extensor pollicis brevis	Radial (posterior interosseous)	C7
IP extension	Extensor pollicis longus	Radial (posterior interosseous)	C7
Opposition	Opponens pollicis	Median	C8-T1
	Opponens digiti minimi	Ulnar	C8

Key: MCP, metacarpophalangeal; PIP, proximal interphalangeal; DIP, distal interphalangeal; IP, interphalangeal.

Table 5. Innervation of the primary muscles of movement for the lower extremity

Joint movement	Primary muscles	Peripheral nerves	Nerve root
Hip			
Flexion	Iliopsoas	Femoral	L1-3
Extension	Gluteus maximus	Inferior gluteal	S1
Abduction	Gluteus medius	Superior gluteal	L5
Adduction	Adductor longus	Obturator	L2-4
Knee			
Flexion	Semimembranosus	Tibial	L5
	Semitendinosus	Tibial	L5
	Biceps femoris	Tibial	S1
Extension	Quadriceps	Femoral	L2-4
Ankle			
Dorsiflexion	Tibialis anterior	Deep peroneal	L4
	Extensor hallucis longus	Deep peroneal	L5
	Extensor digitorum longus	Deep peroneal	L5
Plantarflexion	Peroneus longus and brevis	Superficial peroneal	S1
	Gastrocnemius and soleus	Tibial	S1-2
	Flexor hallucis longus	Tibial	L5
	Flexor digitorum longus	Tibial	L5
	Tibialis posterior	Tibial	L5

Table 6. Deep tendon reflexes

Reflexes	Nerve roots
Biceps	C5
Brachioradialis	C6
Triceps	C7
Patellar	L4
Achilles	S1

H. **Special tests.** There are tests specific to each of the joints. Listed below are some of these tests. Please see the appropriate chapters for more details on the examination of specific joints.

1. **Shoulder**
   a. **Drop-arm test.** Purpose: To test for tears in the rotator cuff. Technique: Have patient fully abduct the arm to 90 degrees and then slowly lower it. The test is positive if the arm falls to the patient's side as he or she is lowering it.
   b. **Impingement syndrome test.** Purpose: To test for rotator cuff tendinitis. Technique: With the patient's elbow in full extension, forcibly flex the arm against resistance. Reproduction of pain is the positive sign.
   c. **Yergason test.** Purpose: To determine if biceps tendon is stable in the bicipital groove. Technique: Have the patient flex the elbow to 90 degrees. Then grasp the patient's elbow and wrist and attempt to rotate the arm externally against resistance while pulling downward on the elbow. If it is unstable, the biceps tendon should pop out.

2. **Elbow**
   a. **Tennis elbow test.** Purpose: To test for lateral epicondylitis. Technique: Stabilize the patient's forearm and have the patient make a fist and extend his or her wrist. Pain will occur at the lateral epicondyle when the examiner attempts to force the wrist into flexion against resistance.

3. **Wrist and hand**
   a. **Tinel's sign.** Purpose: To test for carpal tunnel syndrome. Technique: Percuss over the transverse carpal ligament on the palmar surface of the wrist. The test is positive if reproduction of paresthesia occurs in the median nerve distribution.
   b. **Phalen's test.** Purpose: To test for carpal tunnel syndrome. Technique: Have patient flex both wrists maximally and hold for 1 minute. Development of paresthesia is a positive test.
   c. **Allen test.** Purpose: Test for intact radial and ulnar artery blood flow to the hand. Technique: Have the patient open and close his or her fist several times. While the patient holds the fist closed, the examiner applies pressure to the radial and ulnar arteries to occlude them at the wrist. As the patient opens the fist, the examiner notes its pale color, then releases one of the arteries. If the hand does not immediately flush, partial or complete arterial occlusion should be suspected. The other

artery should be checked in a similar fashion, as should the other hand.

d. **Flexor digitorum superficialis test.** Purpose: To establish an intact flexor digitorum superficialis. Technique: Hold all the patient's fingers in full extension except the finger being tested. Have the patient attempt to flex the finger in question at the proximal interphalangeal joint (PIP). If he or she can flex the finger, the superficialis tendon is intact.

e. **Flexor digitorum profundus test.** Purpose: To establish an intact flexor digitorum profundus. Technique: The examiner holds the patient's PIP joint in extension while the patient flexes the distal interphalangeal (DIP) joint of the finger in question. Flexion of the DIP joint confirms an intact profundus tendon for the tested finger.

4. **Hip**
   a. **Trendelenburg test.** Purpose: To test the strength of the gluteus medius muscle. Technique: Have the patient stand on one leg. A strong gluteus medius on the supported side will elevate the pelvis on the unsupported side. If the gluteus medius is weak, the pelvis on the unsupported side drops and the Trendelenburg test is positive.

   b. **Thomas test.** Purpose: To detect fixed flexion contractures of the hip. Technique: With the patient in a supine position on the examining table, bring the patient's unaffected leg into maximum flexion. Try to extend the contralateral leg fully while the patient maintains the lumbar spine flat upon the table. Failure to fully extend the affected leg is indicative of a flexion contracture.

   c. **Ober test.** Purpose: To test for iliotibial band contraction. Technique: Place the patient on his or her side with the affected leg on top. Put the hip joint in the neutral position with the knee flexed to 90 degrees and bring the leg into full abduction. Release the abducted leg. It should drop to an adducted position if normal. However, if the leg stays abducted, the test is positive for an iliotibial band contraction.

5. **Knee**
   a. **Anterior drawer test.** Purpose: To test for anterior cruciate ligament (ACL) instability. Technique: The patient lies supine with the knee flexed to 90 degrees and the foot on the examining table. While steadying the patient's foot by sitting close to it, the examiner grasps the leg just below the knee and at-

tempts to move the tibia anteriorly with respect to the femur. Greater than 2 cm of anterior mobility suggests ACL rupture.

b. Posterior drawer test. Purpose: To test for posterior cruciate ligament (PCL) instability. Technique: Same as anterior drawer test except that the examiner attempts to move the tibia posteriorly with respect to the femur. Greater than 2 cm of posterior mobility suggests PCL rupture.

c. Lachman's test. Purpose: To test for rupture of the ACL. Technique: This is just like the anterior drawer test except that the knee is flexed less than 30 degrees with the patient supine. This position is more comfortable for a patient with an acute knee injury. The examiner stabilizes the patient's femur with one hand and attempts to move the tibia forward with respect to the femur. Again, increased movement is indicative of ACL damage.

d. McMurray test. Purpose: To test for a torn medial meniscus. Technique: With the patient supine and the knee flexed, the examiner rotates the patient's foot internally and externally to loosen the knee joint. Then the examiner rotates the foot externally with one hand, places a valgus stress on the knee with the other hand, and extends the patient's knee. A "click" palpated or heard in the medial joint line is indicative of a torn medial meniscus.

e. Collateral ligament test. Purpose: To test for rupture of medial or lateral collateral ligaments (MCL and LCL). Technique: Place the patient in a supine position with the knee in slight flexion (15–25 degrees). For the medial collateral ligament, place one hand around the patient's knee with your palmar surface on the fibular head and your fingers along the medial joint line. Place the other hand around the patient's ankle. Apply a valgus stress by pushing the knee medially and the ankle laterally. If there is a rupture of the MCL, an opening in the joint space will be palpable. To test for integrity of the LCL, reverse your hands and apply a varus force to the knee joint. Opening of the joint space suggests damage to the LCL.

f. Ballottement. Purpose: To test for knee joint effusion. Technique: Place the patient's knee in extension and "milk" fluid from the distal thigh into the space between the patella and femur. Tap the patella while maintaining pressure on its lateral margins. If an effusion is present, the tap will be palpable to the hand holding the margins of the patella.

6. **Foot and ankle**
    a. **Anterior drawer test.** Purpose: To test for a tear of the anterior talofibular ligament (ATFL). Technique: With the patient's legs hanging over the examining table and feet in minimal plantarflexion, place one hand on the lower tibia and grasp the calcaneus in the palm of the other hand. Attempt to pull the hindfoot anteriorly while pushing the tibia posteriorly. The test is positive if there is forward motion of the hindfoot.
    b. **Posterior drawer test.** Purpose: To test for a tear of the posterior talofibular ligament (PTFL). Technique: Same as that for anterior drawer test except that the hindfoot is moved posteriorly while the tibia is pulled anteriorly. The test is positive if there is backward motion of the hindfoot.
    c. **Inversion stress test.** Purpose: To test for tear of the calcaneofibular ligament (CFL). Technique: Grasp the patient's calcaneus in one hand and stabilize the tibia with the other. Invert the hindfoot. If there is increased motion, suspect a tear of the CFL.

III. **Orthopaedic definitions**
  A. **Joint movement**
      1. **Abduction.** Movement away from the midline.
      2. **Adduction.** Movement toward the midline.
      3. **Eversion.** Turning in an outward direction.
      4. **Inversion.** Turning in an inward direction.
      5. **Pronation.** Turning of the palmar surface downward or posteriorly.
      6. **Supination.** Turning of the palmar surface upward or anteriorly.
  B. **Anatomy**
      1. **Coxa.** Hip.
      2. **Cubitus.** Elbow.
      3. **Genu.** Knee.
      4. **Hallux.** Great toe.
      5. **Pes.** Foot.
      6. **Pollex.** Thumb.
      7. **Talipes.** Ankle plus foot (talus plus pes).
      8. **Volar.** Palmar surface of hand or sole of foot.

BIBLIOGRAPHY

Chipman, C, ed. *Emergency department orthopaedics.* Rockville, MD: Aspen Systems, 1982.

Hoppenfeld S. *Physical Examination of the Spine and Extremities.* Norwalk, CT: Appleton-Century-Crofts, 1976.

Lhowe DW. Musculoskeletal injuries: general principles of assessment and management. In: May HL, Aghababian RV, Fleisher GR, eds. *Emergency medicine.* Boston: Little, Brown, 1992.

Mallon WJ, McNamara MJ, Urbaniak JR. *Orthopaedics for the house officer.* Baltimore: Willims & Wilkins, 1995.

Mercier LR. *Practical orthopedics.* St. Louis: 4th ed. Mosby, 1995.

Ruiz E, Cicero JJ, eds. *Emergency management of skeletal injuries.* St. Louis: Mosby, 1995.

Swartz MH. *Textbook of physical diagnosis: history and examination.* Philadelphia: WB Saunders, 1994.

Diagnostic Imaging

Charles Pattavina

Although it is not appropriate for every acute orthopaedic problem, well-chosen imaging is the cornerstone of diagnosis for most injuries. The most commonly employed technique is plain radiography, or "x-ray" imaging. Newer modes such as nuclear medicine, ultrasound, computed tomography (a computerized variation on x-ray), and magnetic resonance imaging have increasing roles. They have largely replaced procedures such as myelography and conventional tomography. Improvements in each technique are constantly providing more and better images.

Emergency physicians are called upon to read a wide variety of films in the emergency department at all hours. In most cases, the emergency physician's reading is the only interpretation that will affect the patient's care while he or she is in the emergency department. It is therefore important to develop and improve one's skills, especially for reading plain x-rays.

I. **General principles**
   A. **Viewing the films.** Films that can be viewed in the emergency department (plain radiographs, CT films, etc.) are generally hung or placed against a view box that is back-lit by fluorescent bulbs. Typical intensity is 2000 to 2500 nits, but many boxes can be 3500 nits or even higher. Good intensity makes using the "hot light" less often necessary. Unlike the film in your 35-mm camera, conventional x-ray film has emulsion on both sides. This allows one to enhance the image by lifting the film off the board to view it obliquely, i.e., at a 45-degree angle instead of perpendicularly (at 90 degrees).
   B. **Characteristics of acutely broken bones**
      1. **Adults.** A cortical break is usually a complete one.
      2. **Pediatric.** There may be partial cortical break (greenstick fracture), buckling of cortex on one side (torus fracture), or bending without a cortical defect (plastic fracture).
      3. **Impacted fracture.** This may show only increased area of bone density, but usually there is some disruption of cortex.
      4. **Fracture margins** are sharp and not corticated, in contrast with sesamoid bones or accessory ossification centers (or old fractures), which are smooth and well corticated.
      5. **Associated soft tissue signs** of acute fracture would not be present with an old fracture or nonfracture.
      6. **Orthopaedic texts and atlases** of normal radiographic anatomy and normal variants should be available and referred to in order to describe

fractures accurately and to determine when an unusual finding is not a fracture.

C. **What views to obtain**

1. **Standard views.** It is essential to obtain correctly done views that show the area(s) of interest adequately. This usually means an anteroposterior (AP), a lateral (at a 90-degree angle to the AP), and, in some body parts, one or more oblique films. Generally, films of long bones should show at least the adjacent joint on either side. There are special views for just about any area one would want to image, and unusual obliques or unconventional views can be improvised when needed.

   In any unusual circumstances, however, one must communicate the area and extent of interest directly to the technicians to minimize the need to return a patient for additional views. In some instances, however, the return of a patient is unavoidable.

   It should go without saying that the best way to order the correct films is by thoroughly examining the patient first. Abnormalities including fractures can be missed when the wrong areas are radiographed (e.g., foot versus ankle), when radiographs do not include enough area, or when the angles are not correct.

   Because of the body's bilateral symmetry, we have the advantage of a contralateral "normal" for comparison, especially in pediatric cases. It is rarely necessary to order a comparison view before examining the views of the affected side. If there is an obvious fracture or dislocation, comparison views are usually unnecessary; if there is a questionable finding on only one or two views, one can limit the number of comparison films to the one or two corresponding views. Comparison views are most needed in some pediatric cases because of variable growth rates and variable appearance of growth plates.

2. **Additional views.** These may be needed when a fracture is not visualized. Any nondisplaced fracture can be difficult to see on a routine radiograph performed the day of the injury. Sometimes *indirect* evidence of a fracture is apparent on the initial set of films.

   Perhaps the best-known example is the **fat-pad sign** (also referred to as a **sail sign** because of its abnormal appearance, which resembles that of a well-trimmed spinnaker on a sailboat, depending on the amount of fluid or blood in the joint). A positive fat-pad sign may be the *only* manifestation of a radial head fracture in an adult. An uneven ankle mortise can be a sign of a severe sprain or occult fracture. Soft tissue swelling seen as frank swelling and/or obliteration of normal fascial planes is often associated with an underlying fracture.

Special additional views can also be done of such bones as the scaphoid (carpal navicular views) or patella ("sunrise" view) when indicated by point tenderness. Other modes such as computed tomography or Panorex can be used for some areas.

3. **Postreduction views** should always be obtained after any dislocation is reduced. They not only allow one to identify associated fractures but also document the improvement.

Clinically suspected fractures not demonstrated by any of the above methods or by other methods such as computed tomography should be splinted (treated as fractures) and arrangements made for repeat films in 7 to 10 days. It is far better to find a fracture by signs of healing a week after initial treatment.

III. **Imaging modalities**
   A. **Plain radiographs**
   B. **Computed tomography (CT).** Since its initial development, improvements and refinements in CT have brought it into a number of areas where it is either used primarily or to prove or disprove a fracture or other deformity when plain films are equivocal (e.g., cervical spine, mandible, pelvis, hip) or when soft tissues need to be examined (e.g. lumbosacral spine, knee). CT is excellent for demonstrating complex joint fractures as well.
   C. **Arteriography.** Plain films and/or fluoroscopy with injected contrast may be needed to evaluate for vascular injury associated with a dislocated joint (e.g., knee) or high-velocity injury to the torso (e.g., complex shoulder fracture or sternal fracture).
   D. **Nuclear medicine.** While generally unhelpful on the day of the injury, a bone scan can identify occult fractures once they have begun to heal and can also identify osteomyelitis and metastases causing bone pain.
   E. **Ultrasound.** This noninvasive mode is used in emergency orthopaedics mainly to locate foreign bodies, sometimes even when they are seen on plain films (to facilitate removal). Doppler ultrasound to evaluate for deep venous thrombosis (DVT) may be useful in the diagnosis of leg pain when orthopaedic problems have been ruled out.
   F. **Magnetic resonance imaging (MRI).** This relatively new technique has represented a great advance in the imaging of soft tissues but is often inferior to CT in identifying fractures. One exception may be occult fractures of the hip. Its usefulness in the acute setting is also limited by the difficulty of placing an immobilized trauma victim into a narrow tube

with a strong magnetic field for a long period of time. Soft tissue injuries of joints, osteomyelitis, avascular necrosis, and suspected tumors of bone are all well imaged by this technique.

IV. **Anatomic location**
  A. **Spine**
    1. **Cervical spine.** One of the most critical areas to evaluate properly before discontinuing immobilization.
      a. **Plain films.** One must obtain **AP** and **lateral** views, which, taken together, show the entire cervical spine. This requires at least three films, usually four or more.
        (1) **Anteroposterior (AP) views.** In addition to a routine AP view, an **odontoid** or **open-mouth** view must be obtained to show the C1-C2 joint. This view must often be repeated to fully show the lateral masses of C1, their articulation with C2, and the symmetry of all spaces. A **Waters view** can be helpful when the patient's jaw or teeth continue to inhibit imaging of the C1 or C2 joint.
        (2) **Lateral views.** This is the most critical film in the case of trauma. *First, always count the vertebrae.* One must be able to see all seven lateral vertebrae of the cervical spine to the C7-T1 joint, inclusive. Unfortunately, this is most difficult when it is most critical—in the immobilized trauma patient. The first views are obtained through the radiolucent immobilization devices. The **horizontal-beam lateral** (**cross-table lateral** or **shoot-through**) is taken without moving the patient's head or neck in any way. Often, this view will not adequately demonstrate the C7-T1 joint or perhaps not even the lower three or four cervical vertebrae in very large or obese patients. Donning a lead apron and pulling down on the patient's arms may be enough to enhance visualization. Prevertebral swelling is also assessed on these views.
          (a) **Swimmer's (lateral) view.** Often, the arm traction is not enough, and a view focusing on the lower vertebrae is done with one arm elevated above the head and the other deviated caudally to distribute the bulk of the shoulders more evenly. If the view does not show C2, a lower vertebra must be definitely identifiable to permit accurate counting of the remaining lower

vertebrae. *Immobilization must be maintained until bone injury is ruled out.*

  (b) **Flexion and extension views** are obtained only in the stable patient and only when needed to rule out a subtle subluxation or when the patient has an unusual curvature. These views are limited to the active and voluntary motions made by the patient (i.e., unassisted).

  (3) **Oblique views.** These views are used mainly to show the neuroforamina between the cervical vertebrae and are not usually needed to evaluate the trauma victim. When available, they may offer the added opportunity to identify fractures and dislocations.

  When there is clinical suspicion of a rotatory subluxation of C1-C2 and the *AP odontoid views* do not demonstrate normal symmetry of the spaces on either side of the odontoid, CT may be needed. If both *oblique odontoid views* are obtained and they demonstrate that the asymmetry shifts from one side to the other, CT *may* be avoidable.

 b. **CT** is useful in imaging cervical vertebrae and interspaces when there is too much surrounding tissue for plain films to "clear" the spine. CT scanning is also useful to accurately define fractures and dislocations (e.g., Jefferson's fracture of C1 or rotatory subluxation of C1-C2).

 c. **MRI** is less accurate than CT for bone injury; indeed, it often misses fractures of the vertebral arch. It is superior in every other way, especially in finding and identifying soft tissue abnormalities. It is indicated mainly for viewing contents of the spinal canal. Unfortunately, the usefulness of MRI is limited by the fact that it may be very difficult to perform on a trauma victim, owing to the confining tube and magnetism.

 d. **Myelography** can be useful in demonstrating the spinal cord and disk protrusions but is mainly used only when MRI and CT are not available. This technique is also limited by the need to move the patient to inject contrast.

B. **Lumbar spine**

 1. **Plain films.** The hazards and limitations of plain x-rays should be remembered when one is considering whether to order any views at all in the ab-

sence of significant trauma. According to the World Health Organization (WHO), one set of L-S films provides approximately the same amount of gonadal radiation as one chest x-ray every day for 3 years. Combine this knowledge with the fact that L-S films rarely contribute anything to the acute management of back pain or strain, and one will seldom order them. AP and cross-table lateral views can be useful prior to CT or MRI to rule out unstable injury in victims of significant trauma.

  a. AP and lateral views. Generally, two *lateral* views are performed, one of which demonstrates the entire lumbar and sacral spines and a "spot" film of the L5-S1 interspace. (The angle from the beam's origin to the higher and lower portions of the film tends to clutter the interspaces through which the radiation passes obliquely.) In a victim of severe trauma, the first back film should be the *horizontal-beam* (cross-table) *lateral* to "clear" the lumbar spine before moving the patient. These films can identify compression fractures of the vertebral bodies, either spontaneous/pathological or those sustained in a fall or jump landing on the feet. In the elderly, it may be impossible to determine whether a compression fracture is acute without recent old films or a bone scan.

  b. Oblique views. These views are rarely needed in the injured patient and only result in added radiation exposure and expense.

 2. CT requires movement of the patient to the scanner but is very useful to identify subtle or complex fractures, to image soft tissues, and to localize bone or metal fragments. CT can be enhanced with water-soluble contrast to demonstrate the cord and nerve roots and show dural tears.

 3. MRI is superior to CT for the evaluation of soft tissues but is not as good for visualizing bone. It is also better than myelography for evaluating the spinal cord.

 4. Myelography. This is indicated only when neither MRI nor CT with contrast is available to evaluate the spinal cord. Myelography is also limited by the need to move the patient to introduce contrast.

C. Lower extremity
 1. Pelvis
  a. Plain films
   (1) The standard pelvic film is the AP. This film must be examined very meticulously, as a fracture may initially be

nondisplaced and very subtle and there are almost always bowel contents overlying parts of the bone. Remember that the pelvis is a ring structure, and if a fracture is noted there could be a second fracture or a disruption of an S-I joint or the symphysis pubis. Similarly, the superior and inferior pubic rami (where most fractures are found) are ring structures within a ring structure.

(2) In trauma, **45-degree oblique (Judet) views** can be helpful in identifying fractures and disruptions.

b. **CT** is excellent but not indicated for stable fractures due to radiation and cost. CT is very useful for identifying unstable fractures and sacral and S-I joint fracture-dislocations.

c. **MRI** or follow-up **bone scan** or even old or follow-up **plain films** can also be used if it is important to identify a fracture.

2. **Hip**
   a. **Plain films**
      (1) Standard views—**AP pelvic** (with hip in slight internal rotation) and **true (groin) lateral** of the hip—are generally adequate to find and define hip fractures and dislocations.
      (2) A **frog-leg lateral** may be useful in confirming a subtle subcapitular fracture, slipped femoral capital epiphysis, or avascular necrosis (AVN). Early diagnosis of hip fractures and dislocations is imperative because of the risk of AVN.
   b. **CT** or **MRI** can be useful in identifying the unusual fracture not visible on plain films, and it is also useful in hip dislocations or acetabular fractures to locate loose bodies in the joint. MRI would not be suitable for patients with ferrous metal prostheses or implants.

3. **Femur**
   a. **Plain films.** The standard films are **AP** and **lateral,** and the entire bone (including the joints above and below) must be imaged. Hip dislocations often accompany femoral shaft fractures and may be overlooked because of the obvious shaft fractures. Stress fractures may not be visible on the initial plain films, so CT or MRI may be needed.
   b. **CT** is superior to MRI in vertical stress fractures of the shaft.
   c. **MRI** is superior for stress fractures of the medial femoral neck, which present as vague hip or groin pain.

4. **Knee.** Most knee injuries are limited to soft tissue involvement, but fractures of the tibial spines and plateaus (80% lateral) may also be seen, as well as fractures of the femoral condyle.
   a. **Plain films.** Standard views include **AP** and **lateral** and, in cases of trauma, the **sunrise** view. On the AP, the patella usually overlies the lower femur, so fractures of this small bone may not be seen. Although horizontal fractures of the patella are easily seen on the lateral view (due to displacement by the powerful quadriceps muscle), stellate or longitudinal fractures may only be seen with a sunrise view. The anterior tibial tubercle apophysis may have multiple ossification centers and appear irregular and fragmented, especially on the lateral view. When accompanied by soft tissue swelling and pain at the tibial tubercle, this suggests Osgood-Schlatter disease. Proximal fibular fractures may be associated with ankle fracture/dislocations.
      (1) **Sunrise view.** The x-ray beam is directed over the top of the flexed knee (20 degrees). Bipartite or multipartite patella is *usually* bilateral, well corticated, and found at the superolateral border. The sunrise view is the view of choice for patellar dislocation also. Osteochondral "flake" fractures are usually seen on this view near the medial facet of the patella.
      (2) **Horizontal-beam lateral view.** Done with the patient supine, this is useful for identifying a fat/blood level indicating a traumatic lipohemarthrosis and probable fracture.
      (3) **Oblique view.** This may help to identify a tibial plateau fracture.
   b. **Arteriography** is needed following knee *dislocations* to identify associated vascular injuries.
   c. **CT** is useful to identify subtle fractures such as nondisplaced tibial plateau fractures as well as epiphyseal injuries.
   d. **MRI** may be used instead of CT, as above, and is also invaluable in identifying the myriad of soft tissue injuries which occur with or without bone injuries. MRI of meniscal injuries may eliminate 90% of arthroscopies and can also demonstrate chondromalacia (patellar pain syndrome) when necessary.
5. **Tibia** and **fibula.** Because of their close relationship, these bones are imaged together.
   a. **Plain films. AP** and **lateral "tib-fib"** films are the standard, and, again, the entire length

of the bones from knee to ankle must be seen. A Maisonneuve fracture may involve only the most proximal fibula and distal portions. As with any area, an **oblique** view can be tailored to confirm or rule out a possible abnormality seen on a standard view.

   b.   **Other techniques** are rarely needed except **Doppler/ultrasound** when leg pain could represent a DVT.

6.   **Ankle.** Although the ankle is more commonly injured, it resembles the knee in that soft tissue injuries occur far more commonly than fractures. The ankle is a less complex joint. Most orthopaedic problems can be adequately diagnosed by careful physical exam and plain films. This includes examining up to the patient's knee and, when indicated by tenderness, imaging that area to exclude or identify a Maisonneuve's fracture. There is also sometimes confusion over whether ankle or foot films or both are needed. If the patient is examined well, usually only one or the other is needed, keeping in mind that the base of the fifth metatarsal (a site of frequent foot fracture often confused with ankle injury) is included on the lateral ankle view.

   a.   **Plain films**

      (1)   **Standard** views (three), **AP** and **lateral,** will show most fractures from small avulsions to bimalleolar and "trimalleolar" (bimalleolar plus posterior tibial lip) fracture/dislocations.

The **mortise (internal oblique)** view will help confirm the above and also demonstrate the mortise (horizontal space between the plafond or tibial joint surface and the talar joint surface), which should be a very consistent 3 to 4 mm over the talar surface. Widening of 2 mm or more toward either end is abnormal. Old avulsion fractures from prior sprain-type injuries may be seen, distinguished by smooth, corticated edges.

      (2)   **Stress** views may be needed to demonstrate instability secondary to soft tissue injury. These are done with varus and valgus stress and possibly an anterior drawer. Owing to the wide range of acceptable ankle laxity, **comparison stress views** may be needed.

   b.   **CT** can be useful in accurately characterizing complex fractures such as the juvenile triplane and Tillaux fractures.

7.   **Foot.** Fractures and dislocations of the foot are easily missed; one must pay close attention to the normal bone anatomy and alignment. For exam-

ple, the apophysis of the fifth metatarsal is longitudinally oriented and should not be mistaken for a fracture.

a. **Plain films.** The standard views (three) are **AP, lateral,** and **oblique.**

(1) **AP.** The lateral border of the first metatarsal must align with the lateral border of the medial cuneiform, while the medial border of the second metatarsal normally aligns with the medial border of the middle cuneiform.

Lateral. This view may miss tarsal and metatarsal fractures and dislocations but usually shows calcaneal and talar fractures. In suspected calcaneal fractures, Boehler's angle should be measured: an angle of less than 24 degrees or more than 48 degrees strongly suggests a fracture. Calcaneal fractures are often bilateral (10%) or associated with other injuries of the opposite foot or ankle as well as with thoracolumbar spine compression fractures (the so-called boudoir's or Don Juan fracture from jumping or falling from an excessive height and landing on the feet).

Oblique. The lateral border of the third metatarsal must align with the lateral edge of the lateral metatarsal, while the medial edge of the fourth metatarsal normally aligns with the medial edge of the cuboid bone. The fifth metatarsal should also articulate with the cuboid but extend more laterally.

(2) **Weight-bearing** views (patient bears own body weight standing on a film cassette on the floor) are useful in identifying an occult Lisfranc's fracture.

(3) The **axial** view is available for the calcaneus, which is the most frequently fractured tarsal bone.

b. **CT** can be useful in characterizing complex calcaneal fractures, which can involve its three-faceted articulation with the talus.

8. **Toes.** Toes are generally seen on the aforementioned foot films. Other than reducing a dislocation or dislocated fracture, little or nothing therapeutic is ever done about toe fractures, making x-rays of little importance.

D. **Upper extremity**

1. **Sternum and sternoclavicular joint**

a. **Plain films.** Standard views: the sternum most commonly breaks and/or dislocates at the manubrial sternal joint, which is seen well on a **lateral chest x-ray** or coned-down lateral. These are usually high-velocity injuries (e.g., steering-wheel injury), which may be associated with fractures of the spinal column or cardiac and/or pulmonary contusions. For the sternoclavicular (SC) joint, an **AP view with 40 degrees of cephalic angulation** is best, but a limited CT may be cost-effective.

b. **CT.** Two or three axial cuts of the SC joint should be adequate to identify infection (especially in IVDA) or dislocation (anterior more common).

c. **MRI.** As posterior dislocation of the SC joint may compromise the great vessels, MRI may be preferable to obtain the most complete and accurate diagnosis.

2. **Clavicle**
   a. **Plain films**
      (1) **Standard. Straight AP** and **AP with central beam angled cephalad.** Physical findings plus a fracture line on either projection are adequate to diagnose a fracture (most are in the middle third). Often the fracture fragments will be displaced and overriding, making diagnosis very easy. The two APs will show the distal clavicle, a displaced or (high-grade) acromioclavicular (AC) separation, upper humeral fractures, and inferior dislocation of the glenohumeral joint.

3. **Shoulder**
   a. **Plain films**
      (1) The two standard views are both **AP,** one in **internal rotation** and one in **external rotation.**
      (2) In any case of trauma, an **axillary view** (or **Y view**) should also be done as standard. The axillary view is needed to show whether the inferior dislocation is anterior (80%) or posterior or whether there is a direct posterior dislocation (50% of posterior dislocations are missed initially). The axillary view can also demonstrate minimally displaced scapular coracoid fractures, cortical fractures of the anterior (95%) or posterior humeral head, and the degree of angulation of humeral neck fractures. Postreduction views should be obtained to rule out a fracture after reducing a dislocation (e.g., Hill-Sachs or Bankart lesions). Calcium deposits, indicative of an inflammatory process, may be seen near the biceps tendon.

(3) **Oblique.** If the patient cannot rotate internally and externally, he or she should be rotated and two oblique views obtained.

(4) **Weight bearing.** If it is important to demonstrate an AC separation, views may be obtained with the patient erect and holding 15- to 20-lb weights suspended from each wrist. The unaffected shoulder serves as a comparison (normally 3 to 5 mm) while the weight displaces the AC joint on the affected side (no more than 2 to 3 mm difference normally).

b. **Flow studies/arch studies.** When a complex shoulder fracture is the result of high-velocity injury (e.g., a motor vehicle crash) further study is needed to identify any damage to major vessels in the area.

c. **CT** with arthrography may be needed to evaluate an unstable shoulder and should identify a Bankart lesion or rotator cuff injury.

d. **MRI** or **MR arthrography** has the same uses as CT arthrography.

4. **Humerus.** For **plain films,** the standard views are **AP** and **lateral;** 80% of proximal fractures are nondisplaced, held in position by periosteum, joint capsule, and/or rotator cuff. When the "ice cream" (humeral head) is out of the "cone," a displaced fracture is described. Supracondylar fractures are best diagnosed on elbow films.

5. **Elbow**

a. **Plain films.** The elbow is a complex joint that fortunately comes with fat pads, which are extremely helpful in making a fracture diagnosis. With practice, the normally thin, straight, and narrow anterior fat pad can be seen and contrasted with the fat-pad sign: either abnormal billowing of the anterior fat pad or any visualization of the posterior fat pad (which, when visible, is always abnormal). The presence of a fat-pad sign indicates a joint effusion (hemarthrosis in trauma), with approximately a 90% chance of an underlying fracture, especially in children. The fat pads are more clearly seen by tilting the film to view it obliquely.

In the case of "nursemaid's elbow" radiographs are normal or, rarely, show an effusion. Often the defect is reduced in the process of imaging.

In addition to viewing the fat pads on the lateral, the **anterior humeral line** and the **radiocapitellar line** should be drawn or imagined. Both lines should normally pass through the midportion of the capitellum (on any view), even in children (Table 1). Any other result indicates displacement of the capitellum (e.g., supracondylar fracture) or radial head (e.g., dislocation).

(1) **Standard views** (four) include the **AP, lateral,** and **obliques** (two). Except for the lateral, which should be done in 90 degrees of flexion with the thumb pointing upward, all views are done as fully extended as possible.

(2) Other views may be attempted to demonstrate an occult fracture of the radial head (half of all adult elbow fractures, accounting for most fat-pad signs). Some fractures of the radial head are exceedingly difficult to see (half are nondisplaced) and should be presumed to be present in cases of trauma when a fat-pad sign is seen. Isolated radial head *dislocations* are rare in adults; when present, they should raise suspicion of a Monteggia's (ulnar) fracture distally.

b. **MRI** can be useful to identify soft tissue injuries including lateral epicondylitis ("tennis elbow"), medial epicondylitis, ligament tears, tendon tears, and osteochondritis dissecans.

6. **Forearm.** Except for torus fractures and the "nightstick" fracture, forearm fractures usually include at least two breaks or one break and a dislocation (e.g., Monteggia's fracture). **Plain films, standard views,** as with all long bones, are the **AP** and **lateral,** which should include both the elbow and proximal wrist. Several types of fractures and fracture/dislocations occur in the radius/ulna ring structure.

7. **Wrist.** This group includes distal forearm fractures, which are considered with wrist joint injuries. The wrist is injured with great frequency, especially by falls on the outstretched hand. There are definite patterns of injury related to

Table 1.   Epiphyseal maturation sequence (CRITOE)

C̲apitellum, 1 year
R̲adial head, 3–6 years
I̲nternal (medial epicondyle), 5–7 years
T̲rochlea, 9–10 years
O̲lecranon, 9–10 years
E̲picondyle (lateral epicondyle), 9–13 years

the patient's age—i.e., Colles' fracture tends to occur in older patients.

a. **Plain films**

(1) **Standard views** (four) include the **PA, lateral,** and **obliques** (two). The PA view allows identification of the carpal bones according to one's favorite medical school mnemonic and the three arcs they form:

(a) Along the proximal articular margins of the proximal row

(b) Along the distal articular margins of the proximal row

(c) Along the proximal articular margins of the distal row (capitate and hammate)

Normally, the cortical integrity of all bones should be intact, and the intercarpal joint spaces should all be about 2 mm. The hook of the hammate is seen en face on the PA view. A **true lateral view** is needed to evaluate carpal dislocations and fracture displacements (e.g., lunate, perilunate). On a true lateral, the radius lunate, capitate, and third metacarpal should all be coaxial. Dorsal chip fractures may be seen, usually from the triquetrum, and sometimes small dorsal bony flakes are seen in a simple sprain.

(2) **Navicular views** elongate the profile of the scaphoid (carpal navicular) and *may* demonstrate an acute fracture. These fractures, sustained in a *fall on the outstretched hand* (FOOSH) may not be visible at all until healing is obvious by callus formation in 7 to 10 days. They should, therefore, be presumptively diagnosed and treated on clinical grounds.

(3) **Stress views** or **radial** and **ulnar deviation views** can be used to demonstrate scapholunate dissociation by showing an abnormal widening of the space between those two bones. This has been called the Terry Thomas sign, after the late English actor with a prominent separation between his two upper front teeth. Intercarpal joint spaces should be about 2 mm.

(4) A **supinated oblique view** may help show a fracture of the hook of the hamate, as may a **carpal tunnel view,** but the latter is usually impossible in an acutely injured wrist and provides little other information.

b. **Fluoroscopy** can be helpful in undiagnosed wrist instability.

c. **CT** can be used for scaphoid fractures, hook of hamate fractures, and distal radioulnar dislocations.

d. **MRI** is useful to diagnose AVN, which can occur following injury to the scaphoid or lunate bones.

8. **Hand**

a. **Plain films** are generally adequate to diagnose acute hand injuries other than those involving nonopaque foreign bodies.

(1) **Standard views** include the **AP** and **oblique** of the hand. **Lateral views** of the digits as well as **AP** and **lateral views** of the thumb are ordered as needed.

(a) An **AP view** of the hand prominently shows normal nutrient artery canals on the phalanges, which should not be confused with fractures. They may, similarly, appear on more than one digit or on both hands. Tuft fractures of the distal phalanges are well seen, as are midshaft fractures of various types.

(b) The **oblique view** of the hand is used, in exception to the general rule of two views at a 90-degree angle, because the **hand lateral** superimposes at least four metacarpal bones (although it is useful for the carpometacarpal area and fingers when properly positioned). For the oblique view, the fingers must be spread apart (almost fanned) to prevent their overlap.

(c) **Lateral views** of the *digit(s)* may be obtained by tightly flexing all the uninvolved fingers or by positioning each finger in a different degree of flexion (e.g., index finger only slightly flexed, with each more medial finger more flexed and the little finger in the greatest flexion). Tuft fractures, avulsion fractures, and isolated flexion of an interphalangeal joint (indicating a complete extensor tendon rupture or avulsion) are well seen on the lateral.

(d) **Thumb AP** and **lateral views** are required when the thumb is the area of interest because none of the above positions allows either the true frontal or lateral aspect to be seen.

(2) **Special views**
   (a) The **reversed oblique view** offers an additional angle for identifying occult avulsion fractures (usually at tendon insertions) and for assessing the position of radioopaque foreign bodies. Other oblique angles may be helpful.
   (b) **Stress views** can be useful to identify a volar avulsion **(lateral)** or side avulsion, as in gamekeeper's thumb **(AP).** Comparison stress views may be needed.
   (c) **Carpometacarpal (CMC) PA** for dislocations in that area is done with hand and fingers flat on the cassette. The CMC joint spaces should be of consistent width and the opposing articular surfaces should be parallel and in a zig-zag pattern.
   b. **MRI** can be useful to identify tendon retraction and positioning, but it is rarely needed in the emergency department's management of hand injuries.

BIBLIOGRAPHY

Harris JH, Harris WH. *The radiology of emergency medicine,* 2nd ed. Baltimore: Williams & Wilkins, 1981.

Manaster BJ. Handbook of skeletal radiology, 2nd ed. St. Louis: Mosby-Yearbook, 1997.

Squire LF. *Fundamentals of radiology,* 3rd ed. Cambridge, MA: Harvard University Press, 1982.

Wiest PW, Roth PB. *Fundamentals of emergency radiology.* Philadelphia: WB Saunders, 1996.

4

Principles of Anesthesia for Orthopaedic Procedures

Mary Jo Wagner

The use of pharmacological agents for pain control, anesthesia, and sedation is a vital part of the proper treatment of patients with urgent or emergent orthopaedic problems. Successful completion of an orthopaedic procedure is often dependent upon adequate reduction of pain and muscle spasm.

I. **Regional blocks using local anesthesia**
   A. **Historical information.** Until the beginning of this century, the only local anesthetic agent available for pain control during any type of orthopaedic procedure was cocaine. Procaine was first synthesized in 1905 as an alternative to this toxic local anesthetic. In 1943, lidocaine, the first amide derivative, was synthesized and found to be useful in patients allergic to the ester class of medications (procaine, cocaine). These two classes of pharmacological agents have been used as local and regional anesthetics since that time.
   B. **Pharmacological agents.** In choosing a pharmacological agent for anesthesia, several properties should be considered: onset of action, duration of action, and potency. In most settings, the more rapid the onset of action, the more comfortable the patient will be. However, generally, the faster the onset of action, the shorter the duration of action; therefore a trade-off must often be evaluated. In the emergency department, two predominant classes of pharmacological agents are used for regional blocks: amides and esters. A comparison among the three properties of common anesthetics is listed in Table 1.

   Most patient-reported "allergic" reactions to the local anesthetic occur as the results of pain from the injection causing a vasovagal reaction or the stimulation caused by the epinephrine included in some anesthetics. Some patients are allergic to the preservative added to the anesthetic; preservative-free lidocaine and bupivacaine are available if this allergy exists. True IgE-mediated allergic reactions are rare; most are due to agents in the ester class. If there is a question about a reported allergy to the classical anesthetics, a few studies show that use of 1% diphenhydramine (Benadryl), at least locally, will provide some anesthesia. Extensive studies have not been done using this medication in regional blocks and there have been some case reports about the risk of local necrosis, particularly in tissues that receive end arteries (fingers, nose, etc.) (1). Other techniques for anesthesia may need to be considered in these rare cases.

Table 1. Local and regional anesthetics

Pharmacological agent	Pharmacological class	Onset	Duration	Maximum dose	Maximum dose with epinephrine	Normal concentration for peripheral nerve blocks
Tetracaine	Ester	3–8 min	30–60 min	0.75 mg/kg	—	Used on mucous membranes
Procaine	Ester	2–5 min	1–1-1/2 hr	7 mg/kg	9 mg/kg	1%
Lidocaine	Amide	2–5 min	1–2 hr	4–5 mg/kg	7 mg/kg	1%–2%
Mepivacaine	Amide	3–5 min	2–3 hr	5–6 mg/kg	—	1%–2%
Bupivacaine	Amide	2–10 min	4–8 hr	2 mg/kg	3 mg/kg	0.25%–0.5%
Benadryl	Antihistamine	2–5 min	30–60 min	2 mg/kg	—	1%–2%

Most reactions to local anesthetics are likely to be systemic toxic reactions. Such toxic reactions are usually related to higher doses, more potent drugs, or from inadvertent intravascular injection resulting in systemic administration. Calculating the toxic dose and administering less than this, while carefully following the correct technique for injection, is the best way to reduce the chance of systemic toxic reaction (see table 1 for toxic doses and Section I.G. "Technique"). Recognition of the early signs of toxicity can help prevent serious reactions (see Table 2 for common symptoms of toxicity). Supportive treatment—including airway management, benzodiazepine therapy for seizures, and intravenous (IV) fluids and vasopressors for cardiovascular support—may be needed in the case of severe toxicity.

C. **Indications.** The primary indication for the use of a regional block is to control the pain of injury without causing the patient systemic effects such as drowsiness. There are other advantages to using a regional block, including minimizing tissue distortion at the site of injury and providing an analgesic for the patient that lasts longer than a local block.

D. **Contraindications.** There are few contraindications for using a regional block for anesthesia of local injury to an extremity. Allergy to local anesthetic agents may preclude this procedure. A proximal injury may be difficult to block well with a nontoxic dosage of medication. The practitioner's inexperience with blocks may make this technique less appealing, but the blocks described should be within the scope of most practitioners after careful review of the anatomy and techniques.

E. **Patient history.** Prior to using any anesthetic on a patient, several aspects of the patient's history should be clearly delineated. As with any injury, the mechanism and timing of the injury should be determined. Specific information about prior allergies to any medication, specifically any anesthetic, should be identified. Significant past medical history, including prior

Table 2.   Common signs of toxicity of local anesthetics

Tinnitus

Drowsiness, light-headedness

Tingling of the lips

Slurred speech

Tonic/clonic seizures

Hypotension

Cardiac rhythm disturbances (bradycardia, ventricular tachycardia, asystole)

neurovascular abnormalities (Raynaud's disease, prior vascular occlusion, or previous frostbite) or any previous muscular or tendinous injuries (reimplantation, chronic dislocations, congenital malformations) should be elicited and evaluated.

F. **Physical examination.** A careful physical exam of the entire region that will be affected by the anesthetic procedure should be performed. Thus, if a digital block is to be done to reduce a dislocated distal phalanx, not only the phalanx but also the surrounding fingers and hand should be evaluated, since the block may affect all of these areas. Special care must be taken to evaluate the motor and neurological status of the area in question. Documentation of neurovascular abnormality due to the injury should be made; this should not preclude the use of anesthetic agents. To be accurate about any possible sensory loss, particularly at distal extremities, this documentation generally requires the testing of two-point discrimination. Specific exams can be found in other sections of this textbook.

G. **Technique.** The general purpose of a nerve block is to cause anesthesia of the nerve proximal to an injury at a point along the nerve as it runs from the spine to the periphery. To do this, a small volume of anesthetic is placed immediately adjacent to a peripheral nerve, avoiding direct injection into the nerve or into the vascular structures that generally surround peripheral nerves. To avoid the former, the needle should be withdrawn slightly if the patient develops parasthesias during the injection process. To avoid intravascular injection, the syringe should be aspirated prior to injecting any anesthetic solution. Since most of the nerves that are blocked lie contiguous to an artery, use of epinephrine is contraindicated to prevent the complications of arterial spasm.

The actual injection can be made less painful by using an injection needle that is small in diameter, using warmed and possibly buffered anesthetic solution and a slow rate of injection, with as little volume as possible to minimize tissue distention.

Prior to performing the anesthetic block, the patient's anatomical landmarks should be reviewed and identified. In cases with some difficulty or irregularity, actually marking the skin with a marker or in ink may be useful to help guide the practitioner. The patient should be placed in a supine position if possible. The area to be injected should be prepped with an antiseptic solution and sterilely draped as indicated.

H. **Specific regional blocks**
  1. The **digital block** is used when anesthesia for a procedure is needed on the phalanges of the hand or of the foot. Examples of this might include repair of a distal digital tendon or reduction of a phalanx. The dorsal and volar digital nerves are found

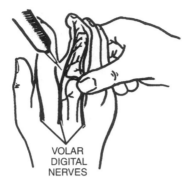

Fig. 1. Digital nerve block.

in a consistent pattern around the phalanges, as shown in Fig. 1. The finger is punctured with a small (27- or 30-gauge) needle on one side of the dorsal surface just lateral to the bony phalanx. The nerve is adjacent to the bone, just under the skin on the *dorsal* surface; 0.5 to 1.0 mL of anesthetic should be placed there, after aspirating to ensure against intravascular injection. The needle is then advanced until it is barely tenting the skin on the palmar surface. It is then withdrawn dorsally by 1 mm, and 0.5 to 1.0 mL of anesthetic is deposited. This is repeated on the opposite side of the finger so that *all four* digital nerves are blocked. Since the vascular supply here is provided by end arteries, only anesthetic *without* epinephrine should be used to avoid vasoconstriction and ischemia. The anatomy and technique are the same with the toes on the foot.

2. The **metacarpal block** is used in place of the digital block by some providers. In theory, there is the smaller chance of injuring the digit, since the arteries at the level of the metacarpal heads are dividing into deep and superficial branches, making the possible injury to one vessel less critical. The injection on the palmar surface is considered more painful, but only one injection is needed. The skin is punctured with a small (27- or 30-gauge) needle on the palmar surface over the metacarpal head. The needle is advanced to one side of the metacarpal just volar to the bone along the path of the digital nerve and 2 to 3 mL of anesthetic is deposited. The needle is withdrawn almost all the way, then it is advanced again (to the left or right) along the other digital nerve and more anesthetic is deposited. This will not anesthetize the proximal dorsal surface of the middle phalanges nor the tip

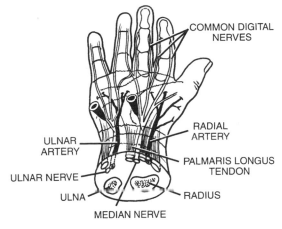

Fig. 2. Median and ulnar, nerve block.

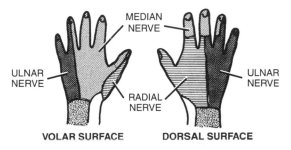

Fig. 3. Innervation pattern of wrist and hand.

of the thumb or little finger, since sensation to
these areas is supplied by the dorsal nerves. In order to anesthetize these areas, a local block should
be made over the dorsal nerves by creating a small
skin wheal along the dorsum of the proximal digit
as shown.

3. The **wrist block,** which involves combining the
   median, ulnar, and radial blocks, can be helpful in
   patients with extensive hand injuries requiring repair or reduction. If only one area of distribution is
   involved (see Fig. 3), each block can be used separately.

   a. The **median nerve block** is useful for repair-
      ing wounds on the palm and fingers supplied
      by this nerve (see Fig. 2). Since this technique
      involves infusion of fluid into the carpal tun-

nel, carpal tunnel syndrome is a relative con-traindication. Identification of the palmaris longus and the flexor carpi radialis tendons at the proximal wrist crease defines the point of injection. After creating a small wheal on the surface, the needle is advanced to the depth of the palmaris longus tendon and 2 to 5 mL of an-esthetic is injected. If parasthesias are elicited, the needle should be withdrawn 1 to 2 mm to prevent intraneural injection. Anesthesia gen-erally occurs within 10 minutes.

b.   The **ulnar nerve** is also easily identified at the proximal wrist crease between the ulnar artery and the flexor carpi ulnaris tendon (see Fig. 2). After a skin wheal is raised, the needle is advanced approximately 1 cm and aspi-rated. A total of 5 mL of anesthetic is injected in this region, taking care to prevent injection into the ulnar artery. If anesthesia of the dor-sum of the hand is needed, the dorsal cuta-neous branch of the ulnar nerve arises proxi-mal to the wrist and can best be anesthetized by placing a 3-mL wheal of anesthetic around the medial edge of the wrist just distal to the ulnar styloid.

c.   The **radial nerve** can only be anesthetized by both a nerve block and a field block due to its multiple branches. The nerve can be found at the proximal wrist crease just lateral to the ra-dial artery at the same depth as the artery. Up to 5 mL of anesthetic is placed in this region (after aspirating to ensure against intraarter-ial injection). The field block can be done using an additional 5 mL of anesthetic locally. The anesthetic is injected from this point dorsally around the radial styloid to the dorsal midline following the wrist crease.

4.   **Intraarticular shoulder anesthesia** has been shown to be very effective for the reduction of sim-ple dislocations. The concerns caused by the use of parenteral analgesics or sedatives are eliminated, and the patient spends considerably less time in the emergency department owing to the briefer re-covery time. After the lateral shoulder is sterilely prepped, the glenohumeral joint is identified by the lateral sulcus formed by the absent humeral head. A needle is introduced 2 cm inferior and lat-eral to the acromion and directed slightly caudad. Identification of the joint is confirmed by the aspi-ration of joint fluid; complete aspiration of the ex-cessive fluid may be useful. A total of 20 mL of an-esthetic (1% lidocaine) is slowly injected into the joint. Generally, anesthesia occurs within 15 min-utes and lasts for several hours (2).

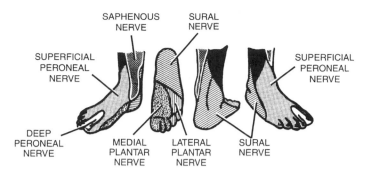

Fig. 4. **Innervation pattern of ankle and foot.**

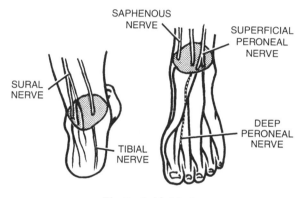

Fig. 5. **Ankle block.**

5. The **ankle block** can be useful in reducing foot
    fractures or dislocations or in treating extensive
    skin or tendon lacerations on the foot. Two individual blocks may be useful for more isolated injuries
    located on one specific nerve distribution (see Fig.
    4). This is particularly useful in repairing sole lacerations where local injection is extremely painful
    and can be technically difficult due to the closely
    adherent fascia.

    a. The **anterior ankle block** is used to anesthetize the superficial peroneal, deep peroneal
        and saphenous nerves, which innervate the
        dorsum of the foot (see Fig. 5). The affected ankle should be supine, in plantarflexion. The
        deep peroneal nerve is blocked initially. Using the extensor hallucis longus and the tib-

ialis anterior tendons as landmarks, a needle is placed at the level of the medial malleolus. After a large superficial wheal is raised, 1 mL of anesthetic is placed at the depth of the tendons; some providers advance the needle until it hits the tibia and then withdraw 1 mm to locate this nerve. To anesthetize the **saphenous nerve,** the same needle can be redirected prior to withdrawal from the skin and another 5 mL of anesthetic placed. This should be done subcutaneously toward the top of the medial malleolus. Finally, the **superficial peroneal nerve** is blocked by injecting 5 to 10 mL more of anesthetic superficially from the lateral malleolus to the extensor hallucis longus.

    b. The **posterior ankle block** of the posterior tibial and sural nerves may be used for repairs of lacerations of the sole and is best achieved with the patient in the prone position with the foot slightly dorsiflexed. The **posterior tibial nerve** is blocked by first locating the tibial artery posterior to the medial malleolus (see Fig. 5). The needle is placed at the level of the proximal edge of the medial malleolus and is advanced to approximately 1.5 cm in depth, where 5 mL of anesthetic agent is injected. The nerve is just posterior to the artery, so care should be taken to avoid intraarterial injection. Another 5 mL of anesthetic should be injected as the needle is withdrawn. The **sural nerve** is more subcutaneous, posterior to the lateral malleolus. The needle should be placed just lateral to the Achilles tendon and advanced to the proximal edge of the lateral malleolus. Injection of 5 mL of anesthetic should be placed in a wheal while withdrawing the needle.

6. A **hematoma block** is occasionally used for reduction of fractures since it is quick and easy, however it does not provide anesthesia as well as some of the other techniques described. There is also the potential of transmitting infection into the fracture, since, theoretically, it converts a closed fracture into an open one; thus this block should not be used with an epiphyseal fracture, nor should the injection be made through broken or contaminated skin. The skin over the fracture site is sterilely prepped and a small needle is placed into the hematoma. After blood is aspirated to help decrease swelling, 5 to 10 mL of anesthetic (usually 2% plain lidocaine) is injected into the hematoma and surrounding periosteum. Generally, anesthesia occurs within 5 minutes and, as with other blocks, may last as long as several hours.

7. The **Bier block** is a true regional anesthetic technique, using an IV anesthetic to block an entire extremity distal to the area of an applied tourniquet. This block is useful for any injury below the shoulder in the upper extremity and below the knee in the lower extremity. Reduction of fractures is the most common indication, but it can provide anesthesia for debridement, exploration, and laceration repair. As with the other blocks, allergy to the anesthetic agent is the only absolute contraindication, though most providers would avoid using this procedure in patients with sickle cell disease and severe hypertension. Toxicity of the anesthetic is the most likely complication with this technique, since patients are more apt to become symptomatic when the bolus of anesthetic is released from the tourniqueted extremity. In order to eliminate much of the toxicity previously associated with this block, the minidose Bier block is now more frequently used. This dosing regimen, using half of the dose of lidocaine, which was originally recommended by August Bier in 1908, has been proven effective in 95% of patients (3). There have been some recent reports of cardiac arrests with use of bupivicaine in IV regional anesthesia, and use of this agent is not advocated. Because of the potential side effects with this technique, resuscitative equipment should be available, and many providers place a precautionary IV line in an unaffected arm in order to facilitate prompt resuscitative therapy if needed.

A pneumatic cuff (preferably not a standard blood pressure cuff) is placed on the affected extremity with some padding around the arm under the cuff. A small IV catheter should be placed in the distal extremity; it has been found that the more distal the placement, the better the success rate of the block. The extremity should be elevated above the heart for at least 1 to 3 minutes to extravasate the venous blood, then the cuff is rapidly inflated to 50 mm Hg above the systolic blood pressure, 200 mm Hg on the average adult. The arm is then lowered and injected with the anesthetic.

Lidocaine is the recommended anesthetic agent; the dose should be precalculated and mixed prior to starting this procedure. Standard dosing now used in the emergency department is 1.5 mg/kg of 1% lidocaine or a total of 100 mg in an adult. This amount should be diluted to a 0.5% mixture with normal saline (10 mL of lidocaine and 10 mL normal saline for an adult) prior to injection. Note that this equals only the standard IV dose given to patients in a bolus for cardiac dysrhythmia. Maximum anesthesia should occur in 15 minutes, though some sensation may still be present with adequate anesthesia. If this procedure does not provide adequate anesthesia, an additional 0.5 mg/kg of the diluted 0.5% lidocaine can be injected. No more than 3 mg/kg should ever be used in any given patient.

When the block is effective, the manipulation or procedure may proceed. Postreduction radiographs should be obtained while the cuff is still inflated. The tourniquet can then be released; many providers release it in cycles, releasing for 5 seconds and then reinflating for 1 to 2 minutes and repeating this three or four times to help decrease the bolus effect of the anesthetic agent. If the procedure was completed very rapidly, it is recommended that the tourniquet remain inflated for at least 20 minutes to allow for enough tissue fixation of the lidocaine. If the full dose of 3 mg/kg was used, it is recommended that a minimum of 30 minutes elapse prior to deflating the cuff. The small catheter can be removed from the affected arm at this time. The tourniquet should not remain in place for longer than 90 minutes so as to avoid complications of ischemia. The patient should be observed for 20 minutes after the cuff is removed, at which time the anesthetic effects should be gone.

Discussion here is directed at the arm, though the same procedure can be used for the lower extremity. Care must be taken to avoid placing the tourniquet over the peroneal nerve just below the knee, and patients do not tolerate a tourniquet placed above the knee, so this limits the technique to ankle and foot problems. Review of this technique is found in Table 3.

Table 3.   The minidose Bier block

Calculate anesthetic dosage of 1% lidocaine (1.5 mg/kg or 100 mg in an adult).

Dilute lidocaine: 1:1 with normal saline to equal 0.5% concentration.

Place cuff proximal to injury after padding.

Place intravenous catheter in distal injured extremity.

Elevate extremity and extravasate, then inflate cuff (200 mm Hg in adult).

Inject lidocaine mixture into intravenous line—wait up to 15 minutes for maximum anesthesia.

Perform procedure or manipulation, including x-rays.

Release tourniquet in cycles (tourniquet should remain inflated >20 minutes before initial deflation).

After cuff deflation, observe until anesthetic effects are gone (20 minutes).

I. **Complications.** The complications of any regional nerve block include those associated with any injection—local infection, excessive bleeding, and toxic reactions—all of which are quite rare. More specifically, injection directly into small nerves can cause prolonged disability. Even with only a small volume of anesthetic infused, chemical irritation or ischemia may occur from injection directly into the nerve. To prevent this, if paresthesias are obtained during the injection, the needle positioning should be changed slightly prior to further injection. Second, if an artery is punctured and a hematoma is formed locally, it may cause prolonged pain or the compression from the resultant reduction of blood flow may cause continued damage.

J. **Disposition.** The patient should be made aware of the expected length of time of the anesthesia or paresthesias to the region involved. Blocks using bupivacaine may last for up to 8 hours, whereas nerve blocks performed with lidocaine may become sensate again after only 1 to 2 hours. Instructions for pain control after the resolution of the analgesia should also be given, e.g., elevating and icing the affected extremity. The patient should be warned to be careful of further injury during the time the extremity is insensate (this could be from excessive heat or cold, pressure from a dressing, or inadvertent reinjury). Other instructions specifically related to the injury should also be given.

II. **Conscious sedation**

A. **Historical information.** Conscious sedation is the use of pharmacological agents to produce a lessening of a patient's anxiety and perception of pain while maintaining all protective reflexes. The first formal contemporary use of an anesthetic to achieve conscious sedation for a painful medical procedure occurred at Massachusetts General Hospital in 1845. Horace Wells used nitrous oxide while extracting a patient's tooth; unfortunately, the patient woke too early, and it was 20 years before this procedure was used regularly in dentistry. Since then, several pharmacological agents have been produced that may cause sedation, analgesia, amnesia, or muscle relaxation (see Table 4 for definitions). The use of therapeutic agents

Table 4.   Definitions of anesthesia

Anesthesia—total loss of sensation to touch of the skin

Sedation—decrease in activity, excitability, and anxiety

Analgesia—relief from pain without sedation

Amnesia—inability to recall events or experiences

Conscious sedation—use of pharmacologic agents to produce a lessening of a patient's perception of pain and anxiety while maintaining all protective reflexes with some or all of these effects may be helpful in providing treatment for a patient with an acute orthopaedic emergency.

B. Pharmacological agents. Several agents given by several different routes are available to help provide anesthesia. The easiest to administer are the inhalants, of which nitrous oxide is the only one commonly used in the emergency department. Many parenteral medications can be given via either the IM or the IV route; some are limited to IV administration. For more precise control of conscious sedation, only IV administration of the agents should be used. The properties of these pharmacologic agents are reviewed first and then a practical protocol for their use is described.

1. **Inhalants.** Nitrous oxide is the only common inhalant used in the emergency department in patients requiring some sedation and dissociative effects. The rapid onset, short half-life, ease of administration, and lack of significant side effects make this an ideal agent for emergency department use. Nitrous oxide must be used in a mixture, generally 50% nitrous oxide with oxygen to prevent hypoxia. It is best used by self-administration, with the patient holding the mask and allowing it to fall off as sedation increases. Nitrous oxide is not a very good analgesic and is often used with local anesthesia to provide pain control.

2. **Analgesics.** Numerous analgesics are available for controlling pain. Some of the more common agents with their usual dosing are listed in Table 5. These generally come in two classes, those of the narcotic agonists and the mixed agonist-antagonists. The latter class is supposed to offer less respiratory depressive effect, the primary side effect of concern with these agents. Two commonly used agonist-antagonists are nalbuphine and butorphanol. Other complications from narcotic agonists include sedation, nausea and vomiting, and hypotension. Morphine and meperidine can also cause histamine release, which may produce bronchospasm and hypotension. Fentanyl does not release histamine but may cause muscle rigidity with rapid administration of high doses—a side effect not generally seen with the usual emergency department dosage.

3. **Sedatives and amnestics** (see Table 6). Sedatives can be used in combination with narcotic analgesics to prevent some gastrointestinal side effects and respiratory depression. The neuroleptic droperidol can accomplish this as well as add some minimal amnestic and anxiolytic effects. Phenothiazines have also been used for these effects but can produce extrapyramidal reactions.

Chloral hydrate is a sedative without analgesic properties that has little respiratory or cardiovascular effect when used at normal doses; however, it

Table 5. Narcotic analgesics

Pharmacological agent	Onset*	Duration*	Dose IV	Dose IM	Comments
Butorphenol (Stadol)†	2–5 min	2–4 hr	0.015–0.02 mg/kg	—	Usual adult dose: 1 mg intranasally
Fentanyl (Sublimaze)	1–3 min	30–60 min	0.5–1.0 ug/kg	0.5–1.0 µg/kg	May cause muscle rigidity
Merperidine (Demerol)	5–15 min	2–4 hr	1.0–2.0 mg/kg	1.0–2.0 mg/kg	Do not use in patients taking MAO‡ inhibitors
Morphine	2–3 min	1–2 hr	0.1 mg/kg	0.1 mg/kg	
Nalbuphine (Nubain)†	2–3 min	3–6 hr	0.1–0.2 mg/kg	0.1–0.2 mg/kg	

*Onset and duration are listed for IV dosing. Generally the onset and duration are approximately double with IM dosing.
†Narcotic agonist-antagonist (all others are narcotic agonists).
‡Monoamine oxidase.

Table 6.   Sedative and amnestic agents

Pharmacological agent	Onset*	Duration*	Dose IV	Dose IM	Comments
Chloral hydrate (Noctec)	20–60 min	1–4 hr	—	—	50 mg/kg; oral only
Diazepam (Valium)	3–10 min	2–4 hr	0.04–0.2 mg/kg	Erratic absorption	Rectal 0.5 mg/kg
Droperidol (Inapsine)	3–10 min	2–4 hr	0.02–0.10 mg/kg	0.02–0.10 mg/kg	
Lorazapam (Ativan)	5–10 min	2–6 hr	0.02–0.10 mg/kg	0.02–0.10 mg/kg	
Midazolam (Versed)	3–5 min	1–2 hr	0.03–0.05 mg/kg	0.05–0.15 mg/kg	0.2–0.4 mg/kg intranasally or 0.5–0.7 mg/kg orally
Pentobarbital (Nembutal)	4 min	30–60 min	2.0–5.0 mg/kg	4.0–6.0 mg/kg	
Ketamine	1–3 min	30–120 min	1.0 mg/kg	4.0 mg/kg	Use with atropine 0.01 mg/kg (max. 0.5 mg)
Propofol	1–2 min	15–30 min	0.5–2.0 mg/kg	—	Continue sedation with infusion 25–130 mg/kg/min

*Onset and duration are listed for IV dosing. Generally the onset and duration are approximately double with IM dosing.

is available only in an oral solution, making titration of the dosage difficult. Some providers use it for children to avoid the trauma of an intramuscular or IV injection.

Ketamine is a sedative often used in children; it provides analgesia as well as dissociative and amnestic effects. This agent seems to produce few of the respiratory depressant or cardiovascular side effects of other analgesics. Postemergence delirium has been observed (much more often in adults), which has been found to be tempered by concurrent use of a benzodiazepine. Ketamine causes a sensitization of the gag reflex and an increase in upper airway secretions. These effects can cause laryngospasm; therefore ketamine is commonly given with atropine, which decreases the secretions. Ketamine should be avoided in those patients with an upper respiratory illness.

The most common class of agents that produce substantial amnestic effects in addition to sedation are the benzodiazepines. This includes midazolam, diazepam, and lorazepam, which provide some dissociative effects for patients as well as muscle relaxation. When any of these is used with narcotic analgesia, the patient will have little pain, little recall, and minimal concern about the procedure performed. This class of drugs does produce respiratory depression and hypotension and therefore should be titrated to produce the effect needed without hemodynamic or respiratory compromise.

One of the newer sedatives is propofol, used in place of benzodiazepines for sedation and amnesia. It has significant cardiovascular effects and causes respiratory depression when administered rapidly as a bolus; propofol has been used as an induction agent. When it is used slowly as an infusion, these effects are minimized. Propofol's very short half-life makes it ideal for quick, painful procedures, but care must be taken to monitor the patient's respiratory status, since up to 40% of patients have apnea at these therapeutic doses.

Pentobarbital is a short-acting barbiturate that is occasionally used for sedation; barbiturates have no analgesic effects. Care must be taken, since pentobarbital can cause respiratory depression and loss of protective respiratory reflexes.

C. **Indications.** The indications for use of conscious sedation include the need to perform a procedure or manipulation that may be painful to the patient, requires cooperation, or for which muscle relaxation is necessary. Useful combinations for patients requiring conscious sedation are listed in Table 7.

D. **Contraindications.** The only absolute contraindication for the use of any pharmacologic anesthetic for

Table 7.   Useful combinations for conscious sedation

Recommended for IV sedation (adults or children):

Give: 1. Fentanyl—Give 0.5–1.0 µg/kg IV over 30–60 seconds. May repeat dose every 2–3 minutes to a total of 5 µg/kg to achieve desired analgesia.

2. Midazolam—Give 0.02–0.04 mg/kg IV. May repeat dose every 2–3 minutes to a total of 0.1 mg/kg to achieve desired sedation.

Recommended for IM sedation (children <10 years old):

Combine in one syringe: 1. Atropine—Give 0.01 mg/kg IM. Use a minimum of 0.1 mg to a maximum of 0.5 mg.
2. Midazolam—Give 0.1 mg/kg IM.
3. Ketamine—Give 3.0 mg/kg IM. May repeat ketamine with 2 mg/kg IM in 10 minutes to achieve desired analgesia and dissociation.

conscious sedation is a known allergy to the medication. Relative contraindications include any respiratory problems [sleep apnea, severe chronic obstructive pulmonary disease (COPD), or even a recent upper respiratory infection (URI)] in which even minor respiratory depression may cause significant hypoxia or hypoventilation. Prior to using these medications in patients with anatomically abnormal airways, one should consider whether they would make ventilation or intubation difficult or impossible.

E. **Patient history.** Specific historical information not relating to the immediate orthopaedic injury is important to obtain prior to using analgesia and sedation. Allergies and current medications should be determined, as well as significant past medical history, including a history of asthma, laryngospasm, or prior anesthetic complications. A brief review of systems, taking special note of recent respiratory illnesses, is important to elicit, as this may require an alteration of the pharmacologic agent used. History of the last meal should be obtained, but since every patient should be treated as if he or she had a full stomach, this should not preclude anyone from receiving adequate analgesia and sedation.

F. **Physical examination.** A screening physical exam should be performed as well as careful examination of the region of the orthopaedic injury. Evaluation of the oropharynx and neck should include a check for possible obstruction or difficulty with airway management. Any abnormal lung sounds, particularly wheezing or a cardiac murmur, should be evaluated prior to using any systemic pharmacologic agents. Evaluation of possible vascular access should be done if none is to be used as part of the procedure.

G. **Technique.** Any patient who will be given a systemic pharmacologic agent to alter the level of consciousness also has the potential for developing an altered hemodynamic and respiratory status. The provider who is supervising the sedation should be capable of identifying signs of instability and of providing all phases of advanced life support, including airway management and cardiovascular resuscitation.

Prior to initiating any therapy, at least a minimal level of patient monitoring should be maintained, the degree being based upon the level of sedation and analgesia (see Table 8). At least one care provider who is not actively performing the procedure should be at the bedside, monitoring the patient's status. All patients should have their routine vital signs checked frequently, including blood pressure, pulse, and respiratory rate. All patients should have their ventilation continuously monitored by an oxygen saturation monitor if given a medication that will decrease respiratory drive. Level of consciousness should be evaluated frequently. A flow sheet to record this is recommended for accurate documentation.

The patient should not be discharged until there is evidence that he or she can perform necessary motor activity (walking) and minimal cognitive activity and has been hemodynamically stable for at least 1 hour.

H. **Complications.** The physician providing sedation/analgesia should be capable of reacting to all possible

---

Table 8. Routine monitoring for patients with conscious sedation

The following should be documented during the procedure:

1. Oxygen saturation via pulse oximetry (patient should be on oxygen at least by nasal cannula).

2. Blood pressure and/or pulse rate.

3. Level of consciousness.

An assistant who is not involved in the procedure should be present to observe vital signs and respiratory status.

The following should also be present at the bedside during the procedure:

1. Appropriate bag and mask.

2. Suction apparatus.

3. Reversal agents—naloxone, flumazenil as appropriate.

complications of the use of these medications. This should include the knowledge and technical skills to manage an airway, acquire vascular access, and use reversal and supportive pharmacological agents. Most complications of all the agents used for sedation and analgesia involve hemodynamic instability, notably hypotension and respiratory depression. Hypotension can be avoided in most cases by decreasing the rate of delivery of the medication, although there are some dose-related effects. Respiratory depression is dose-related and can be avoided by careful titration of the agent during the procedure.

I. **Reversal agents.** All discussions of the use of systemic analgesia should include mention of the reversal agents for these medications.

1. **Naloxone,** a narcotic antagonist, can be used to reverse many of the effects of most narcotic medications. Improvement of such side effects as respiratory depression, hypotension, and loss of protective reflexes can be achieved. Unfortunately, this will also reverse the analgesic effects for which the medication was used. In order to titrate this better, naloxone (0.4 to 2.0 mg) should be diluted with normal saline in a 1:10 mixture and given intravenously, using only the amount needed to reverse a patient's respiratory depression but not to completely reverse the pain control that has been achieved.

2. **Flumazenil** can serve to reverse the effects of benzodiazepines, but it should be used with some caution. It has been found to improve alertness, reverse respiratory depression, and decrease the duration of amnesia, but it has little effect on the hypotension caused by benzodiazepines. The usual dosage is 0.2 mg IV given over 15 to 30 seconds, with repeat doses of 0.1 mg/min given IV, until a total of 1 mg has been administered. Flumazenil can cause seizures in patients who have been using benzodiazepines chronically or who take tricyclic antidepressants; it should be used carefully in these patients and be administered by a provider who is familiar with the treatment and supportive therapy needed should such side effects arise.

J. **Disposition.** Patients should be back to their baseline levels of motor control and should follow and verbalize directions well prior to discharge. Continued sleepiness only is not a reason to observe a patient further. Clear instructions that describe the normal reactions and the common and serious complications from these medications should be given to the patient and an accompanying responsible person. Most providers would warn a patient not to drive or use heavy machinery for the rest of the day. See Table 9 for a sample outline of discharge instructions.

Table 9.   Discharge instructions for patients having conscious sedation

No eating or drinking for the next 2 hours. No drinking alcohol for the next 24 hours.

No driving or operating of equipment that requires coordination for the next 12 hours.

The patient should be observed by a responsible adult for the next 8 hours.

The patient should be awakened every 2 hours for the first 4 hours after discharge.

The patient should return to the emergency department if he or she has any difficulty breathing, if the breathing seems too slow or shallow, if the patient cannot be awakened, or if there are any signs of an allergic reaction such as a rash or throat swelling.

REFERENCES

1. Green SM, Rothrock SG, Gorchynski J. Validation of diphenhydramine as a dermal local anesthesia. *Ann Emerg Med* 1994;23: 1284–1289.
2. Matthews DE, Roberts T. Intraarticular lidocaine versus intravenous analgesic for reduction of acute anterior shoulder dislocations: a prospective randomized study. *Am J Sports Med* 1995; 23(1):54–58.
3. Farrell RG, et al. Safe and effective IV regional anesthesia for use in the emergency department. *Ann Emerg Med* 1985;14: 288–292.

BIBLIOGRAPHY

Murphy MR. Regional anesthesia in the emergency department. *Emerg Med Clin North Am* 1988;6:783–810.

Orlinsky M, Dean E. Local and topical anesthesia and nerve blocks of the thorax and extremities: emergency medicine procedures. In: Roberts JR, Hedges JR, eds. *Clinical procedures in emergency medicine.* Philadelphia: WB Saunders, 1991.

Sacchetti A, et al. Pediatric analgesia and sedation. *Ann Emerg Med* 1994;23:237–250.

Tintinalli JE, Krome RL, Ruiz E. *Emergency medicine: a comprehensive study guide,* 4th ed. New York: McGraw-Hill, 1996.

5

Principles of
Orthopaedic Reductions

Valerie Neylan and Matthew Wols

Dislocations are named according to the relation of the distal articulating surface to that of the proximal (e.g., *anterior shoulder dislocation* means the humeral head lies anterior to the glenoid fossa). A knowledge of relevant joint anatomy and reduction techniques is essential. Unless neurovascular compromise is present, radiographs should be obtained prior to reduction to check for associated fractures. Use proper and adequate analgesia/muscle relaxation and a slow, gentle technique to accomplish the reduction. If conscious sedation is used, an intravenous line should be established with continuous monitoring of the patient. Always do postreduction radiographs after immobilizing the patient. The joint must be properly splinted after a reduction, with a clear understanding of possible complications. Inability to reduce the dislocation does not necessarily mean that an improper technique was used. It may indicate soft tissue entrapment or a fracture fragment in the joint space. After several unsuccessful attempts at reduction, refer to the orthopaedic surgeon for possible open reduction or closed reduction under anesthesia. If the joint was reduced prior to the patient's arrival, always treat the dislocation (splint/immobilize appropriately). Recurrent dislocations of a joint should be treated in the same way as an initial event but may eventually need surgical intervention.

- I. **Shoulder dislocation.** The shoulder is a ball-and-socket joint with a large range of motion that predisposes it to instability. It is the most common site of major joint dislocation (50%) in adults seen in the emergency department.
  - A. **Anterior shoulder dislocation.** The most common (>95%) of all shoulder dislocations.
    1. **Classification.** This lesion can be classified by mechanism (traumatic versus nontraumatic), frequency (primary versus recurrent), or anatomic position of the dislocated humeral head (in order of frequency: subcoracoid, subglenoid, subclavicular, and intrathoracic). The subcoracoid and subglenoid positions represent 99% of all anterior dislocations.
    2. **Mechanism of injury.** The cause is usually an indirect force applied to the shoulder in forced abduction, extension, and external rotation but may rarely occur with a direct blow to the posterior aspect of the shoulder. In younger patients, this most commonly occurs during sports; in older patients, it is usually due to a fall on an outstretched arm.

3. **Physical examination.** The acutely dislocated shoulder is painful and the dislocated arm is held in slight abduction and external rotation. The shoulder is incapable of complete internal rotation and adduction. There may be a loss of the deltoid contour, with the shoulder appearing squared off; the humeral head may be palpable anteriorly. A complete neurovascular exam should be done with special attention to injuries to the brachial plexus, axillary nerve, radial nerve, or axillary artery. The incidence of axillary nerve injury is between 2.8% and 4%; such injury can be evaluated by assessing sensation to pinprick or two-point discrimination over the lateral aspect of the deltoid insertion and comparing it to sensation on the uninjured side.

4. **Radiography.** This is necessary to determine the direction of the dislocation, associated fractures, and possible barriers to reduction. A true anteroposterior (AP) view or AP in the scapular plane is preferred. If any overlap exists on the true AP view, there is a dislocation. The scapular lateral or scapular Y view reveals the direction of dislocation. The humeral head should be in the center of the Y overlying the glenoid fossa. The axillary view is useful in showing associated fractures. The **Hill-Sachs deformity** is a compression or impaction fracture of the posterolateral humeral head that results from the forceful impingement of the humeral head on the anterior rim of the glenoid fossa. This occurs in approximately 25% of acute dislocations and over 75% of recurrent dislocations.

5. **Treatment.** Four general principles apply to the reduction of anterior shoulder dislocations: traction, leverage, scapular manipulation, or a combination of these. The leverage techniques are associated with a higher incidence of associated injuries and should be discouraged. A successful reduction is indicated by decreased pain, the physician or patient feeling the humeral head slip back into place, or return of a normal contour. After the reduction, the shoulder should be moved through 10 to 15 degrees of the range of motion to ensure appropriate alignment.

   a. **Stimson technique.** The patient is placed prone with the dislocated arm hanging free over the edge of the cart and a folded sheet or pillow placed under the shoulder. Using a strap, a 10- to 15-lb weight is suspended from the wrist or lower forearm for 20 to 30 minutes. Muscle relaxation is essential and the patient should be closely monitored at all times. If spontaneous reduction does not occur, slight traction to the arm with gentle external and then internal rotation should complete the reduction.

b. **Scapular manipulation.** This is a safe and effective method of reduction and differs from other methods in that it manipulates the glenoid rather than the humeral head. It can be done either in the prone or sitting position. In the prone position, begin as in the Stimson technique with a weight or gentle downward traction applied to the dislocated arm for 5 to 10 minutes to stabilize the humeral head. Then the inferior tip of the scapula is rotated medially by applying pressure with one hand while simultaneously fixing the superior and medial edge with the opposite hand. This technique is reported to have a very high rate of success (>92%) and often calls for little to no sedation. No complications have been reported using this technique. It is the author's preferred method of reduction. With the patient in the sitting position, the dislocated arm is held in forward flexion with an assistant applying mild traction with one hand and supporting the humeral head with the other while the scapula is rotated.

c. **Traction/countertraction.** This method can be used with the patient sitting up or supine. Countertraction is applied by an assistant holding a folded sheet placed around the upper chest and pulling it toward the center of the opposite shoulder. In-line traction is gently applied to the injured arm and gradually increased against the countertraction. Lateral traction may be added in a difficult reduction by an assistant, using a pillowcase folded and wrapped around the proximal humerus. This should be applied only after disimpaction of the humeral head is achieved. **Matsen's** preferred technique is a variation of this. The patient is supine and an assistant applies countertraction as described while the physician stands near the waist on the injured side and places a folded sheet around the patient's forearm just distal to a flexed elbow. With the sheet tied around the patient's waist, in-line traction is applied by gently and steadily leaning back against the sheet and grasping the forearm against countertraction. If difficulty is encountered, lateral traction or gentle rocking of the humerus with external/internal rotation can be added.

d. **External rotation method (Hennepin or Liedelmeyer technique).** This method is safe and fast, may not call for an anesthetic, and has a high success rate. The patient is supine with the injured arm adducted to the side and the elbow flexed to 90 degrees. The forearm is then gently and steadily rotated externally to 90 degrees. If reduction is not achieved at this point, the arm is then abducted while held in 90 degrees of external rotation. This reduction should not be forced but done slowly and gently, with intermittent pauses in the event of excessive pain.

e. **Milch (Cooper) technique.** The patient is supine at about 30 degrees with the elbow flexed to 90 degrees. The patient is told to abduct and externally rotate the injured arm up slowly so that he or she can pat the back of the head. The physician lightly supports the arm for guidance while this is accomplished and places a thumb over the humeral head to push it back into place gently. Once the arm is in this position, gentle traction may be applied to it to complete the reduction.

The Hippocratic method and Kocher technique are not recommended owing to the higher incidence of associated neurovascular complications.

The neurovascular examination should be repeated after the reduction and documented. Postreduction radiographs should be done to confirm reduction and identify associated fractures. The reduced shoulder is placed in a shoulder immobilizer or sling and swathe with the arm adducted and rotated internally. The patient is referred to the orthopaedist for early follow-up, usually in 5 to 7 days. Younger patients generally require longer immobilization, while older patients require shorter periods because of increased risk of joint stiffness. Early surgical indications are unsuccessful closed reduction, a large fracture of the glenoid fossa on prereduction films, or a displaced fracture of the greater tuberosity after reduction.

6. **Complications.** Injuries to the ligament and capsule are frequent and may lead to the most common complication, recurrent dislocations. Rotator cuff injuries may occur in 10% to 15% of cases and increase in incidence with advanced

age. Nerve injuries occur in 5% to 12%; they are usually neurapraxias and will recover in time. The incidence increases with advanced age, duration of the dislocation, and amount of trauma. Fractures can occur, especially avulsion of the greater tuberosity, humeral head, or glenoid rim.

B. **Posterior shoulder dislocations.** These are rare and represent 2% to 4% of all shoulder dislocations. The anatomy of the glenoid offers natural protection against posterior dislocations because of the shape of the bony rim and the heavy rotator cuff muscles on the posterior aspect. This is, however, the most frequently missed dislocation in the emergency department.

1. **Classification.** The anatomical position of the humeral head is subacromial, subglenoid, and subspinous, in order of frequency. The subacromial represents 98% of all posterior dislocations.

2. **Mechanism of injury.** This injury most often results from violent muscle contractions, as with epileptic seizures or from an electric shock and is frequently associated with unilateral or bilateral posterior dislocations. It may also occur indirectly from a fall on the outstretched hand with the arm held in flexion, adduction, and internal rotation or, rarely, a direct blow to the anterior shoulder.

3. **Physical examination.** The shoulder is held in a sling position, adducted, and internally rotated. These dislocations are usually locked with the humeral head on the edge of the glenoids, so there is limitation of external rotation (<10 degrees) and abduction (often <90 degrees). There may be a posterior prominence and flattening of the anterior aspect of the shoulder, with a prominent coracoid process. The best position to view these asymmetries is by standing behind the seated patient and viewing from above, looking downward. These injuries are frequently missed and misdiagnosed as frozen joints.

4. **Radiography.** The standard AP view may appear deceptively normal, as the most common dislocation, the subacromial, is at a right angle to the plane of the film, with only subtle findings. Additional views—such as the scapular lateral or Y view as well as the axillary view—are needed. Findings on the standard AP film may be absence of the normal elliptical overlap shadow, the vacant glenoid sign with the glenoid fossa appearing partially vacant, a loss of the normal humeral neck profile appearing like a cone of light, an increased distance between

the anterior glenoid rim and the humeral head greater than 6 mm (rim sign), and a trough line or reverse Hill-Sachs deformity (compression fracture of the anteromedial humeral head). An isolated lesser tuberosity fracture should arouse suspicion of an associated posterior dislocation.

5. **Treatment.** Closed reduction may be difficult and complications such as associated fractures are high, so consult the orthopaedist early and prior to reduction. In-line traction should be applied using adequate sedation and analgesia. The patient is placed supine and traction is applied to the adducted arm with gentle direct pressure on the posterior humeral head. Closed reduction under general anesthesia may be needed. Many possible immobilization techniques are described. Most recommended that the arm be positioned in abduction, external rotation, and extension with a shoulder spica cast.

6. **Complications.** There is a high incidence of fractures of the posterior glenoid rim, proximal humeral head, and greater and lesser tuberosities. Neurovascular injuries are rare. There may be rotator cuff detachments, such as that of the subscapularis muscle at its insertion site on the lesser tuberosity. Dislocations recur in up to 30% of patients.

C. **Inferior shoulder dislocations (luxatio erecta).** This is a rare type of dislocation, occurring in 0.5% of all shoulder dislocations. The humeral head is displaced inferior to the glenoid fossa with the humeral shaft pointing overhead.

1. **Mechanism of injury.** The majority are due to indirect forces from a hyperabduction of the humerus. This causes impingement of the humeral neck on the acromion, ruptures the capsule, and dislocates the head inferiorly. This can also occur with a direct axial load to an abducted shoulder, forcing the humeral head downward.

2. **Physical examination.** The patient presents with the arm overhead locked between 110 and 160 degrees of abduction, with the elbow flexed and the forearm resting on top of the head. The humeral head may be palpable along the lateral chest wall. This is a locked dislocation, so movements are limited and cause significant pain.

3. **Radiography.** The standard AP view will demonstrate the dislocation, with the humeral head located inferiorly to the glenoid fossa. Associated fractures are frequently present and should be looked for.

4. **Treatment.** A closed reduction should be done using a traction/countertraction technique. In-

travenous sedation and analgesia should be given. In-line traction is applied to the humeral shaft while countertraction is applied, using a folded sheet across the top of the injured shoulder and pulling toward the opposite side. Traction is applied upward initially, then into less abduction; finally, the arm is brought to the patient's side. Orthopaedic consultation is necessary because of the high incidence of complications. Apply a shoulder immobilizer.

   5. **Complications.** Severe soft tissue injuries with tears of the rotator cuff and associated fractures are common. Neurovascular injuries may occur, such as thrombosis of the axillary artery and neurapraxias of the brachial plexus. Adhesive capsulitis is a possible long-term complication.

D. **Superior shoulder dislocations.** These injuries are extremely rare.

   1. **Mechanism of injury.** An extreme forward and upward force to an adducted arm is generally the cause.

   2. **Physical examination.** The humeral head lies above the level of the acromion and the arm is shortened and adducted.

   3. **Radiographs.** AP and lateral scapular views.

   4. **Treatment options.** Closed reduction is indicated with close orthopaedic follow-up.

   5. **Complications.** Soft tissue damage and neurovascular injuries are very common.

II. **Elbow dislocations.** The elbow is a hinge-like joint subject to mechanical instability and is the second most frequently dislocated major joint. The highest incidence occurs in 10- to 20-year-olds, usually while playing sports. Dislocations may be posterior, anterior, medial, lateral, or divergent, and most occur at the ulnohumeral joint. These dislocations need to be reduced promptly, not only to relieve pain but to prevent circulatory compromise and cartilaginous damage. A significant force is needed to dislocate the joint, and 30% to 40% of these injuries are associated with fractures. They often involve severe damage to ligaments and soft tissues and may develop marked swelling, causing a compartment syndrome.

A. **Posterior elbow dislocations.** This is the most common type of elbow dislocation.

   1. **Mechanism of injury.** A fall on an outstretched arm with the elbow extended or hyperextended.

   2. **Physical examination.** The affected arm is held at the side with the elbow in 30 to 40 degrees of flexion, with a prominent olecranon process. The neurovascular exam is important, especially checking the brachial artery, median, and ulnar nerves.

3. **Radiography.** Lateral and AP views are needed. Check for associated fractures, especially of the epicondyles, which could impede the reduction.

4. **Treatment.** Several methods can be used, all based on traction followed by anterior translation. It is important to avoid hyperextension or full extension during the reduction. With the patient in the supine position, an assistant applies countertraction to the humerus while gentle steady traction is applied to the wrist. The wrist should be held supinated with the elbow maintained in slight flexion. Any medial or lateral displacement is corrected first, then distal traction is continued as the elbow is gently flexed. If this maneuver is unsuccessful, downward pressure may be applied on the proximal forearm to disengage the coronoid or pressure may be applied behind the olecranon while maintaining traction. This same principle can be applied with the patient in the prone position on the cart with the either the forearm or arm hanging off the cart and either weights suspended from the wrist or steady downward traction applied. The elbow is then gently flexed or forward pressure to the olecranon may be applied to complete the reduction.

   After the reduction, it is important to repeat the neurovascular exam and gently test the elbow's range of motion passively for stability. If range of motion is decreased, check carefully for associated fractures or entrapment of the medial epicondyle. The elbow should be maintained in 90 to 120 degrees of flexion (as much as the circulation will tolerate) and immobilized in a posterior long arm splint with the wrist in the neutral position and suspended in a sling. Frequent neurovascular checks should be done over the first 24 to 36 hours to assess for vascular compromise and potential, compartment syndrome.

5. **Complications.** A compartment syndrome may develop from the severe soft tissue swelling. The brachial artery as well as the median and ulnar nerves may be injured. Severe disruption to the elbow joint results in brachial artery injury in 8% of cases and should be suspected with a wide opening palpable on exam or seen on the radiograph. Medial epicondylar fractures may occur and may become entrapped during the reduction. Ectopic calcifications or myositis ossificans may develop as a late complication.

B. **Anterior elbow dislocations.** These injuries are rare but constitute the second most common elbow dislocation.

1. **Mechanism of injury.** A fall with a force striking the posterior forearm while in a flexed position is generally the cause. This requires a tremendous amount of force.

2. **Physical examination.** The arm appears shortened with the forearm elongated. The forearm is in supination and elbow is in full extension. The patient will resist any movement of the arm.

3. **Radiography.** AP and lateral views are adequate. Always check for associated fractures.

4. **Treatment.** The patient is placed in the supine position. An assistant applies countertraction to the humerus and steady in-line traction is applied to the wrist with one hand while the other hand applies steady downward pressure at the proximal forearm. Gentle, passive movement through the range of motion should be attempted to check for stability and the neurovascular exam should be repeated. A posterior long arm splint with the elbow in 45 degrees of flexion should be applied once the reduction is achieved. An orthopaedic surgeon should be consulted early for probable admission or close observation for neurovascular checks.

5. **Complications.** This injury is often associated with fractures and neurovascular injuries. These injuries cause a much higher incidence of vascular injury than the posterior dislocations.

III. **Wrist dislocations.** The wrist joint includes the distal metaphyseal portions of the radius and ulna, the carpal bones, and the surrounding soft tissue–supporting structures. Because the wrist is supported by numerous ligaments, great force is required to disrupt it.

   A. **Lunate and perilunate dislocations.** These are midcarpal dislocations, occurring between the two rows of carpal bones.

   1. **Mechanism of injury.** Most often extreme dorsiflexion forces, as due to a fall from a height, are the cause.

   2. **Physical exam.** There is limitation of normal wrist movement and palpable fullness may be appreciated volarly or dorsally. The median nerve may be compressed in the carpal canal, resulting in signs of median nerve injury.

   3. **Radiology.** Lunate dislocations reveal foreshortening of the wrist on AP projection, with overlap of the capitate and lunate. On lateral view, the radius, capitate, and lunate normally align, with a straight-line traversing at the midline of each bone. In lunate dislocations, the lunate lies volar or dorsal to this line. In perilunate dislocations, the lunate remains aligned with the distal radius on lateral view and the capitate and the metacarpals are dislocated,

usually dorsally. Perilunate dislocations can be associated with carpal bone fractures and are described as transradial, transscaphoid, transcapitate, or transtriquetrum perilunate, depending on which carpal bones are fractured.

4. **Treatment.** Immobilize the wrist in neutral position in a volar splint and refer immediately for reduction and definitive care.

5. **Complications.** Joint stiffness, pain, instability of the wrist, degenerative arthritis, and avascular necrosis are major complications.

B. **Scapholunate dissociation and rotary subluxation of the scaphoid.** These are injuries that involve the ligaments supporting the scaphoid.

1. **Mechanism.** The mechanism of injury is forceful hyperextension of the wrist.

2. **Physical examination.** There is pain with dorsiflexion of the wrist, a clicking sensation with radial or ulnar deviation, and local tenderness distal and radial to Lister's tubercle.

3. **Radiology.** AP and lateral views. The AP shows a gap between the scaphoid and the lunate greater than 3 mm, or the scaphoid may appear shortened, with a dense ring-shaped image around its distal perimeter as it rotates volarly. On lateral projection, the scapholunate angle is greater than 60 degrees.

4. **Treatment.** Splint wrist in neutral position with a volar splint and refer for either closed reduction with percutaneous pinning or possible open reduction.

5. **Complications.** If treated improperly, this condition may produce a weak, painful wrist with early degenerative arthritis.

IV. **Hand dislocations**

A. **Carpometacarpal (CMC) joint dislocations excluding the thumb.** The metacarpal bones interlock with the distal row of carpal bones with complex ligamentous attachments. CMC dislocations often result in fractures of the carpals or metacarpals.

1. **Mechanism.** The mechanism of injury is one of extreme violence—crush injuries, blows from heavy falling objects or from punching an object with a closed fist.

2. **Physical examination.** The deformity that one might expect to see is often obscured by marked swelling of the hand.

3. **Radiology.** AP, lateral, and oblique views. Oblique views with the hand pronated and supinated 30 degrees respectively from the true lateral view may be helpful.

4. **Treatment.** Longitudinal traction (finger traps) and direct pressure over the metacarpal bases is the method of reduction. Hand surgery

consultation is essential, as operative management is often necessary.

5. **Complications.** CMC dislocations may result in ulnar or median nerve damage, extensor tendon injury, vascular compromise, or posttraumatic arthritis.

B. **CMC joint dislocations of the thumb.** Complete dislocations are rare and dislocation without fracture is uncommon.

1. **Mechanism.** The mechanism of injury is a longitudinally directed force with the metacarpal in slight flexion. Because of the strong attachment of the anterior oblique ligament, this mechanism is more likely to fracture the volar surface of the metacarpal, resulting in a Bennett's fracture/subluxation.

2. **Physical examination.** The base of the metacarpal is usually dislocated in a dorsoradial direction.

3. **Radiology.** AP and lateral views. A true AP view (Robert view) is necessary to show the CMC joint adequately; it is taken with the hand in maximum pronation.

4. **Treatment.** These dislocations are easily reduced but unstable after reduction. Thumb spica splints and referral to hand surgery for possible operative repair is appropriate management.

5. **Complications.** Capsular or small bone fragments may be interposed in the joint after reduction and the metacarpal will not sit properly on the trapezium, leading to joint instability. Degenerative changes and chronic pain may also result.

C. **Dorsal metacarpophalangeal (MCP) joint dislocations excluding the thumb.** Dorsal dislocations are divided into simple and complex. Simple dislocations are easily reduced and complex ones are not reducible.

1. **Simple dorsal dislocations**
   a. **Mechanism.** These injuries occur with hyperextension stresses applied to the MCP joint.
   b. **Physical examination.** The proximal phalanx rests in 60 to 90 degrees of hyperextension.
   c. **Radiology.** AP and lateral views.
   d. **Treatment.** The proximal phalanx is hyperextended 90 degrees on the metacarpal and direct pressure is applied to the dorsum of the base of the proximal phalanx, reducing the dislocation. The MCP joint should be splinted in 50 to 70 degrees of flexion for 10 days.

e. **Complications.** Incorrect manipulation may result in conversion to a complex dislocation.

2. **Complex dorsal dislocations**

a. **Mechanism.** These injuries also result from hyperextension stresses.

b. **Physical examination.** The MCP joint is only slightly hyperextended, with the proximal phalanx lying on the dorsum of the metacarpal head. Puckering of the skin in the proximal palmar crease is pathognomonic of a complex dislocation.

c. **Radiology.** AP and lateral views. A widened joint space and interposition of sesamoid indicates a complex dislocation.

d. **Treatment.** A single attempt at reduction may be warranted, but open repair is usually indicated because the volar plate is interposed within the joint. Complex reductions must be referred for operative reduction.

e. **Complications.** Decreased range of motion of the MCP joint may result.

D. **Volar MCP joint dislocations excluding the thumb.** These injuries are very rare, and the pathological anatomy is not well understood. The volar plate, collateral ligament, and dorsal capsule have all been implicated in irreducibility.

E. **Lateral MCP joint dislocations excluding the thumb.** These are uncommon injuries because of the protected position of the joint.

1. **Mechanism.** An ulnar-directed force against the MCP joint causes the dislocation.

2. **Physical examination.** The most specific clinical sign is pain on lateral stress when the MCP joint is held in full extension, regardless of instability.

3. **Radiology.** AP and lateral views.

4. **Treatment.** Splint the MCP joint in 50 degrees of flexion, usually for 3 weeks. Refer the patient to a hand surgeon for possible operative repair of grossly unstable joints or an associated intraarticular fracture.

5. **Complications.** Chronic pain and instability may result from improperly treated injuries.

F. **Dorsal dislocations of the MCP joint of the thumb.** Dorsal dislocations are divided into simple and complex. Simple ones are easily reduced and complex ones cannot be reduced.

1. **Simple dorsal dislocations**

a. **Mechanism.** The mechanism of injury is an extreme hyperextension or shearing force.

b. **Physical examination.** In a simple dislocation (subluxation), the phalanx usually rests on the head of the metacarpal in nearly 90 degrees of hyperextension.

c. **Radiology.** AP and lateral views.

d. **Treatment.** Closed reduction is accomplished by first hyperextending the proximal phalanx on the metacarpal and then applying dorsal pressure at the base of the phalanx. Flexing of the wrist and interphalangeal joint aids in the reduction. Attempting to reduce the deformity with traction alone may entrap the volar plate. The thumb is splinted in a thumb spica with the MCP joint in 20 degrees of flexion for about 3 to 6 weeks. After reduction, the collateral ligaments should be tested. The patient should be referred to a hand specialist for possible operative repair.

e. **Complications.** Complications include hyperextension, instability, and chronic pain on pinching.

2. **Complex dorsal dislocations**

a. **Mechanism.** The mechanism, as in simple dislocations, is an extreme hypertension or shearing force.

b. **Physical examination.** The proximal phalanx is nearly parallel to the metacarpal with only slight hyperextension. Another important clinical sign is a skin dimple over the thenar eminence.

c. **Radiology.** AP and lateral views. Demonstration of a sesamoid within the widened joint space is pathognomonic of complex dislocation.

d. **Treatment options.** A single attempt at closed reduction under adequate anesthesia should be made. If reduction fails, a hand surgeon should be consulted for open reduction.

e. **Complications.** Complications include hyperextension, instability, and chronic pain on pinching.

G. **Lateral dislocations of the MCP joint of the thumb**

1. **Mechanism.** A sudden varus or valgus stress probably combined with hyperextension is responsible for this injury.

2. **Physical examination.** Lateral dislocations typically present with only swelling and local tenderness to the radial or ulnar aspect of the metacarpal head, depending on the ligament involved. Rupture of the ulnar collateral ligament (gamekeeper's thumb) may be easily diagnosed if the joint opens up while being stressed. Unless gross instability is easily demonstrated, ab-

duction and adduction stress tests under local anesthesia should be done with the interphalangeal (IP) joint in flexion and extension. The affected joint is compared to that on the unaffected side.

3. **Radiology.** AP and lateral views. Stress views may be helpful.
4. **Treatment.** Place in the spica splint and refer for possible surgical repair.
5. **Complications.** Chronic pain and instability of the thumb MCP joint are complications.

H. **Proximal interphalangeal (PIP) joint dislocations.** The PIP joint is the most commonly dislocated joint in the hand.

1. **Dorsal PIP joint dislocations.** These are the most common of the PIP dislocations
   a. **Mechanism.** These are hyperextension injuries, as occur when an outstretched finger is struck by a ball.
   b. **Physical examination.** Gross deformity is usually present on exam. After reduction of the joint, the stability of the volar plate should be assessed by stressing the joint.
   c. **Radiology.** AP and lateral views.
   d. **Treatment.** After a digital block has been completed, traction and hyperextension are applied while dorsal pressure is placed on the base of the middle phalanx. The digit is immobilized in 15 to 20 degrees of flexion.
   e. **Complications.** Irreducible dislocations are uncommon, but they have been reported to result from entrapment of the volar plate or flexor tendons. Joint laxity and a swanneck deformity are other complications.

2. **Lateral PIP joint dislocations**
   a. **Mechanism.** These injuries are due to abduction or adduction forces on an extended digit.
   b. **Physical examination.** One should assess the active and passive stability of the ligaments of the joint after reduction. There will be pain on lateral stressing of the joint and tenderness over the lateral joint.
   c. **Radiology.** AP and lateral views. Stress views may be taken.
   d. **Treatment.** These dislocations usually reduce spontaneously on examination in the emergency department. The affected digit is buddy-taped to the adjacent digit and the patient is referred to a hand surgeon for possible operative repair.
   e. **Complications.** If the patient is treated improperly, pain, instability, or limitation of joint motion may result.

3. **Volar PIP joint dislocations.** These are relatively rare and result from disruption of the central slip.

   a. **Mechanism.** These result from varus or valgus forces combined with an anteriorly directed force.

   b. **Physical examination.** Dislocation may be reduced on presentation to the emergency department.

   c. **Radiology.** AP and lateral views. Dorsal chip fractures are often associated.

   d. **Treatment.** Volar dislocations are reduced by gentle traction with the MCP and PIP joint flexed. The PIP should be immobilized in extension. Prompt referral is important if joint surfaces are incongruent or if dislocation is irreducible.

   e. **Complications.** Inadequately treated volar dislocations may result in a boutonnière deformity or in a flexion contracture of the PIP with limited, painful motion.

V. **Hip dislocations.** The hip is a stable ball-and-socket joint and great force is needed to dislocate it; therefore other injuries should be sought on examination. Motor vehicle accidents are the most common cause of hip dislocations. On examination, these injuries should be obvious from the patient's position unless there is an ipsilateral extremity fracture that obscures the clinical deformity. Hip dislocations are often associated with fractures of the femoral head, femoral neck, acetabulum, or pelvis as well as significant soft tissue injury. These injuries should be considered true orthopaedic emergencies and should be reduced promptly, usually within 6–12 hours, to reduce avascular necrosis of the femoral head. There are numerous classifications of hip dislocations, but they are generally grouped into posterior, anterior, and central.

A. **Posterior hip dislocations.** These are the most common hip dislocations.

   1. **Classification.** One method is that of Thompson and Epstein.

      Type I: With or without minor fracture

      Type II: With a large single fracture of the posterior acetabular rim

      Type III: With comminution of the acetabular rim with or without a major fragment

      Type IV: With acetabular floor fracture

      Type V: With fracture of the femoral head

   2. **Mechanism of injury.** Motor vehicle injuries are the most common cause. A force is applied to the flexed knee with the hip in varying degrees of flexion, as when the knee strikes the car's dashboard, forcing the femoral head posteriorly.

3. **Physical examination.** The leg is shortened, internally rotated, and adducted (PID = posterior, internal, adducted). Sciatic nerve function needs to be assessed for injury and is involved in 10% to 14% of cases. Other life- and limb-threatening injuries should be sought. If it is associated with a femoral shaft fracture, the dislocation may go unrecognized because the classic position may not be present.

4. **Radiography.** AP and lateral views of the hip and pelvis should be obtained. The AP view should be adequate to diagnose the dislocation but additional views are necessary to search for associated fractures of the femur and pelvis. There are clues on the AP film to help distinguish a posterior from an anterior dislocation. With a posterior dislocation, the femoral head will appear smaller than the one on the normal side because it lies closer to the film cassette; in an anterior dislocation, the opposite is true. In a posterior dislocation, the lesser trochanter will not be seen on the AP view, as the hip is in adduction and internal rotation; but it will be seen in an anterior dislocation. Knee films should be done if clinically indicated. Special attention should focus on the femoral head, femoral neck, and acetabulum. Special views such as the Judet view may be needed to rule out associated fractures.

5. **Treatment options.** These dislocations ideally should be reduced by an orthopaedist with the patient under general or spinal anesthesia. Under certain circumstances, a simple dislocation can be treated with closed reduction using conscious sedation and analgesics. Multiple attempts are discouraged, as is the use of excessive force, as a simple dislocation can be converted to a fracture/dislocation.

    a. **Stimson's maneuver.** The least traumatic method. The patient is placed in the prone position with the hip flexed over the end of the cart. An assistant stabilizes the pelvis by putting pressure on the sacrum or by extending the opposite limb. The injured hip and knee are flexed to 90 degrees and downward traction is applied behind the flexed knee. A gentle internal and external rotation of the femur while traction is maintained may help the reduction. It may not be possible to use this method in a patient with multiple injuries. The assistant can push the greater trochanter toward the acetabulum.

    b. **Allis's maneuver.** The patient is supine while an assistant stabilizes the pelvis by applying pressure on both anterior iliac spines. Traction is then applied to the injured limb in direct line of the deformity, and this is followed by gentle hip flexion to 90 degrees. The hip is then gently rotated internally and externally in this position with continued longitudinal traction until the reduction is completed. The assistant can push the greater trochanter toward the acetabulum. Light skin or buck traction should be applied after the reduction with the hip extended and the leg slightly abducted and externally rotated.

6. **Complications.** Early complications include associated fractures, sciatic nerve injury, tearing of the iliofemoral ligament, and damage to the articular surface. Late complications include avascular necrosis of the femoral head, posttraumatic osteoarthritis, and pulmonary embolism.

B. **Anterior hip dislocations.** These account for 5% to 15% of all traumatic hip dislocations.

1. **Classifications.** There are three general types: superior iliac, superior pubic, and inferior obturator. These are determined by the final position of the femoral head in relation to the acetabulum.

2. **Mechanism of injury.** These injuries result from a forced abduction of the thigh, usually in a car accident with the knee striking the dashboard while the thigh is abducted. The femoral neck or greater trochanter impinges on the acetabular rim and levers the femoral head out through a tear in the anterior hip capsule. The degree of hip flexion at the time of the injury determines whether it is in the superior or inferior position.

3. **Physical examination.** In the superior iliac and pubic dislocations, the hip is held in external rotation, extension, and a variable degree of abduction. In the obturator dislocation, the hip is externally rotated, abducted, and markedly flexed. The femoral neurovascular status should be assessed repeatedly for any injury.

4. **Radiography.** AP and lateral views of the hips and pelvis. Careful examination for associated fractures of the acetabulum, femoral head, and femoral neck is important.

5. **Treatment.** These injuries are best treated with early closed reduction under spinal or general anesthesia. Emergent referral to the orthopaedic surgeon is recommended. Open reduction may be required.

6. **Complications.** There is a significant risk of femoral artery and vein injury as well as associated fractures.

C. **Central dislocations.** There is a medial displacement of the femoral head into the pelvis. The femoral head remains contiguous with the severely comminuted fragments of the fractured acetabulum. This injury occurs from a blow to the lateral aspect of the trochanter that transmits the force to the acetabulum. The diagnosis is made radiographically on AP and internal and external oblique views. Life-threatening skeletal and visceral injuries are commonly associated with this injury, and the diagnosis may be delayed or overlooked. These injuries require surgery.

D. **Prosthetic hip dislocations.** There is an increased incidence of these types of injuries because of the increasing numbers of patients with hip prostheses. These injuries may occur with minimal trauma. The examiner must check for the direction of the dislocation, dislodgement of the acetabular or femoral prosthesis, and associated pelvic or femoral fractures.

VI. **Knee dislocations.** The knee is a stable joint reinforced by strong ligaments. Dislocations are extremely rare and require a tremendous amount of force to the knee, as in a motor vehicle accident. They are often associated with major life- and limb-threatening injuries. Many will reduce spontaneously prior to the patient's arrival in the emergency department. Neurovascular injuries are common, with 30% to 40% being associated with a popliteal artery injury. They are classified as anterior, posterior, medial, lateral, and rotatory, according to the relationship of the tibia to the femur.

A. **Anterior knee dislocations.** Knee dislocations are most commonly anterior.

1. **Mechanism of injury.** A hyperextension force that results in a tear of the posterior capsule, anterior cruciate, and posterior cruciate ligaments.

2. **Physical examination.** These injuries are usually obvious clinically, with a grossly deformed or unstable knee joint. Neurovascular injuries are frequent, especially involving the popliteal artery and peroneal nerve. A peroneal nerve injury would cause decreased sensation to the dorsal foot and decreased foot dorsiflexion. Absent pulses despite a warm foot indicate a vascular injury until proven otherwise.

3. **Radiography.** AP and lateral knee views are indicated unless vascular compromise is present, in which case immediate reduction is indicated. Consider radiographs of the hip and pelvis to rule out associated injuries. Never delay reduction to obtain radiographs if neurovascular compromise is present. Angiography should be considered in all patients with this injury.

4. **Treatment.** Reduction may be done with an assistant placing longitudinal traction on the leg while the femur is lifted anteriorly into the reduced position. This can also be done with an assistant applying traction to the distal femur while traction is applied to the leg with posterior pressure over the proximal leg. These are relatively easy reductions, but are unstable and need immobilization in a posterior long leg splint at 15 to 20 degrees of flexion to stabilize the knee and prevent further neurovascular injury.

All of these patients need hospitalization, most will need surgery, and all should have immediate orthopaedic referral. Temporary immobilization with a posterior long leg splint with knee in 20 to 30 degrees of flexion is required. Angiography should be considered in all cases. Prognosis depends on extent of injury and operative intervention. Patients with operative intervention have a better prognosis than those without.

5. **Complications.** Major neurovascular injuries include popliteal artery and peroneal nerve injury as well as ligamentous injury. The incidence of popliteal artery injury is 40% to 50%; and up to half of these, will require amputation. Deep venous thrombosis and compartment syndrome, may occur.

B. **Posterior knee dislocations**
    1. **Mechanism of injury.** These injuries result from a direct posterior force to the anterior tibia with the knee flexed. The posterior capsule and anterior and posterior cruciates are injured. Popliteal artery injury is less common.
    2. **Physical examination.** This shows a grossly deformed or unstable knee.
    3. **Radiographs.** AP and lateral views suffice if no neurovascular compromise is present. Angiography should be considered in all patients with this injury.
    4. **Treatment.** An assistant applies longitudinal traction to the femur and in-line traction is applied to the leg while the proximal tibia is lifted anteriorly.
    5. **Complications.** Same as for anterior dislocations. Arthritis is common after these injuries, as well as persistent joint instability from the ligamentous injury.
C. **Patellar dislocations.** These injuries are relatively common but usually reduce spontaneously prior to the patient's arrival in the emergency department. The majority are seen in patients with chronic patellofemoral anatomical abnormalities such as genu valgum (knock-knees) or patella alta (high-riding patella). According to the location of

the patella in relation to the knee joint, these injuries are classified as lateral, superior, medial, and intraarticular.

1. **Lateral patellar dislocations.** These are the most common patellar dislocations.

   a. **Mechanism of injury.** The most common mechanism is an indirect force with sudden flexion and external rotation of the tibia and contraction of the quadriceps, as in a golf swing or dancing. This may also occur from direct trauma. These forces cause the patella to ride over the lateral condyle of the femur.

   b. **Physical examination.** The patient is unable to bear weight and the knee is in slight flexion. There may be pain, swelling, or a mild hemarthrosis. The patella can be palpated laterally. The apprehension test may be positive (pain elicited on an attempt to displace the patella laterally) if the patella had reduced spontaneously prior to examination.

   c. **Radiography.** AP and lateral views initially. These should be obtained to exclude a fracture, even if the dislocation reduced spontaneously. A "sunrise" view should be obtained after reduction to rule out fractures or a loose body. A fat-fluid level is suggestive of a bone or osteochrondral fracture.

   d. **Treatment.** Reduction can be done by flexing the hip and gently extending the knee to 180 degrees while applying medially directed pressure to the patella. Occasionally pressure may need to be applied both anteriorly and medially. The knee should be immobilized in extension with a knee immobilizer or posterior long leg splint. The patient should not bear weight and receive an orthopaedic referral. Surgery is usually recommended for loose bodies or structural abnormalities likely to cause recurrences.

   e. **Complications.** Dislocations will recur in 50% of patients. Osteochondral fractures occur in 5%, and some may also develop degenerative arthritis.

VII. **Ankle dislocations.** Isolated dislocations of the ankle are rare. Stability of the ankle is provided by the tight articulation of the talus with the lower portions of the tibia and fibula.

  A. **Anterior dislocation**

   1. **Mechanism.** This type of dislocation is due to a force that causes posterior displacement of the tibia on a fixed foot or forced dorsiflexion of the foot—as occurs during a fall on a dorsiflexed foot.

2. **Physical examination.** The foot is dorsiflexed and elongated. Almost half of the reported ankle dislocations were open injuries. Check for neurovascular compromise, as it is especially common in open injuries.

3. **Radiology.** AP, lateral, and oblique views.

4. **Treatment.** Dorsiflex the foot slightly to disengage the talus and apply downward traction, pushing the foot posteriorly into its normal position. A short leg posterior mold and immediate orthopaedic consultation are required.

5. **Complications.** Fractures of the malleoli are commonly associated. Residual swelling and a decreased range of motion are complications.

B. **Posterior dislocations.** These are the most common types of dislocations.

1. **Mechanism.** The mechanism of a posterior dislocation involves a plantarflexed foot. The dislocation results from either a forward thrust of the tibia or a backward thrust of the foot.

2. **Physical examination.** The foot is plantarflexed and shortened. Always assess neurovascular integrity.

3. **Radiology.** AP, lateral, and oblique views.

4. **Treatment.** Reduction involves further plantarflexion and manipulation of the foot anteriorly. A posterior mold is applied and orthopaedic consultation is obtained on initial presentation. The patient may require surgery.

5. **Complications.** Irreducibility from a fracture/dislocation may result, as well as residual swelling and a decreased range of motion.

C. **Lateral dislocations.** These are probably the most common ankle dislocations seen in the emergency department and are always associated with malleolar or fibular fractures.

1. **Mechanism.** The medial or lateral ankle receives a forceful direct blow.

2. **Physical examination.** The foot is displaced laterally and the skin is taut medially. Remember to assess neurovascular integrity.

3. **Radiology.** AP, lateral, and oblique views.

4. **Treatment.** While a partner stabilizes the leg, longitudinal traction and medial manipulation of the foot usually reduce the dislocation easily. Place a posterior splint and refer for probable surgical repair.

5. **Complications.** Residual swelling and a decrease in range of motion may result.

VIII. **Foot dislocations**

A. **Subtalar dislocations.** The talus becomes dislocated as the talocalcaneal and talonavicular ligaments are disrupted. Subtalar dislocations occur medially (85%) and laterally (15%).

1. **Mechanism.** A medial dislocation is produced by a combination of a large inversion force along with plantarflexion. It has been reported in basketball players who land on an inverted, plantarflexed foot. A lateral dislocation results from a large eversion force.

2. **Physical examination.** In medial dislocations, the foot will be displaced medially and the talus is prominent laterally. The vascular supply to the skin may be compromised by talar pressure. In lateral dislocations, the calcaneus is displaced lateral to the talus and the talar head is prominent medially.

3. **Radiology.** AP, lateral, and oblique films are difficult to obtain owing to distortion of the foot. The AP film is the most helpful; the head of the talus should articulate with the "cup" of the proximal navicular.

4. **Treatment.** If prompt consultation is not available, an attempt at closed reduction is warranted, because soft tissue pressure may convert a closed injury into an open one. Reduction requires traction on the heel, to disengage the dislocation, combined with a downward force on the talar head, with abduction, pronation, and dorsiflexion of the foot. A lateral dislocation is reduced by longitudinal traction, adduction, and dorsiflexion. Open reduction may be required for either.

5. **Complications.** Complications include avascular necrosis, loss of ankle motion, traumatic arthritis, and ischemic skin loss.

B. **Total dislocations of the talus.** This is a rare injury.

1. **Mechanism.** Extreme inversion first produces a medial subtalar dislocation; if the force continues, a total lateral talar dislocation may result. Extreme eversion produces a lateral subtalar dislocation and, with continuing pronation, a total medial dislocation.

2. **Physical examination.** Most are open injuries.

3. **Radiology.** AP, lateral and oblique views.

4. **Treatment.** Debridement, open reduction, and talectomy are often required.

5. **Complications.** Infection has been reported in up to 89% of cases. Avascular necrosis and degenerative arthritis of the ankle and subtalar joint frequently result.

C. **Tarsometatarsal fracture-dislocation (Lisfranc).** The Lisfranc fracture/dislocation is a dislocation or fracture-dislocation of the tarsometatarsal (Lisfranc) joint.

1. **Mechanism.** This injury may result from direct trauma, as when a foot is trapped under

the wheel of car or a heavy object falls on the foot. An indirect mechanism, such as a fall from a height, may also produce this injury.

2. **Physical examination.** Severe swelling and pain on palpation of the tarsometatarsal area may be present.

3. **Radiology.** AP, lateral, and 30-degree oblique views are essential. Injury is often overlooked (20%). Comparison views are often helpful. The most reliable radiological sign is separation between the base of the first and the second metatarsals.

4. **Treatment.** Closed reduction often results in an unstable foot. Surgical fixation is usually required.

5. **Complications.** Degenerative arthritis and impaired circulation to the distal foot may result.

D. **Dislocation of lesser metatarsophalangeal joints**

1. **Mechanism.** An extreme medial or lateral force displaces a digit on the metatarsal head. This often happens when a bare foot is jammed into a piece of furniture.

2. **Physical examination.** The base of the proximal phalanx is usually displaced dorsally and laterally, overriding the metatarsal.

3. **Radiology.** AP and lateral views.

4. **Treatment.** Reduction is usually accomplished easily with traction and/or application of pressure to the dorsum of the proximal phalanx.

5. **Complications.** Complex (irreducible) dislocations have been reported and require open reduction.

E. **Dislocations of the first metatarsophalangeal joint**

1. **Mechanism.** High-energy automobile collisions are usually responsible for this rare injury.

2. **Physical examination.** Most are dorsal dislocations producing dorsal prominence and shortening of the toe.

3. **Radiology.** AP, lateral, and oblique views. Complex (irreducible) dislocations should be suspected when unfractured sesamoids are seen in the joint space.

4. **Treatment.** Dislocations should be reduced promptly to avoid circulatory compromise to the dorsal skin. Most dislocations are easily reduced with gentle longitudinal traction or hyperextension of the proximal phalanx and dorsal pressure on the base of the proximal phalanx.

5. **Complications.** Occasionally, closed reduction is not possible and these complex dislocations require open reduction.

F. Lesser toe interphalangeal joint dislocations
  1. **Mechanism.** Dorsal or plantar forces may result in dislocation of the dorsal or proximal interphalangeal joints in the dorsal or plantar direction.
  2. **Radiology.** AP and lateral views.
  3. **Treatment.** Manual reduction under digital block using gentle traction is usually stable. The toe should be splinted to the adjacent toe for 10 to 14 days.
  4. **Complications.** Rarely, an entrapped flexor tendon or capsule may require open reduction.
G. Great toe dislocations
  1. **Mechanism.** Dislocation or fracture/dislocation of the interphalangeal joint usually results from an axial load to the digit, as from a kick to a fixed object.
  2. **Physical examination.** Dorsal prominence and shortening are noted clinically.
  3. **Radiology.** AP and lateral views. Sesamoid bone may be seen in the joint space, indicating an irreducible dislocation.
  4. **Treatment.** Most dislocations are dorsal and may be easily reduced with digital anesthesia and traction. After reduction, the toe is usually stable and is splinted to the second toe for 2 to 3 weeks.
  5. **Complications.** A displayed plantar plate may prevent closed reduction, so that open reduction is required.

BIBLIOGRAPHY

Harwood-Nuss AL et al. *The clinical practice of emergency medicine.* New York: Lippincott-Raven, 1996.

Kothari RU, Dronen SC. Prospective evaluation of the scapular manipulation technique in reducing anterior shoulder dislocations. *Ann Emerg Med* 1992;21:1349–1352.

Kothari RU, Dronen SC. The scapular manipulation technique for the reduction of acute anterior shoulder dislocations. *J Emerg Med* 1990;8:625–628.

Roberts Jr, Hedges JR. *Clinical Procedures in Emergency Medicine.* Philadelphia: WB Saunders, 1991.

Rockwood C, Green D, et al. *Fractures.* Vols 1 and 2. Philadelphia: JB Lippincott, 1991.

Rosen P, Barkin RM, et al. *Emergency medicine concepts and clinical practice.* St. Louis: Mosby–Year Book, 1992.

Rosen P, Doris PE, et al. *Diagnosis radiology in emergency medicine.* St. Louis: Mosby–Year Book, 1992.

Simon R et al. *Orthopedics in emergency medicine: the extremities,* 3rd ed. Appleton-Century-Crofts, 1996.

Tintinalli J et al. *Emergency medicine: a comprehensive study guide,* 3rd ed. New York: McGraw-Hill, 1992.

Principles of Splinting

Stephen J. Playe and Wendy S. Filener

I. **Principles**
   A. **Definition.** A splint is an appliance that decreases the mobility of a body part. It consists of padding, a rigid (usually plaster) noncircumferential component, and an outer wrap to hold the splint in place.
   B. **Indications.** Splints provide short-term immobilization of joints and fractures. They provide less secure immobilization than circumferential casts but have the advantages of allowing for continued swelling without risk of ischemic injury and can be removed for bathing, exercise, or wound care. Splints can be used to treat:
      1. **Inflammatory joint pain**
      2. **Wounds** (including lacerations across joints, tendon lacerations, contaminated lacerations, and puncture wounds of extremities)
      3. **Infections** of joints, tendons, or deep spaces of the hand or foot
      4. **Sprains**
      5. **Fractures** (temporary immobilization of unstable fractures and definitive treatment of some stable fractures)
   C. **Design.** A well-designed splint is capable of immobilization nearly equivalent to that of a circumferential cast, with less risk of complications. Options include custom-made, premade, and hybrid splints custom-made from prefabricated padded plaster or prefabricated padded fiberglass.
      1. **Custom versus premade.** There are many forms of premade splints on the market, most of which consist of metal or plastic forms that are attached with Velcro straps. These splints are quick and easy to apply; however, they fit imperfectly, resulting in suboptimal immobilization, and they are expensive. Commercially available prefabricated plaster splint rolls have 10 to 20 layers of plaster sandwiched between a thick foam pad and a thin cloth layer. They are dipped, can be applied quickly, and are secured with an elastic bandage. However, they are also expensive and lack the versatility and excellent fit of a custom-made splint. Thus emergency departments usually use plaster custom splints because they are the least expensive, provide the best fit, and are the most versatile. This chapter concentrates on their use.
      2. **Plaster versus fiberglass.** Whether to use fiberglass or plaster is largely a matter of individual

preference. Fiberglass is lightweight, fast-setting, extremely strong, and resistant to damage by water (although most splint dressings contain other material that should be kept dry). However, fiberglass is expensive, sticky, and awkward to premeasure, and the speed of its setting may not allow enough time to properly shape and mold the splint. For these reasons, plaster is the material most commonly used for emergency department splints.

D. **Equipment**
   1. **Padding.** A single layer of stockinette is often the first part of the splint to be applied. It should extend about 4 in. beyond the splint on both ends. It protects the skin and can be folded back over the ends of the splint for a smooth finish. Stockinette comes in widths of 2, 3, 4, 8, 10, and 12 in. It can also be used as a sling for injuries of the upper extremity. The next layer is Webril, a dense cotton padding that protects the skin and bony prominences. It can stretch and tear, thus allowing for soft tissue swelling. It is available in widths of 3, 4, and 6 in.
   2. **Plaster and its preparation.** Plaster of paris splinting consists of rolls or strips of crinoline-type material impregnated with calcium sulfate. When it comes into contact with water, the plaster incorporates the water molecules to form a crystalline lattice of calcium dihydrate molecules. This is an exothermic reaction, and the amount of heat generated increases with the speed of the reaction. The warmer the water, the faster the reaction and the faster the plaster sets. Thus when plaster comes into contact with very warm water, especially as it approaches 40°C, enough heat is generated to burn a patient severely. To avoid this, use water that is only slightly warmer than room temperature (ideally about 24°C). A slower setting time also allows more time to properly mold the splint. Other factors that increase heat production during setting include increased splint thickness, setting time ("extra fast" formulations of plaster set in 2 to 4 minutes rather than the 5 to 8 minutes of the usual "fast" plaster), and wrapping the extremity in a pillow or towel for support while the plaster dries. Minor variables that speed the setting process are high humidity, high ambient temperature, and reuse of the dip water.
   3. **Elastic bandages.** Elastic (ACE) bandages come in various widths. In general, the 2-in. size works best for the hands and feet; the 3- and 4-in. sizes do well for the upper extremities; and 4- and 6-in. widths are used for the lower extremities.
   4. **Tape.** Cloth or silk tape, 1/2 in. in width, tears easily, sticks well to splint media, and is of a practical size.

5. **Cutters.** Standard trauma shears can be used to cut anything from elastic bandages to dry plaster to premade aluminum finger splints.

6. **Bucket.** A stainless steel or plastic 3-gal bucket is needed; it should be half filled with water that is slightly warmer than room temperature.

7. **Protective gear.** Gloves make cleanup faster and plaster easier to mold because it does not stick to them. They can be removed after dipping and applying the splint to avoid getting plaster on the elastic bandage. Aprons or gowns protect clothes. Protective eyewear should also be worn, especially when cutting hard materials.

E. **Application**
  1. **Patient preparation.** If possible, the patient should be protected by a sheet or gown during the splinting procedure. The area to be splinted must be carefully examined for soft tissue injuries. Wounds should be treated and dressed appropriately, including applying sterile saline dressings over open fractures. Neurovascular status should be assessed before and after splint application.

  2. **Stockinette.** The first layer applied is often stockinette. If it is decided to use stockinette, care must be taken to prevent wrinkles. In areas of flexion creases, the stockinette should be slit and overlapped to avoid pressure points (or use two separate pieces that overlap at the crease). In general, the 3-in. width is best for the upper extremities and the 4-in. width for the lower extremities. Leave 3 or 4 in. of stockinette extending beyond the ends of the splint. After the splint is applied, fold these ends over the splint edges and secure with elastic bandage for a smooth finish. Although stockinette creates a polished-looking splint, it is not essential, and many argue that avoiding stockinette and applying Webril as the first layer results in better immobilization and speeds application.

  3. **Padding.** Cotton padding (Webril) should be applied smoothly and evenly over all areas to be covered by the splint, extending about 1 in. beyond the ends of the splint. Extra strips can be placed over bony prominences and between any splinted digits to avoid skin maceration. There are two general methods by which Webril may be applied.
     a. **Circumferential wrap.** Webril should be wrapped circumferentially when the splint is to be worn continuously. It should be two or three layers thick and each wrap should overlap the previous by 50%. Extra strips of padding are applied to protect bony prominences. As the Webril is unrolled to cover the extremity, it can be stretched or torn to facilitate even application. In areas where joints that are at

sharp angles must be covered, continuous wrapping may be combined with vertical and horizontal strips until the padding is evenly distributed. Tear off any loose or excess Webril to avoid wrinkles that can cause pressure sores. Position the limb *before* applying stockinette and Webril.

In general, the 2-in. width is used for the hands and feet and the 3- and 4-in. widths for upper extremities. The 4- and 6-in. widths are reserved for the lower extremities. This varies with patient size, and the narrower widths may be preferred in awkward regions because they are easier to apply evenly. After the splint is applied, a layer of Webril is wrapped over the splint (again circumferentially) before the elastic bandage is applied as the final layer. The second layer of Webril prevents the elastic bandage from sticking to the splint, which would make removal much more difficult and painful due to increased movement of the extremity. This use of circumferential Webril provides very secure immobilization and discourages patients from removing the splint.

b. **Incorporation into removable splint.** Webril may also be used to line the splint longitudinally in situations that do not demand the most secure stabilization or to allow splint removal for bathing, dressing changes, or wound inspection.

Choose Webril that is 1 in. wider than the plaster (to pad sharp edges). Measure out a strip of Webril the length of the splint plus 1 in. extra at each end. Double back twice to make a three-layer stack of Webril. Unroll one final layer over the stack and tear off the excess roll. Now peel back that final layer so that the stack is open, like a book. After the plaster is dipped, lay it on the stack of three layers, smooth out the bubbles, and remove your gloves. Close that final layer over the plaster so it is completely encased in a Webril "sandwich," with three layers on one side and one layer on the other. The splint is then applied with the three-layer side against the skin.

Prior to application, smaller splints (i.e., volar wrist splints) can be encased in stockinette for a neater appearance. Measure stockinette of the same width as the Webril and several inches longer than the splint you have constructed. Insert your right arm through the stockinette, then grasp the assembled splint and padding with your right hand. Stabilize the distal end of the stockinette with your left hand while pulling the splint back until it is inside the stockinette. The stockinette is then folded back and tucked inside itself at each end of the splint. The unit is now applied directly to the extremity. While this method provides less secure immobilization than the circumferential wrap method, application is quicker and the splint can easily be removed and reapplied by the patient. It is a less convenient but less expensive alternative than that of the commercially available padded splinting material.

4. **Plaster.** Plaster comes in strips or rolls that are 2, 3, 4, and 6 in. in width. It is most easily measured by laying out dry plaster next to the area to be splinted. Allow some extra length, because the splint will shrink a bit when wet; if it is too long, the ends can easily be folded back. In general, you should choose a width that is slightly greater than the diameter of the limb being splinted. If the limb is to be wrapped circumferentially in Webril, measure out the plaster after wrapping the limb to avoid underestimating splint length.

Unroll the plaster far enough to fold it, creating one layer of the proper length. Hold the fold and drop the rolled end to the floor. You may now create your splint by folding the unrolled plaster over itself with a hand-over-hand motion. This method of folding the plaster around itself is quick and creates a stronger splint than if it is folded back and forth.

Splint thickness will vary. If too few layers are used, the splint will soon break, but thicker splints are heavy and uncomfortable, and they give off more heat while setting (with more than 12 layers, the risk of a significant burn increases). As a general guideline in adults, use 8 layers for an upper extremity and 12 layers (or even up to 15 in a large adult) for a lower extremity.

Activate and apply the splint by taking the following steps:

a. **Dip.** Fully submerge the plaster material in tepid water until the bubbling stops.

b. **Strip.** Fan-fold the strips, squeeze once, then hold up one end with your nondominant hand and strip excess water from the splint between the extended index and long fingers. Repeat from each edge for wide material. Strip toward each end of the splint.

c. **Smooth.** Lay the splint on a flat surface (a towel on a table or counter) and smooth it with a gloved flat hand to remove wrinkles and create a homogeneous mass. Cross-linking within and between layers thus maximizes strength.

d. **Position.** Place the splint over the Webril and gently smooth it with your flat palm to conform with the extremity. Although plaster is somewhat adherent to Webril, an assistant may be needed to hold the splint in place. Support should be provided with the palms, not the fingers, because dents from fingers may remain on the inner surface, potentially causing skin injury, even if they are rubbed smooth on the external edge.

e. **Trim.** Excess plaster can be folded back. Excess Webril can be torn or cut. Excess stockinette can be folded back over the padded splint.

5. **Wrap.** All movement should be avoided after the plaster has reached a thick consistency. Movement at this time disrupts the crystalline network and decreases the strength of the splint.

The splint is secured with elastic bandage (ACE) that is rolled on (flat side of roll against the splint) under slight tension. Each layer of ACE should overlap the previous by 50%. Holes for digits may be cut into the ACE if needed. (One layer of Webril between the splint and the elastic wrap will prevent the bandage from being incorporated into the drying plaster.) The elastic bandage can be secured with the two metal clips covered by tape, or simply by tape.

F. **Complications.** Vascular compromise can result from splints despite the absence of circumferentially applied plaster. While Webril can stretch and tear, there are limits to the degree to which elastic bandages can stretch, and they may cause neurovascular compromise. Splint application can limit observation and care of skin and soft tissue injuries. Patients should be carefully instructed regarding the removal, when necessary, of the splint to provide adequate outpatient care of their injuries. Skin maceration between digits can be avoided by the placement of Webril strips between any digits that are incorporated into splints.

G. **Aftercare.** Patients should receive written and verbal instructions regarding pain control, use of ice or heat, and elevation. Ice should not be in direct contact with the splint, as water will damage plaster splints. Thus patients should be instructed to either cover the splint securely with a plastic bag, or, if the injury permits, remove the splint when bathing. The splint should not be stressed for 24 hours because the plaster does not reach its maximal strength until then. During the 24 hours, the plaster continues to decrease its water content by evaporation ("curing") until it reaches about 21% of its hydrated level and the plaster is strongly set. Follow-up appropriate to the injury should be arranged. Finally, the patient should be advised to be alert for vascular compromise (indicated by a significant increase in pain, numbness or tingling, pallor or decreased capillary refill, or weakness). Any of these signs or symptoms should prompt immediate loosening of the elastic wrap and return for physician evaluation.

H. **Pearls**

1. In applying any rolled material (Webril, ACE), the flat side is kept against the surface so the material unrolls itself along the extremity. This gives more control and a smoother finish.

2. Measure the plaster after the Webril is applied to avoid a splint that is too short.

3. Trim or fold back excess plaster to avoid skin irritation.

4. The tight plastic cases of ACE rolls can be popped open quickly by grasping the roll with your palm over one end (as you would to open a jar) and then striking the other circular end against the palm of your other hand (or against your knee).

5. When you are unsure, splint in the position of function.

6. Generally, splint the joints proximal and distal to the injury.

II. **Specific splints (see Table 1 for indications)**

A. **Upper extremities**

1. **Clavicle: sling**

   a. **Indications.** Injuries to the clavicle and support for a splinted upper extremity.

   b. **Equipment.** Various commercial slings ("large" size for most adults) or a simple triangular bandage.

   c. **Position.** The hand should be higher than the elbow (flexing the elbow a bit beyond 90 degrees). The hand and wrist should be inside the sling, because venous return is restricted if the hand is allowed to protrude.

   d. **Design.** The elbow should be well supported to reduce stress on the shoulder. The sling should immobilize and elevate the hand, forearm, elbow, and shoulder. Figure-of-eight bandages have never been proven superior in the treatment of clavicular fractures and may promote deformity or nonunion.

2. **Shoulder: sling-and-swathe shoulder immobilizer (Fig. 1)**

   a. **Indications.** Shoulder injuries and proximal humeral fractures.

   b. **Equipment.** Two triangular bandages, a commercial sling ("large" for most adults), one triangular bandage or a commercial shoulder immobilizer, Webril (one 4-in. roll).

   c. **Position.** Arm supported by sling (hand higher than elbow), swathe secures the arm to chest wall (immobilizes the shoulder).

   d. **Design.** The hand should not extend beyond the end of the sling, or venous return will be compromised. Pad the axilla with folds of Webril if the patient will be immobilized for more than a few days. Advantages of the commercial immobilizer include ease of removal and reapplication for showering and range-of-motion exercises. The Velpeau bandage is a variation of the sling and swathe that elevates the hand to the opposite (uninjured) shoulder. It is difficult to apply and remove, offers no advantage over standard sling and swathe, and is not well tolerated for long periods.

3. **Upper arm and elbow**
   a. **Posterior mold (Fig. 2)**
      (1) **Indications.** Injuries to the elbow, forearm, or wrist that require immobilization of the wrist and elbow.
      (2) **Equipment.** Two rolls of 6-in. plaster (4 in. in smaller patients), Webril (one 3-in. and four 4-in. rolls), ACE (three 4-in. rolls), sling.
      (3) **Position.** Elbow flexed at 90 degrees, wrist slightly extended at 10 to 20 degrees, forearm in neutral position (thumb up).
      (4) **Design.** Measure plaster from the proximal humerus to the palmar crease. Prepare an eight-layer splint. Apply the splint to the posterior aspect of the upper arm and the ulnar half of the forearm up to the palmar crease (leaving the fingers free). Fold or pinch the excess plaster created at the elbow (due to flexion) against the exterior of the splint. The splint is reinforced by two struts, constructed from double-folded strips of plaster 1 in. wide. Wet the struts and mold them to the splint from midhumerus to midforearm. One strut goes on the lateral side and the other on the medial side of the splint. Secure with ACE wrap. Mold the splint to the above position. When the plaster has hardened, place the arm in a sling.
   b. **Double sugar tong**
      (1) **Indications.** Injuries to elbow, forearm, or wrist; may be used as an alternative to the posterior mold.
      (2) **Equipment.** 4-in. plaster (four rolls), Webril (one 3-in. and four 4-in. rolls), ACE (three 4-in. rolls), sling.
      (3) **Position.** Elbow flexed at 90 degrees, wrist extended at 10 to 20 degrees, forearm in neutral position (thumb up), thumb and fingers free.
      (4) **Design.** Two separate splints are made. The first is an eight-layer splint extending from the metacarpal joints, over the

Table 1.   Splints for specific injuries

Injury	Splint
Clavicular fracture	Sling*
Scapular fracture	Sling*
Shoulder	
Soft tissue injury	Sling*
Rotator cuff injury	Sling*
Acromioclavicular joint injury	Sling*
Dislocation, postreduction	Sling and swathe*
Humerus	
Proximal fracture	Sling and swathe*
Shaft fracture	Coaptation splint
Elbow fracture	
Mild	Sling* or posterior mold*
Moderate	Posterior mold
Severe	Double sugar tong
Forearm	
Shaft fracture	Posterior mold or double sugar tong
Wrist	
Sprain	Volar*
Fracture	
Colles'	Sugar tong
Torus	Volar
Carpal fractures or suspected fracture (i.e., scaphoid, lunate, triquetrum)	Thumb spica*
Hand	
First metacarpal fracture	Thumb spica*
Second or third metacarpal fracture	Radial gutter*
Fourth and fifth metacarpal fracture	Ulnar gutter*
Soft tissue injury (i.e., burns, lacerations, contusions and inflammatory conditions)	Bulky dressing*
Finger	
Proximal phalanx fracture	
First digit	Thumb spica*
Second or third digit	Radial gutter* or dorsal aluminum*
Fourth or fifth digit	Ulnar gutter* or dorsal aluminum*
Middle phalanx fracture	Dorsal aluminum (long)* or dynamic splint (buddy tape)*
Distal phalanx fracture	Fingertip protection* (U-shaped aluminum)
"Mallet" deformity	Dorsal aluminum (short)*
Dislocation (postreduction)	Dorsal aluminum (long)*

Table 1.   *Continued.*

Injury	Splint
Pelvis	
Fracture	Pneumatic anti-shock garment
Femur	
Hip fracture	Hare or Sager traction
Shaft fracture	Hare or Sager traction
Knee	
Soft tissue injury	Knee immobilizer* or compression (Jones) dressing*
Tendon rupture (quadriceps, patellar)	Long leg posterior gutter or knee immobilizer
Patellar dislocation (postreduction)	Knee immobilizer*
Patellar fracture	Knee immobilizer or long leg posterior gutter
Femoral condyle fracture	Long leg posterior gutter
Tibial spine or tuberosity fracture	Knee immobilizer with compression dressing
Tibial plateau fracture	Knee immobilizer with compression dressing
Leg	
Tibial and/or fibular shaft fracture	Long leg posterior gutter
	Long leg sugar tong
Gastrocnemius rupture	Short leg posterior
Ankle	
Sprain	
First degree	Air stirrup* or Unna boot*
Second degree	Air stirrup* or short leg posterior*
Third degree	Short leg posterior or bivalve
Achilles tendon rupture	Short leg posterior (in equinus)
Distal tibial or fibular fracture	Short leg posterior or sugar tong
Severe ankle fracture (i.e., bimalleolar or trimallealor)	"AO" (sugar tong with posterior splint) or bivalve
Dislocation (postreduction)	Short leg posterior, sugar tong with posterior splint or bivalve
Foot	
Soft tissue injuries	Postoperative shoe*
Metatarsal fractures	
Minor/stable	Postoperative shoe*
Major/severe (i.e., multiple or displaced)	Short leg posterior, "AO" (sugar-tong with posterior splint), or bivalve
Calcaneal fracture	Short leg posterior
Talus fracture	
Avulsion	Air splint*
Neck and body	Short leg posterior

Continued.

Table 1. *Continued.*

Injury	Splint
Toe	
Soft tissue injury	Dynamic splint (buddy taping)
Fracture	
Great toe	Postoperative shoe*
Second to fifth toe	Dynamic splint* with, if necessary, postoperative shoe
Dislocation (postreduction)	
Great toe	Postoperative shoe*
Second to fifth toe	Dynamic splint* with, if necessary, postoperative shoe

*This splint may be the definitive immobilization for the specific injury. See text in appropriate chapter for treatment guidelines. See text in this chapter for description of splinting technique.

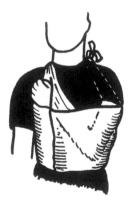

Fig. 1.   **Sling and swathe.**

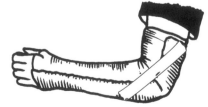

Fig. 2.   **Posterior mold.**

dorsal forearm, around the elbow, up the volar surface of the forearm, and ending at the palmar crease. The second splint (also eight layers) is applied to the medial surface of the upper arm at the proximal humerus. It extends down around the elbow, over the first splint, and on up the lateral surface of the upper arm to the proximal humerus. Secure the splint in the above position with an ACE bandage. When the plaster has hardened, support the arm in a sling.

c. **Coaptation**
   (1) **Indications.** Humeral injuries.
   (2) **Equipment.** 4 in. plaster (two rolls), Webril (one 3 in. and five 4 in. rolls), ACE (four 4-in. rolls), sling.
   (3) **Position.** Elbow flexed at 90 degrees, wrist and hand free, shoulder held in full adduction and internal rotation.
   (4) **Design.** Prepare an eight-layer splint that will extend from the axilla down the medial upper arm and around the elbow, up the lateral upper arm, over the deltoid, and to the middle third of the clavicle. Pad the axilla with folds of Webril and apply the splint. Secure it with ACE wrap in the above position. Be sure the ACE extends well up onto the shoulder. Wrap the forearm and hand with ACE to prevent distal congestion and edema. When the plaster has hardened, support the arm in a sling.

4. **Forearm and wrist**
   a. **Volar**
      (1) **Indications.** Injuries to the wrist or forearm *not* requiring immobilization of the elbow or limitation of supination/pronation.
      (2) **Equipment.** 3-in. plaster (one roll), Webril (one 3-in. and two 4-in. rolls), ACE (two 4-in. rolls).
      (3) **Position.** Wrist in 10 to 20 degrees of extension, thumb and fingers free.
      (4) **Design.** Prepare an eight-layer splint extending from the proximal forearm to the fingertips, cutting a generous crescent notch in one side at the thumb (to allow free movement). Apply the splint to the volar surface of the forearm, from proximal forearm to fingertips. Then roll back the end at the fingertips to the palmar crease. This provides a rounded surface for the fingers to grip without inhibiting movement. Secure it with 3-in. ACE.

b. **Volar/dorsal bivalve**
   (1) **Indications.** Soft tissue injuries to the wrist and forearm not requiring immobilization of the elbow or limitation of supination/pronation (provides more protection than a volar splint alone but not more immobilization).
   (2) **Equipment.** 3-in. plaster (two rolls), Webril (one 3-in. and two 4-in. rolls), ACE (two 4-in. rolls), sling.
   (3) **Position.** Wrist is in slight extension (10 to 20 degrees), thumb and fingers free.
   (4) **Design.** This splint is basically a volar splint with a dorsal slab. Prepare two eight-layer splints. Apply the first from the palmar crease to the proximal volar forearm and the second from the metacarpal joints to proximal dorsal forearm. Secure the slabs with ACE. Mold to the above position and support with a sling (because of the weight of the double slabs). The volar slab may include extra plaster at the palmar end that is folded back on itself to provide a smooth gripping surface for the fingertips.

c. **Sugar tong**
   (1) **Indications.** Injuries to forearm and wrist requiring immobilization with elimination of pronation and supination.
   (2) **Equipment.** 4-in. plaster (two rolls), Webril (one 3-in. and two 4-in. rolls), ACE (two 4-in. rolls), sling.
   (3) **Position.** Elbow flexed at 90 degrees, forearm neutral (thumb up), thumb and fingers free.
   (4) **Design.** Prepare an eight-layer splint that extends from the metacarpal joints up the dorsal forearm, around the elbow, and down the volar forearm to the palmar crease. The thumb and fingers should be left free. Secure the splint in the above position with ACE. When the plaster has hardened, support the arm in a sling.

5. **Hand**
   a. **Ulnar gutter (Fig. 3)**
      (1) **Indications.** Fractures of the fourth and fifth metacarpals or proximal phalanges (or soft tissue injuries to these areas).
      (2) **Equipment.** 4-in. plaster (one roll), Webril (one 3-in. and two 4-in. rolls), ACE (one 3-in. and one 4-in. roll), sling.
      (3) **Position.** Metacarpophalangeal joints flexed to 90 degrees, interphalangeal joints slightly flexed, wrist extended to 15 degrees, first three digits left free.

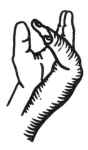

Fig. 3. Ulnar gutter.

(4) **Design.** Place folds of Webril between the fourth and fifth digits to prevent maceration. If both the digits are injured, use 5-in. plaster and incorporate the third digit into the splint as well. Measure out plaster from the elbow to the fingertips. Apply an eight-layer splint to the medial (ulnar) half of the forearm, from elbow to fingertips. Leave the nails exposed so that perfusion can be assessed. Secure with ACE wrap. Using palms only, mold the splint into position.

b. **Radial gutter**
  (1) **Indications.** Fractures of the second and third metacarpals or proximal phalanges (or soft tissue injuries to these regions).
  (2) **Equipment.** 4-in. plaster (one roll), Webril (one 3-in. and two 4-in. rolls), ACE (one 3-in. and one 4-in. roll).
  (3) **Position.** Metacarpophalangeal joints flexed to 90 degrees, interphalangeal joints slightly flexed, wrist extended to 15 degrees, thumb and fourth and fifth digits left free.
  (4) **Design.** Place folds of Webril between the second and third digits to avoid maceration. Measure plaster from the proximal forearm to fingertips and cut a large hole for the thumb. Tear the Webril similarly to accommodate the thumb. Prepare an eight-layer splint. Apply it to the lateral (radial) half of the forearm. The nails should be left exposed to assess perfusion. Secure with ACE, and using only the palms, mold the splint into position.

c. **Thumb spica (Fig. 4)**
  (1) **Indications.** Fractures of the first metacarpal or proximal phalanx, definite or suspected fractures of the carpal navicular (scaphoid), or soft tissue injuries to the thumb.

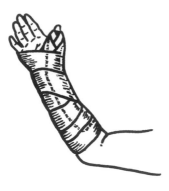

Fig. 4.   Thumb spica.

(2) **Equipment.** 4-in. plaster (one roll), Webril (one 3-in. and two 4-in. rolls), ACE
(one 3-in. and one 4-in. roll).

(3) **Position.** Wrist extended to 15 degrees,
thumb abducted in a position of function
(similar to position hand would assume if
holding a glass); digits two to five are left
free.

(4) **Design.** Measure plaster from thumbnail
to proximal forearm and prepare an
eight-layer splint. Apply the splint to the
lateral (radial) half of the forearm. Plaster edges should meet on the medial aspect of the thumb, encircling it to maintain abduction. One way of helping the
patient maintain this position is by having him or her grasp a can, bottle, or similar object to induce a position of function
as the splint is applied. Secure with ACE
and mold into position.

d. **Bulky hand dressing**

(1) **Indications.** Soft tissue injuries and inflammatory conditions of the hand.

(2) **Equipment.** 4-by 4-in. coarse mesh pads
(about 10), 3-in. Kerlix rolls (two or three),
3-in. ACE wrap (two), 1/2-in. cloth tape.

(3) **Position.** Wrist extended 15 degrees, hand
in position to hold a glass, fingers slightly
separated.

(4) **Design.** 4 by 4 pads are unfolded and
placed between digits (along palm and
back to dorsum of hand). Wad of 4 by 4
pads is placed in palm for the patient to
gently hold. Kerlix is first wrapped circumferentially around the hand, then the
wrist and out to the fingers. Then Kerlix is
applied repeatedly back and forth from the
volar wrist, over the fingers, to the dorsal

wrist. This is anchored by again wrapping the Kerlix circumferentially around the wrist and hand. Tape then secures the end of the Kerlix. The resultant dressing looks like a small thumbless boxing glove. Fingertips can be allowed to protrude for observation of circulation status if indicated. Elastic bandages are optional. They can be slit longitudinally along the midline to permit fingertip exposure. Strips of tape running from the palmar side of the dressing, between the fingers, and then up to the dorsum of the wrist can help to maintain slight wrist extension.

6. **Fingers**
   a. **Dynamic splint (buddy-taping)**
      (1) **Indications.** Soft tissue injuries distal to the metacarpophalangeal joint. Injured finger is stabilized by an adjacent uninjured finger.
      (2) **Equipment.** 1/2-in. cloth tape, Webril (small strip).
      (3) **Position.** Allows motion at the metacarpophalangeal joint, limited motion at the interphalangeal joint.
      (4) **Design.** A strip of Webril is folded in half lengthwise and placed between the two fingers. Then the two fingers are taped together with the tape encircling the fingers between joints.
   b. **Dorsal aluminum splints**
      (1) **Indications.** A *short splint* is used for a mallet finger, and a *long splint* is used for soft tissue injuries to the digits or fractures of the proximal or middle phalanges.
      (2) **Equipment.** 1/2-in. cloth tape, commercially available aluminum splints padded with foam rubber.
      (3) **Position.** Either *short,* distal interphalangeal joint in full extension but not hyperextended, or *long,* interphalangeal joint flexed at 15 to 20 degrees. If the metacarpophalangeal joint is included, it is flexed at 50 degrees, and motion is allowed at the wrist.
      (4) **Design.** The splints come in long strips that may be cut to the desired length with trauma shears. An easier method is to score the edge of the splint with a partial cut with the scissors then bend the aluminum back and forth until it breaks. Corners should be contoured and all cut edges should be covered with tape. The splint is placed over the dorsum of the digit and secured by strips of tape around each

splinted phalanx (between each joint). If the splint includes the metacarpophalangeal joint, it should end just distal to the wrist joint, and tape should be applied circumferentially around the hand both proximal and distal to the thumb. Splints applied on the volar surface are less well tolerated (since volar sensation is functionally more important) and immobilize less well (due to increased subcutaneous tissue over the volar aspect).

   c. **Fingertip protection**
     (1) **Indications.** Distal Phalanx (tuft) fractures and soft tissue injuries. Used to provide protection from contact, not immobilization.
     (2) **Equipment.** Foam-rubber-padded aluminum splints or tube gauze and applicator.
     (3) **Position.** Passive extension.
     (4) **Design.** An aluminum padded splint can be bent into a U shape, placed around the fingertip in either the volar-dorsal orientation (splinting the distal interphalangeal joint and covering the volar pad) or a radial-ulnar direction (allowing motion at the distal interphalangeal joint and exposure for sensation over the volar pad). For less severe injuries, a tube gauze dressing may be adequate.

B. Lower extremities
  1. Pelvis: pneumatic antishock trousers garment
    a. **Indications.** Pelvic or femoral fractures requiring stabilization.
    b. **Equipment.** MAST garment.
    c. **Position.** Maintains both legs in extension when leg compartments are inflated.
    d. **Application.** The patient should be supine. The legs are inflated first, then the abdominal compartment. Pneumatic antishock garment cannot be used longer than 2 hours without concern for increased risk of compartment syndrome. If the patient is in shock, inflation stops at about 100 mm Hg (or inflation may limit itself). Blood pressure must be closely monitored on deflation and good intravenous access secured. The abdomen is deflated first, then the legs, one at a time. Use of the pneumatic antishock garment is an evolving topic, with a number of studies currently in progress.

  2. Hip and femur
    a. **Hare traction**
     (1) **Indications.** Fractures of the femur or hip.

      (2) **Equipment.** Hare traction device.

      (3) **Position.** Holds knee in extension, applies traction to the lower extremity.

      (4) **Application.** Holding the lower extremity at the foot and ankle, traction is applied. The figure-of-eight ankle hitch is applied to the ankle and the splint is slid under the leg. The posterior padded ring should be under the buttocks against the ischial tuberosity. The top strap is secured first; the ankle hitch is then hooked onto the traction strap. Unfold the prop under the splint to elevate the heel. Traction is applied until the extremity appears stabilized. Then the remaining straps are secured (two above and two below the knee). Assess neurovascular status before and after splint placement. The splint must be strapped to bare skin to be effective.

  b. Sager traction

      (1) **Indications.** Fractures of the femur or hip.

      (2) **Equipment.** Sager traction device.

      (3) **Position.** Holds knee in extension, puts traction on the lower extremity.

      (4) **Application.** This device is applied in the same manner as a Hare traction splint; however, it provides some advantages. The amount of traction applied is measured on a gauge and should be 10% of the patient's body weight or 22 lbs, whichever is smaller. There is no posterior ring to cause sciatic compression. The splint may be used in patients with pelvic or groin injuries and may be applied over clothing. Assess neurovascular status before and after placing the splint.

3. Knee

  a. Immobilizer

      (1) **Indications.** Ligamentous or soft tissue injuries to the knee, limited to injuries not requiring immediate surgery or traction.

      (2) **Equipment.** Commercially available knee immobilizer comes in small, medium, large, extra large.

      (3) **Position.** Holds knee in full extension.

      (4) **Application.** Determine size by placing the immobilizer next to the leg. With the patella even with the anterior patellar opening, the wider end should fall a few inches below the buttock crease. Slide the splint under the leg and wrap the edges around the extremity. Secure it firmly

with the Velcro straps. The patella should be exposed through the circular cutout over the knee. The splint can be applied directly over clothing. Crutches may be used but are not essential.

b. **Long leg posterior gutter**
   (1) **Indications.** Knee injuries that require more stabilization or are too large for a simple immobilizer or especially large extremities, angulated fractures, or injuries requiring immediate surgery.
   (2) **Equipment.** 6-in. plaster (three rolls), Webril (five 4-in. rolls), ACE (three 6-in. rolls).
   (3) **Position.** Knee in full extension, ankle and hip freely mobile.
   (4) **Design.** Prepare a 12-layer splint and apply it to the posterior leg from just below the crease of the buttock to 3 in. above the malleoli. Secure the splint in the above position with ACE. Mold the splint edges around the leg in a gutter configuration. As the patient lies supine, have an assistant lift the leg by the heel as the splint is applied or support the heel with a pillow.

c. **Compression dressing (Jones wrap)**
   (1) **Indications.** Short-term immobilization of soft tissue injuries to the knee (allows slight flexion and extension), or may be combined with the immobilizer for unstable injuries such as tibial plateau fractures.
   (2) **Equipment.** 6-in. Webril (three or four), ACE (two or three 6-in. rolls).
   (3) **Position.** Knee in full extension, ankle and hip mobile.
   (4) **Design.** With the patient supine, have an assistant raise the heel (or support it with a pillow). Webril is wrapped from the buttock crease to just above the malleoli. Apply two or three layers of Webril. Finish by wrapping ACE around the Webril (usually two wide ACE bandages are needed). For increased support, the process can be repeated with more Webril and ACE.

d. **Long leg sugar tong**
   (1) **Indications.** Mild or moderate knee injuries, especially those unsuitable for an immobilizer (due to size of extremity, angulated fracture, etc.). Provides better immobilization of lateral and medial collateral ligaments.
   (2) **Equipment.** 6-in. plaster (four), Webril (one 4-in. and three 6-in.), ACE (four 6-in. rolls).

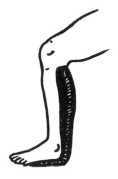

Fig. 5. Posterior short leg.

    (3) **Position.** Knee held in full extension.

    (4) **Design.** Have the patient lie supine with the heel elevated and supported. Measure out plaster from the proximal inner thigh (2 in. below the groin), down the medial surface of the leg, under the heel, and up the lateral surface of the leg until even with the buttock crease. Apply the splint in the above position and secure with ACE. Alternatively, two parallel long leg splints can be applied medially and laterally in a bivalve configuration.

4. **Leg and ankle**
  a. **Posterior short leg (Fig. 5)**

    (1) **Indications.** Second- and third-degree ankle sprains, fractures of the distal tibia and fibula, reduced ankle dislocations, or injuries to tarsals or metatarsals (and other foot conditions).

    (2) **Equipment.** 4-in. plaster (two rolls), Webril (four 4-in. rolls), ACE (three 4-in. rolls).

    (3) **Position.** Ankle at 90 degrees (neutral); for Achilles tendon injuries, the foot is placed in equinus.

    (4) **Design.** Place the patient prone, with the knee and ankle flexed to 90 degrees. Place Webril between the toes and be sure that prominences (particularly the malleoli) are well padded. Apply a 12-layer splint that extends from just beyond the great toe (for protection), along the sole of the foot, and up the posterior calf to the level of the fibular head. Secure with ACE and mold to the desired position. Carefully mold around the malleoli and instep for a secure fit. Pinch the excess plaster at

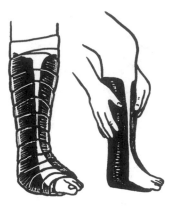

Fig. 6.   Sugar tong (leg).

the ankle and tuck it to the outside for a smooth fit. The splint should not be walked on.

b. **Sugar tong (Fig. 6)**

   (1) **Indications.** Ankle injuries (similar to posterior short leg, but stabilizes the medial and lateral ligaments more effectively).

   (2) **Equipment.** 6-in. plaster (two rolls), Webril (four 4-in. rolls), ACE (three 4-in. rolls).

   (3) **Position.** Ankle at 90 degrees (neutral).

   (4) **Design.** Place the patient prone with the knee and ankle at 90 degrees. Apply a 12-layer splint to the lateral lower leg (starting at the level of the fibular head); extend it distally under the foot (between the heel and metatarsal heads) and back up the medial lower leg to end even with the fibular head. Secure the splint with ACE, using figure-of-eight turns around the ankle. Mold to the above position, fully shaping around the malleoli. The plaster may overlap anteriorly. The splint should not be walked on.

c. **Sugar tong with posterior splint ("AO")**

   (1) **Indications.** Severe injuries to ankle or foot requiring more stabilization than a simple sugar tong (especially trimalleolar fractures); similar to a cast in degree of immobilization.

   (2) **Equipment.** 4-in. plaster (two rolls) for posterior splints, 6-in. plaster (two rolls) for sugar tong, Webril (four 4-in. rolls), ACE (three 4-in. rolls).

(3) **Position.** Ankle at 90 degrees.
(4) **Design.** This is a combination of a sugar tong and modified posterior splint. Place the patient prone with the knee and ankle flexed at 90 degrees. Place Webril between the toes. *Apply the posterior slab first.* It should be a 12-layer splint that extends from halfway up the calf to just beyond the toes. Pinch and fold to the outside any excess at the ankle flexion site. Next, apply the sugar-tong splint over the posterior splint described in the preceding section. Tuck the dorsal edges of the posterior slab *underneath* those of the sugar tong (for a smooth interior). Secure the splint with ACE and mold it into position, carefully shaping the instep and malleoli. This splint should not be walked on.

An optional improvement on this design can be created by folding the posterior splint down over the sugar-tong splint, providing a very secure foot plate. Only six layers are needed for the posterior splint, since it will be doubled over.

d. **Bivalve**
(1) **Indications.** Serious fractures and soft tissue injuries of the foot and ankle.
(2) **Equipment.** 4-in. plaster (two rolls for posterior splint, two rolls for anterior splint), Webril (four 4-in. rolls), ACE (three 4-in. rolls).
(3) **Position.** Ankle at 90 degrees.
(4) **Design.** This is simply a posterior splint with an anterior slab. Place a posterior splint as described previously, but before applying ACE wrap, place a 12-layer anterior slab parallel to the posterior splint. Wrap with ACE and mold into the desired position. This splint should not be walked on.

e. **Air stirrup**
(1) **Indications.** Minor ligamentous and soft tissue injuries of the foot and ankle not requiring complete immobilization.
(2) **Equipment.** Commercially available air stirrup (resembles a sugar tong with inflatable sides).
(3) **Position.** Ankle at 90 degrees but free to flex and extend; inversion and eversion still possible but stabilized.
(4) **Application.** The oval plate is placed under the heel, and the sides are pulled snugly up the medial and lateral calf. The

air bladders are partially inflated and the straps secured. The splint may have anterior and posterior edges that are labeled. A shoe may be worn over the splint with a sock underneath. It is a full-weight-bearing device.

   f. **Unna boot**

     (1) **Indications.** Ligamentous injuries of the ankle, especially with concurrent dermatitis or abrasions.

     (2) **Equipment.** Dome paste or Unna boot (moist rolled dressing impregnated with calamine gelatin–zinc oxide), ACE.

     (3) **Position.** Ankle flexed at 90 degrees.

     (4) **Application.** The Unna boot is rolled onto the ankle using figure-of-eight turns and extends from the metatarsal heads to the distal leg. It is then covered with ACE. Within a few days, it will dry to a leather-like substance. It can be worn under a shoe and permits full weight bearing. It is nonyielding, so perfusion must be routinely assessed.

5. **Foot: postoperative shoe**

   a. **Indications.** Fractures or soft tissue injuries of the foot; can also used with a splint to allow partial weight bearing.

   b. **Equipment.** Commercially available hard shoe or postoperative shoe.

   c. **Position.** Ankle free, sole of foot supported.

   d. **Application.** The shoe simply slips over the foot and fastens with ties or Velcro straps. A single ACE may be wrapped around the foot to prevent chafing, but some of the immobilization is lost. If the patient has a fractured toe, buddy-tape the digit before placing the shoe. The patient may bear weight on the shoe.

6. **Toes**

   a. **Dynamic splint (buddy-taping)**

     (1) **Indications.** Soft tissue injuries or fractures of the toes.

     (2) **Equipment.** 1/2-in. cloth tape, Webril (small strip).

     (3) **Position.** Injured toe is stabilized by an uninjured adjacent toe (second toe is taped to 3rd toe rather than larger, more mobile, great toe).

     (4) **Application.** Place a small piece of folded Webril between the two toes to be taped. Apply one or two pieces of tape circumferentially around the toes, being careful not to pull the tape too tightly.

   b. **Dynamic splint (buddy-taping) with postoperative shoe**

     (1) **Indications.** Fractures of the toes.

    (2) Equipment. 1/2-in. cloth tape, Webril, postoperative shoe.

    (3) Position. Injured toe stabilized by an uninjured adjacent toe, protected by a hard shoe (also described previously).

    (4) Application. Buddy-tape the fractured toe as described in the previous section. Then put the foot into a postoperative shoe (as previously described). The patient may bear weight as tolerated. If ambulation is painful, crutches may be needed.

BIBLIOGRAPHY

Advanced trauma life support. Chicago: American College of Surgeons, 1993.

Howes DS, Kaufman JJ. Plaster splints: techniques and indications. *Am Fam Physician* 1984;30:215–221.

Rittenberry TJ. *Plaster/immobilization lab.* Dallas: American College of Emergency Physicians, 1995.

Roberts JR, Hedges JR. *Clinical procedures in emergency medicine.* Philadelphia: WB Saunders, 1991.

Rockwood CA, Green DP. *Fractures in adults,* 4th ed. Philadelphia: JB Lippincott, 1995.

Simon RER, Koenigsknecht SJ. *Orthopedics in emergency medicine: the extremities,* 3rd ed. Norwalk: Appleton & Lange, 1995.

Tintinalli JE, Ruiz E, Krome RL. *Emergency medicine: a comprehensive study guide,* 4th ed. New York: McGraw-Hill, 1996.

Wu KK. *Techniques in surgical casting and splinting.* Philadelphia: Lea & Febiger, 1987.

7

Principles of Orthopaedic Surgery

Wesley P. Eilbert

With the development of modern anesthesia in the twentieth century, operative intervention for orthopaedic problems has become commonplace. Orthopaedic surgical procedures can be divided into three categories: emergent, urgent, and elective. Injuries requiring emergent intervention are those that may lead to infection, neurological damage, amputation, or possibly loss of life if surgery is delayed. These include open fractures, irreducible dislocations of major joints, spinal injuries with deteriorating neurological deficits, fracture/dislocations that impair the vascularity of the limb, and fractures with compartment syndromes. Urgent procedures are those that can be done within 24 to 72 hours after injury. These include long bone stabilization in multitrauma patients, hip fractures, and unstable fracture/dislocations. Elective operations may be done up to 4 weeks after injury. Such cases include skeletal fractures that have been reduced nonoperatively but require surgery for optimal outcomes, such as fractures of both forearm bones and intraarticular fractures that require further radiographic evaluation for adequate preoperative planning.

I. **Fractures**
   A. **Treatment.** Definitive treatment of any fracture should be delayed until the general condition of the patient has been stabilized. The goal of fracture treatment is to have the bone heal in such a position that function and cosmesis are preserved with minimal soft tissue damage. Several treatment modalities are available to optimize fracture healing.
      1. **Closed reduction with casting.** This time-honored method is typically used for simple, closed, isolated, stable fractures of the upper extremity. However, any fracture for which surgical intervention is contraindicated can be treated in this manner.
      2. **Pin or wire fixation.** These methods are usually combined with bracing or casting and are used for the fixation of small fragments in metaphyseal and epiphyseal fractures. They work particularly well in fractures of the distal foot, forearm, and hand, Colles' fractures, and displaced metacarpal and phalangeal fractures after closed reduction.
      3. **Screws.** Various types of screws exist. They are used to attach plates and prosthetic devices to bone, bone to bone, and ligaments and tendons to bone. Screws play a vital role in compressing

bone fragments to improve the mechanical stability of internal fixation.

4. **Plates.** Plates are used to neutralize deforming forces that cannot be counteracted by screws alone. They offer anatomic reduction of fractures for early resumption of motor activities, but must be protected from premature weight bearing.

5. **Medullary nails.** These are used most often in patients with displaced, closed fractures of the lower extremity with stable fracture patterns, where early rehabilitation and weight bearing are desired.

6. **External fixation.** This method allows fixation of bones when other forms of immobilization are impractical. Open fractures with associated extensive soft tissue injury requiring continuous care and fractures with multiple comminuted fragments are frequently treated in this manner.

B. **Open fractures.** By definition, an open fracture is one in which a break in the integument and underlying soft tissue leads directly into the fracture and its surrounding hematoma. Various classification systems have been proposed to describe open fractures. The most commonly used is the system proposed by Gustilo, Tscherne, and the AO group. It is often difficult to determine if a small wound in close proximity communicates with the fracture. Some authors advocate probing the wound with a sterile, blunt instrument to determine if this is the case. If any uncertainty exists, it is advisable to assume an open fracture and proceed as such. Management of open fractures should proceed without delay. Ultimately the prevention of osteomyelitis is the goal. Gross debris should be removed and then wound cultures obtained. The fracture should be splinted without reduction unless there is vascular compromise. The wound should be irrigated with saline and then covered with saline-soaked sterile gauze. Tetanus prophylaxis should be administered as appropriate. Intravenous antibiotics should be given as soon as possible. Most authorities agree that a first-generation cephalosporin with the possible addition of an aminoglycoside provides adequate antimicrobial coverage. Definitive management of open fractures involves debridement of the wound, copious irrigation, and removal of any foreign bodies. While rare minor wounds overlying open fractures may be debrided in the emergency department, the operating room is the appropriate place for treatment of most open fractures.

C. **Closed fractures.** Many closed fractures can be treated with closed reduction and immobilization.

1. **Indications for open reduction with internal fixation**
   a. When closed methods of reduction have failed.
   b. When it is known from experience that closed methods will be ineffective, as in the case of femoral neck fractures and Monteggia and Galeazzi fracture/dislocations.
   c. When articular surfaces are fractured and displaced. This is especially true for joints in the lower extremities.
   d. Displaced fractures secondary to tumor metastasis in patients not imminently terminal.
   e. When there is an associated arterial or nerve injury. While there is some controversy concerning this, many believe fixation of the fracture is necessary to protect the arterial or nerve repair.
   f. When multiple injuries are present and conservative measures, such as traction and casting, will hinder appropriate nursing and rehabilitation.
   g. Major avulsion fractures associated with disruption of important musculotendinous or ligamentous groups that are known to do poorly with nonoperative treatment.
   h. Displaced fractures with epiphyseal injuries known to have a propensity for growth arrest (Salter-Harris types III and IV).
   i. Fractures with compartment syndromes requiring fasciotomy.
   j. When the cost and time of treatment may be substantially reduced.

2. **Contraindications to surgical reduction and stabilization**
   a. Osteoporotic bone that is too fragile for stabilization by internal or external fixation.
   b. Significant damage of overlying skin caused by scarring, burns, dermatitis, or active infection, so that internal fixation would result in loss of soft tissue coverage or exacerbation of infection.
   c. Active infection or osteomyelitis.
   d. Severe fracture comminution to a degree that successful reconstruction is unlikely.
   e. Unstable medical conditions where the risks of surgery and anesthesia would outweigh possible benefits.

II. **Muscle and tendon injuries.** The common causes of partial or complete rupture of a muscle or a tendon include sudden overload of the muscle tendon unit, a sharp blow to a contracting muscle, and open lacerations of the muscle or tendon.

A. **Muscle ruptures.** While most muscle strains can be treated conservatively with rest, ice, and anti-inflammatory medication, functionally important muscles that have been disrupted or lacerated should be treated with early surgical repair. Closed muscle ruptures should be repaired surgically on an urgent basis. Open lacerations to muscle units can be treated with debridement, irrigation, and primary repair. Interrupted, nonabsorbable mattress sutures placed close together at regular intervals around the circumference of the muscle, including the muscle sheath, should be used. Immobilization of the muscle after repair is of obvious importance. Open muscle lacerations associated with other local injuries requiring emergency surgery are best repaired in the operating room

B. **Tendon ruptures.** Most partial tendon ruptures require only immobilization, with the affected extremity or digit splinted in a position to allow least tension on the tendon. Complete ruptures ultimately require some intervention for repair. Tendon repair after rupture or laceration need not be done on an emergent basis. Open tendon ruptures may be treated with cleaning, irrigation and primary closure of the wound, with delayed primary repair of the tendon 7 to 10 days later. The affected extremity or digit should be splinted in a position to allow maximal relaxation of the severed muscle-tendon unit until definitive repair occurs. Other than a few select extensor tendon injuries of the hand, most tendon repairs require operative intervention by an orthopaedist or hand surgeon. *A disproportionate number of tendon injuries occur in the hand;* their management warrants special discussion.

1. The **flexor tendons** of the hand require extensive exploration for definitive treatment, and primary repair in the emergency department should not be attempted.

2. The **extensor tendons** of the hand can be divided into five specific zones.

    a. Open **zone I** and **III** injuries may be repaired primarily in the emergency department. Popular methods of repair include the roll-type suture or the figure-of-eight. With both methods, 4-0 or 5-0 nonabsorbable suture should be used. The affected finger should be splinted in extension after the repair.

    b. **Extensor tendon lacerations in zones II, IV,** and **V** usually require extensive exploration and therefore are best repaired in the operating room.

    c. Any extensor tendon injury associated with other local injuries requiring surgical treatment should be repaired in the operating room.

III. **Ligamentous injuries.** Ligamentous injuries can occur in any joint, with the knee, ankle, and hand joints being the most commonly affected.

    A. **Classification.** Classification of ligamentous injuries varies by author and joint described, but in general the types are as follows:

        1. **First-degree sprain:** a tear of a minimum number of fibers in the ligament with localized tenderness and no instability.

        2. **Second-degree sprain:** greater disruption of ligamentous fibers with mild to moderate instability.

        3. **Third-degree sprain:** complete disruption of the ligament with resultant marked instability. It should be noted that complete rupture of isolated ligaments is rare without damage to other local structures, given the extreme joint displacement required to disrupt a ligament.

    B. **Treatment.** The goal of treatment is to restore the stability of the joint. Most first-degree sprains can be managed with rest, ice, and a compression bandage. Second-degree sprains require rest and some degree of immobilization to protect the injured ligament. Third-degree sprains often require primary repair of the ligament or surgical fixation of the ligament to bone to regain joint stability. This is done ideally within 1 week of the injury.

IV. **Dislocations.** A joint is said to be dislocated when its articular surfaces are completely out of contact with one another. While any joint may dislocate, those most commonly dislocated include the knee, hip, elbow, shoulder, acromioclavicular, and finger joints. Acute dislocations should be reduced as soon as possible.

The urgency to reduce dislocated joints stems from two main considerations. One is that the longer the joint remains dislocated, the more difficult it usually is to reduce. The second is that any neurovascular deficit involved with a dislocation may go from temporary to permanent if treatment is delayed. With delays in treatment, a hip dislocation carries the added risk of the increasing incidence of avascular necrosis of the femoral head. All patients with traumatically dislocated joints should be advised of the risk of posttraumatic arthritis. Most dislocations can be reduced by closed methods with intravenous analgesia and sedation. Those that cannot be reduced in the emergency department may require anesthesia in the operating room before closed reduction can be achieved. Open reduction of acute dislocations is usually indicated in the following circumstances:

    A. Open dislocations, which require extensive irrigation to reduce the risk of joint infection.

B. When proper reduction cannot be achieved by closed techniques. This often occurs because of interposed soft tissues or osteochondral fragments.

C. When a stable reduction cannot be maintained. Fractures of the articular surfaces are often unstable and require open reduction and fixation to ensure the stability of the reduction.

D. When exam before closed reduction reveals no neurological deficit and after reduction a complete motor and sensory nerve deficit.

E. When a circulatory deficit distal to the dislocation is found and persists after closed reduction. Further assessment of the vasculature should include arteriography, and vascular repair, if indicated, should proceed on an emergent basis.

V. Joint infections. Septic arthritis is an orthopaedic emergency requiring prompt treatment to avoid permanent joint damage.

A. Diagnosis. Diagnosis is made by joint aspiration and treatment involves intravenous antibiotics, with repeated joint aspirations and irrigation as needed.

B. Treatment. Indications for arthrotomy and surgical drainage are controversial. Most agree that any joint infection that does not improve with appropriate therapy, usually within 48 hours, should be treated with open drainage. Likewise, most authors advocate prompt surgical drainage for any deeply situated joint, such as the hip or shoulder. Infection in a prosthetic joint can present either in the immediate postoperative period, with an intraoperative contaminant being the most likely source, or later as septic arthritis, usually caused by hematogenous spread of bacteria. In either situation, prompt open irrigation and debridement is indicated. Any malfunctioning prosthetic devices should be removed and intravenous antibiotics begun. With this aggressive treatment, up to 50% of prosthetic joints may be saved. However, continuing evidence of joint infection after treatment warrants prosthetic removal.

VI. Amputations. With the development of modern microvascular surgical techniques in the 1960s, **replantation** of digits and limbs after traumatic amputation has become commonplace. Fingers and the thumb are most effectively replanted. Replantation of a lower extremity is rarely indicated owing to the high frequency of crush injuries in these severed limbs and the benefit of a prosthesis as compared with the long rehabilitation period associated with replantation. Any severed part that may be replanted should have gross debris removed and then gently cleaned with normal saline irrigation. It should be wrapped in sterile gauze moistened with saline and placed in a plastic bag. The bag should then be placed on ice. When replantation is being considered, several factors must be taken into account.

A. Ischemia time. Most digits can be successfully replanted after 8 hours of warm ischemia and up to 24 hours if cooled. Amputations containing significant amounts of muscle, such as those of the forearm, are less tolerant of ischemia; such limbs must be replanted within 6 to 8 hours.

B. Patient characteristics. Hand dominance, occupation, and likely compliance with rehabilitation must be considered. The elderly, patients with chronic illnesses—such as peripheral vascular disease and diabetes mellitus, and patients with other life-threatening injuries are poor candidates for replantation. Most replantations in children do well.

C. Characteristics of the amputation
1. **Characteristics favoring replantation**
   a. All thumb amputations
   b. Multiple digit amputations
   c. Wrist and forearm amputations
   d. Single-digit amputations in which the amputation occurs distal to the insertion of the flexor digitorum superficialis
   e. Sharp amputations with minimal to moderate avulsion proximal to the elbow
2. **Characteristics unfavorable to replantation**
   a. Multiple-level amputations
   b. Single-digit amputations proximal to the flexor digitorum superficialis insertion
   c. Severe crush injuries

VII. Injuries of the spine. The goals of treatment of spinal injury are to (a) realign the spine, (b) prevent progression of neurologic damage, (c) improve neurologic recovery, (d) assure spinal stability, and (e) maximize functional recovery.

Spinal instability is defined as the loss of the spine's ability under physiologic loads to maintain relationships between vertebrae in such a way that the cord and nerve roots are not damaged or irritated and deformity or pain does not develop. Several surgical implants are available for use in establishing spinal stability, including wires, mesh, screws, clamps, plates, and rods. In addition, spinal fusion, often using bone-grafting techniques, can be used.

A. Cervical spine. Many stable cervical spine injuries can be treated nonsurgically with rigid cervical immobilization, usually with a halo vest device. Malalignment of the cervical spine can be treated initially with skeletal traction with the use of tongs in the skull. Failure to achieve realignment with traction is an indication for open reduction and stabilization. Patients with injuries that jeopardize the stability of the spine or compress the neural elements require surgical intervention, although the timing of this intervention is controversial. Most authors agree that any progression of neurologic signs or radiographic evidence of spinal cord compression despite optimal alignment warrants urgent surgical intervention. Open fractures and penetrating injuries also require immediate irrigation and debridement in the operating room.

B. **Thoracic and lumbar spine.** Treatment of unstable fractures and fracture/dislocations in the thoracolumbar spine is controversial, with some advocating nonoperative treatment and others emphasizing the advantages of open reduction and internal fixation. Most authors agree, however, that emergent surgical intervention is indicated for gunshot wounds and if a progressive neurological deficit exists.

VIII. **Soft tissue injuries associated with orthopaedic trauma**

A. **Peripheral nerve injuries** are classically described as one of three types.

1. **Neurapraxia:** a mild injury producing nerve dysfunction without gross anatomic disruption. Full functional recovery usually occurs with time.

2. **Axonotmesis:** more extensive damage to the nerve with interruption of axons and myelin sheaths but preservation of the endoneural tube. Total loss of neurological function occurs, but spontaneous recovery is possible.

3. **Neurotmesis:** complete severance of the nerve or damage to the point where spontaneous regeneration is impossible. Surgical repair is indicated in these situations. While several microsurgical techniques may be used to repair peripheral nerves, only the indications for and timing of surgery are discussed here.

a. **Indications for surgical exploration of a peripheral nerve deficit:**

(1) When a sharp injury has obviously severed a nerve. Repair of the nerve can be done at the time of exploration or at a later date. Repair may be delayed in grossly contaminated wounds.

(2) When avulsion or blast injuries have rendered the condition of the nerve unknown. Exploration is required to identify the extent of the nerve injury. Severed nerve ends can be identified and tagged to aid in future repair.

(3) When there is a nerve deficit after a closed fracture, dislocation, or blunt injury and no clinical or electrical evidence of regeneration has appeared after an appropriate lapse of time.

(4) When a nerve deficit was not present before closed reduction or casting of a fracture and is apparent afterward.

(5) When a nerve deficit follows penetrating trauma, such as a low-velocity gunshot wound, and evidence of regeneration does not appear after an appropriate lapse of time.

b. The optimal *timing* of nerve repair remains controversial. Most authors agree that early repair is preferable in clean wounds with adequate soft tissue coverage. Repairs done more than 2 weeks after injury have diminishing rates of success because of muscle atrophy and fibrosis in the nerve stumps.

B. **Arterial injury with fractures and dislocations** as well as *penetrating trauma* must always be considered.

1. **Hard signs of vascular injury** include massive external bleeding, a rapidly expanding hematoma, a palpable thrill or bruit over a hematoma, and the other classic signs of arterial occlusion: pulselessness, pallor, paresthesia, pain, paralysis, and poikilothermia. In these patients, immediate surgical exploration and vascular repair are indicated if significant external bleeding, impending limb loss, or the need for emergent surgery for another injury is present. Other, more stable patients may undergo angiography prior to surgery to help define the specific location of the vascular injury **Patients with pulse deficits distal to fractures and dislocations** should undergo immediate reduction. .

2. **Soft signs of vascular injury** include a questionable history of arterial bleeding; proximity of a penetrating wound to an artery; a small, nonpulsatile hematoma; or a neurological deficit. These patients can be managed with arteriography or observation alone.

3. **Complete occlusion of one of the major arteries distal to the elbow or knee** may be observed with reliance on Collateral flow as an alternative to arterial repair. Relative indications for arterial repair in these situations include inadequate collateral flow, previous injury to the collateral artery, and associated major nerve injury (e.g., median or ulnar nerve).

C. **Compartment syndromes**

1. **Diagnosis and assessment.** A compartment syndrome is a condition characterized by increased pressure within a closed fascial space that causes decreased perfusion of the enclosed tissues or tissues distal to the area with poten-

tially irreversible damage. Compartment syndromes most commonly occur in the forearm and lower leg but can also occur in the hand, foot, upper arm, shoulder, thigh, and buttocks.

a. **The most common causes** of compartment syndromes are as follows:

   (1) **Fractures.** Tibial fractures are the most common cause.

   (2) **Soft tissue injuries** such as contusions.

   (3) **Arterial injury** or **thrombosis** causing postischemic swelling.

   (4) **Prolonged limb compression.** This is often seen in patients with altered mental status.

   (5) **Burns**

   (6) Other causes such as **venous obstruction** or **excessive exercise. External compression** caused by ill-fitting casts or bandages can increase already elevated compartmental pressures in any of the above conditions.

b. The **clinical features** of compartment syndrome can be remembered using the mnemonic of the six P's.

   (1) **Pain** greater than would be expected for the primary injury is the most important symptom of an impending compartment syndrome. Unfortunately, this may not be evident in those patients with altered mental status or a coexisting sensorineural deficit.

   (2) **Pain with stretch** of the involved muscle groups is usually present, but this can be a nonspecific finding.

   (3) **Paresis** or weakness of involved muscles may be present, but this may be due to unrelated nerve damage or guarding secondary to pain.

   (4) **Paresthesias** in the distribution of the nerve in the involved compartment. This eventually progresses to complete anesthesia if the pressure is not relieved.

   (5) **Pulses intact.** Unlike arterial injuries, which can present with similar symptoms, distal pulses as well as capillary refill and extremity color are typically preserved with compartment syndromes.

   (6) **Pressure.** This is the only reliable objective finding with compartment syndromes. Several catheters and monitoring systems are available to measure compartmental pressures. In-

dications for measurement of intra-compartment pressures include confirmation of a clinically suspected compartment syndrome, observation in unreliable patients such as children and patients with an altered mental status, and nerve deficits attributable to another cause.

2. **Treatment.** The only effective way to treat an acute compartment syndrome is with surgical fasciotomy to relieve the pressure. The intracompartmental pressure threshold for fasciotomy is controversial. Some authors recommend that fasciotomy be performed when the intracompartmental pressure has risen to within 20 to 40 mm Hg of the diastolic pressure. Others believe that any intracompartmental pressure greater than 30 mm Hg with positive clinical findings warrants treatment.

BIBLIOGRAPHY

Browner BD, Jupiter JB, Levine AM, Trafton PG, eds. *Skeletal trauma.* Philadelphia: WB Saunders, 1992.

Chapman MW, Madison M, eds. *Operative orthopedics,* 2nd ed. Philadelphia: JB Lippincott, 1993.

Connolly JF, ed. *Fractures and dislocations: closed management.* Philadelphia: WB Saunders, 1995.

Crenshaw AH, ed. *Campbell's operative orthopedics,* 8th ed. St Louis: Mosby–Year Book, 1992.

Schlenker JD, Koulis CP. Amputations and replantations. *Emerg Med Clin North Am* 3:11, 1993.

Long-Term Care and Rehabilitation of Orthopaedic Injuries

Wesley P. Eilbert

I. Treatment modalities

A. Casts. Placement of a full-circumference cast prevents any observation or examination of the underlying tissues. Because of this, several complications may arise.

1. The tight cast. This is typically caused by swelling under the cast. Pain is the first and most reliable symptom and there should be no hesitation to bivalve a cast when a patient presents with this complaint. The cast should be cut longitudinally on opposite sides and half removed. The underlying cast padding may be cut if symptoms persist after the bivalving. In some cases, complete removal of the cast and padding is needed. If relief is obtained by bivalving the cast, it can be replaced and held in position with an elastic bandage. However, a bivalved cast should not be used as a permanent immobilizing device, and a new cast should be applied in 1 to 3 days.

2. Cast sores. Any indentations in the cast or lack of adequate padding may lead to cast sores. Patients typically present with a localized burning pain or discomfort. Prompt removal of the cast with inspection of the involved area is indicated.

3. Cast cuts. These occur at the ends of the casts, especially at the fold of the buttock. The cast causes excoriations due to the continual rubbing of its unflared end. Treatment entails bending the border of the cast away from the skin with pliers.

4. Itching under the cast. This frequently occurs and can usually be controlled with oral antipruritic agents or by blowing hot air under the cast with a blow dryer. The patient should be instructed not to attempt to relieve the itching by pushing a coat hanger or similar device under the cast.

B. External fixation devices. A main goal of outpatient care with these devices is to prevent pin-track infections. Daily care of the pin sites should include cleaning with a mild soap and saline or possibly tap water. Exposed portions of the pins should be wrapped with bulky gauze. Excessive drainage from pin sites, alone or with mild cellulitis, can be treated with an oral first-generation cephalosporin and aggressive pin-site hygiene. Any cellulitis larger than only mild erythema around the pin should be treated with parenteral antibiotics. Any loose pins should be removed. Clinical loosening of pins with radiographic evidence of osteomyelitis should be treated with pin removal and 10 to 14 days of parenteral antibiotics.

C. **Ambulatory aids**
  1. **Crutches.** Crutches offer an inexpensive and readily available aid for those lower extremity injuries that require no or partial weight bearing. The crutches should be adjusted so that a hand breadth of space exists between the crutch pad and axilla. Pressure on the axilla can cause a "crutch palsy" of the brachial plexus. The handpiece should be adjusted to allow the elbow to be partially flexed while bearing weight. Discharge with a single crutch should be discouraged. It should be realized that crutch walking is an exercise that requires a significant amount of upper extremity strength and coordination as well as cardiovascular conditioning. Many elderly or debilitated patients will be better served by a walker if partial weight bearing is the goal.
  2. **Walkers.** Walkers provide an excellent ambulatory aid for those patients requiring partial weight bearing on a lower extremity (e.g., after fixation of a hip fracture). Walkers should not be used for non-weight-bearing ambulation.
  3. **Canes.** Canes can be used for partial weight bearing but are less efficient than walkers or crutches for this purpose.

D. **Applications of cold and heat**
  1. **Cryotherapy.** Use of ice or cold packs is a time-honored treatment for musculoskeletal injuries. Cold decreases pain by impairing neuronal function and decreases inflammation by various mechanisms. The recommended application of cold is for 10 to 20 minutes at 2-hour intervals. The maximum benefits of cryotherapy are obtained if it is used within the first 72 hours after injury.
  2. **Heat.** Forms of heat can be divided into superficial (hot packs, heating pads, and whirlpool baths) and deep (ultrasound, short wave, and microwave). Heat is used in various musculoskeletal conditions for analgesia and muscle relaxation and to facilitate the reduction in chronic inflammation. Heat also increases blood flow as well as soft tissue extensibility. Heat should be used later (after the first 24 to 36

hours) in the treatment course of a musculoskeletal injury.

E. **Electrical stimulation**
   1. **Wound healing.** Several different methods of
      electrical stimulation have been used to en-
      hance healing in musculoskeletal injuries. Heal-
      ing of lower extremity fractures in particular
      has been proven to be enhanced by electrical
      stimulation.
   2. **Transcutaneous electrical nerve stimula-
      tion (TENS).** This form of electroanalgesia has
      become popular in the past 25 years. TENS
      can be defined as the application of low-voltage
      electrical pulses to the nervous system by pass-
      ing electricity through the skin. TENS is fre-
      quently used to control acute and chronic pain
      caused by musculoskeletal injuries and other
      painful conditions.

F. **Therapeutic exercise and massage**
   1. **Exercise** is essential in the rehabilitative pro-
      cess following musculoskeletal injuries. Proper
      exercise strengthens injured bone and soft tis-
      sues, increases mobility, and prevents the detri-
      mental effects of prolonged immobilization.
      Specific exercises used in the rehabilitation of
      specific injuries are discussed later in this
      chapter. Exercising in water can be extremely
      useful. The buoyancy effects of water can sup-
      port ambulation after lower extremity injuries
      and assist initial strength training in weakened
      muscle groups.
   2. **Massage** is an age-old technique used for
      its mechanical, neurological, and psychological
      benefits. Some authors advocate the use of mas-
      sage in conjunction with exercise for the re-
      habilitation of musculoskeletal injury. The
      exact benefits of massage, however, remain
      controversial.

G. Pharmacological agents. Patients treated and released from the emergency department with musculoskeletal injuries frequently require treatment
   with analgesic agents. While many can obtain adequate pain relief with RICE (rest, ice, compression,
   and elevation) therapy, pharmacological agents are
   frequently indicated. Most soft tissue injuries can
   be managed with nonsteroidal anti-inflammatory
   drugs (NSAIDs). These medications have the added
   benefit of decreasing inflammation associated with
   injury. Their side-effect profile (gastric irritation, renal impairment), however, can limit their use.
   Narcotic analgesics [acetaminophen/codeine, (Tylenol
   #3), hydrocodone/acetaminophen (Vicodin), and
   others] can be used to treat more painful conditions,
   such as fractures. There is theoretical concern that

patients may overmedicate themselves with these agents and mask the early symptoms of a compartment syndrome. However, most pain research indicates that physicians routinely undertreat pain. Caution should be used when prescribing these agents, as prolonged use can be habit-forming.

II. **Reflex sympathetic dystrophy (RSD).** RSD is a syndrome of chronic pain, neurovascular disturbance, and dystrophic changes of the skin and bones that frequently follows orthopaedic injuries of the upper extremity. Other names for this entity include *major causalgia, posttraumatic painful osteoporosis, Sudeck's atrophy, posttraumatic dystrophy,* and *shoulder-hand syndrome.* The exact pathogenesis of this condition is unknown; however, it results in a dysfunction of the sympathetic nervous system in the involved extremity.

A. **Clinical features.** RSD is frequently misdiagnosed in its early stages as symptoms of disuse caused by immobilization. The disease process typically progresses through three stages.

1. **Stage I** lasts a few weeks to 6 months and is characterized by pain in the extremity that is out of proportion to the severity of the injury. Increased blood flow results in redness, warmth, and pitting edema. Decreased range of motion begins as a result of pain avoidance.

2. **Stage II** can develop as soon as 3 months after the onset of symptoms and typically lasts another 3 to 6 months. At this stage, the affected extremity often becomes cold, with glossy skin, and hair and nail growth may be diminished. Pain and decreased range of motion are prominent features, and atrophy of muscle and subcutaneous tissue develops. X-ray examination shows osteoporotic changes.

3. **Stage III** begins approximately 1 year after the onset of symptoms and can last up to several years. This stage is marked by progressive and irreversible atrophic changes of muscle and soft tissue with marked loss of range of motion and extensive osteoporosis.

B. **Treatment.** Initiation of treatment prior to the onset of the trophic changes seen in stages II and III is of paramount importance to obtain functional recovery. Blocking of the associated sympathetic ganglion with a local anesthetic is both diagnostic and therapeutic and may be repeated multiple times. Several other pharmacological interventions have been advocated, including corticosteroids, NSAIDs, anticonvulsants, tricyclic antidepressants, beta blockers, and calcium channel blockers. A surgical sympathectomy may provide relief in recalcitrant cases when local anesthetic blockades have been effective but temporary. The cornerstone of the treatment of RSD is the establishment of a progressive exercise program for the affected limb. The treatments mentioned above serve only to allow for the initiation of such a program.

III. **Fractures**

A. To better understand long-term fracture treatment, comprehension of the stages of healing is necessary.

1. **Inflammation.** This begins at the time of injury and lasts 3 to 4 days. Clinically, this stage ends when pain and swelling begin to subside. During this stage, fracture hematoma formation occurs and inflammatory cells predominate at the fracture site.

2. **Soft callus.** This begins immediately after the inflammation stage and lasts approximately 1 month. This stage is marked by clinical union of the fracture by fibrous and cartilaginous tissue. Clinically, this stage ends when the fracture is no longer grossly mobile.

3. **Hard callus.** This begins 3 to 4 weeks after the fracture and lasts 2 to 3 months. During this stage, the fibrocartilaginous union initially formed is replaced by a fibroosseus union. At the end of this stage, the fracture is clinically and radiographically healed.

4. **Remodeling.** During this stage, the newly formed fibrous bone is reshaped and reorganized so that it more closely resembles the original bone. This process takes months to years to complete. Children have a much greater capacity to remodel bone than adults. For this reason, angular deformities after initial reduction are not as much of a concern in children.

B. **Long-term management.** All fractures require observation throughout the healing period to ensure proper union. Repeat radiographic evaluations are done early in the treatment course to assure maintenance of proper reduction. Repeat exams can be performed less frequently later, as the union becomes more stable over time. Casts should remain in place until clinical union has occurred. This varies with the type of fracture, the age of the patient, and the specific bone involved. It should be noted that radiographic evidence of union often lags behind true clinical union. If the fracture has no motion and is not tender to palpation or stress, enough healing has probably occurred to leave the cast off. If any question exists, a removable splint may be used for 2 to 3 weeks while some limited activity is allowed. External fixation devices, like casts, should remain in place until clinical union has occurred. The amount of time an internal fixator should remain is a matter of controversy. While some advocate removal of the implant after adequate fracture healing has occurred, many believe that removing the implant significantly increases the chance of refracture. These clinicians believe that the implant may be left in place indefinitely unless it begins to cause complications such as pain or fibrosis.

1. **Delayed union** occurs when an adequate amount of time has passed since initial fracture and neither clinical nor radiographic evidence of osseous union has appeared, as would be expected for that particular fracture. It should be noted that individual patient characteristics (age, systemic illness, nutritional status, etc.) lead to varied healing rates in different patients. Several factors may be responsible for delayed union, including inadequate reduction, extensive soft tissue disruption associated with the fracture, inadequate immobilization, excessive distraction of the fracture ends, inadequate internal fixation, and overly aggressive debridement of comminuted fractures, leading to a large osseous defect. A change in the management of the fracture is indicated in these circumstances in order to stimulate healing and prevent nonunion.

2. **Nonunion** is said to have occurred when all healing processes have ceased yet bone continuity has not been restored. The diagnosis is based on clinical and radiographic findings. Infection and poor vascular supply as well as any of the disruptive factors listed above may lead to nonunion. Fractures with a tendency for nonunion include comminuted, open fractures of the tibia, comminuted fractures of the distal femur, fractures of the femoral neck, and fractures of the scaphoid. Pseudoarthrosis is a relatively rare form of nonunion described in fractures of the clavicle, humerus, and tibia. Dense scar tissue forms at the nonunion site, with formation of a false joint. Management of fracture nonunion involves aggressive treatment of any associated infection and frequently surgical intervention, such as internal fixation or bone grafting.

3. **Malunion** describes the healing of a fracture in an unsatisfactory position. Surgical correction of malunion deformities is indicated if they cause unacceptable cosmetic or functional deformity. Three main types of malunion occur.

   a. **Angulation.** A significant amount of angulation will correct itself during the remodeling stage of fracture healing. A greater degree of fracture angulation is permissible near epiphyseal centers in children because of the extensive amount of corrective remodeling and growth at the epiphyseal line after the fracture. Angulation is less acceptable in the proximal portion of an extremity or digit, given the effect of projection of the angulation. For example, 2 to 3 degrees of angulation is of minimal cosmetic importance in a distal phalangeal fracture. However, the same degree of angulation in a proximal phalangeal fracture causes significant deformity, given the projection of the angulation over the length of the digit.

b. **Rotation.** Rotational deformities are frequently not recognized until the fracture has healed. This is especially true for fractures involving digits.

c. **Shortening.** Loss of length has much greater functional significance in a weight-bearing bone of the lower extremity than in the upper extremity. Shortening of the tibia in an adult by as little as 1 cm will result in the need for a shoe lift to maintain proper gait. Loss of length in the upper extremity is primarily of cosmetic concern. Some shortening of weight-bearing bones is acceptable if the bone can be expected to make up for this discrepancy as healing occurs. This is true in children, who will compensate with overgrowth at the epiphyseal center of the involved bone.

4. **Ischemic necrosis** occurs when the vascular supply to the bone is permanently disrupted, leading to resorption of the dead bone. The bone eventually collapses. This long-term complication usually occurs in bones with a limited vascular supply. Fractures at risk for ischemic necrosis include those of the femoral neck, the neck of the talus, and the scaphoid.

C. **Rehabilitation.** Many of the rehabilitative problems encountered after a fracture are secondary to the immobilization imposed to treat the fracture. The main goals of rehabilitation in the fracture patient are (a) to enhance fracture healing through activity, (b) to preserve muscle strength and endurance, (c) to maintain or restore range of motion of joints, and (d) to return the patient to his or her prior level of functioning. It must be emphasized that the rehabilitative process should begin as soon as feasible, which is often immediately after injury. While the extensive literature on fracture rehabilitation cannot be reviewed here, some key points should be emphasized.

1. **Muscle strength and endurance.** To increase strength, a muscle should be exercised against increasing resistance. For improved endurance, the number of contractions against a relatively constant resistance should be increased. **Isometric exercises** are those in

which the muscle contracts without producing any motion in the joint. These exercises are useful when the involved joint is immobilized or when movement would be detrimental, as with incompletely healed fractures. **Isotonic exercises** involve contraction of the muscle against a constant resistance with resultant movement at the joint.

2. **Maintenance of joint motion.** Range-of-motion exercises should be performed on all non-immobilized joints to prevent contracture. Passive exercise can be used when the muscles are paralyzed or too weak for active exercise or when the patient cannot cooperate with an exercise regimen. In severe cases, manipulation under anesthesia may be done when intraarticular adhesions or other soft tissue limitations prevent any other means of exercise. Referral to physical therapy is indicated in any fracture requiring more than simple strength and range-of-motion exercises (e.g., lower extremity fractures requiring gait training). Referral to an occupational therapist is indicated in fracture patients who require assistance or special training to return to their routine daily activities. Consultation with a physiatrist should be obtained for those patients requiring extensive rehabilitation (e.g., spinal injury with paralysis).

IV. **Dislocations**
  A. **Healing.** Varying lengths of time are required for healing of the joint capsule and other soft tissues after joint dislocation. Healing of specific ligaments and fractures associated with dislocations varies depending on which specific structure is involved.
  B. **Long-term management of common dislocations**
    1. **Acromioclavicular.** Most can be treated with simple shoulder support and early active range-of-motion exercises. Most patients will be able to return to full activities by 2 weeks. If surgical repair is performed, immobilization with a sling and swath for 4 weeks is indicated, with initiation of exercise thereafter.
    2. **Shoulder.** Patients below 40 years of age should have the arm immobilized in a sling for 4 to 6 weeks; in older patients, immobilization should last only until the pain subsides (typically 7 to 10 days). Exercises to strengthen the rotator cuff and scapular musculature should begin immediately after the end of immobilization.
    3. **Elbow.** The elbow can be immobilized in a posterior splint, and active exercise can usually begin by 3 to 5 days, as the swelling subsides. The

splint should remain in place between exercise sessions until 10 to 14 days, when it can be discarded. Unstable dislocations require longer immobilization to allow for ligamentous healing.

4. **Lunate and perilunate.** Lunate dislocations require immobilization for 8 to 12 weeks, with casts changed every 2 to 3 weeks as swelling subsides. If stabilization with wires is used, the wires should be removed at 4 to 6 weeks. Active exercise of the joint may begin immediately after the end of immobilization. Perilunate dislocations are immobilized by a cast and/or percutaneous pins for 3 to 4 weeks, after which active exercise can begin.

5. **Metacarpophalangeal (MCP) and interphalangeal (IP) joints**
   a. **Finger.** With simple MCP and IP dislocations, the reduced joint can be buddy-taped to the adjacent digit, allowing for active flexion and extension for 3 to 5 days.
   b. **Thumb.** Reduced MCP and IP dislocations can be immobilized in a thumb spica cast for 5 to 7 days, followed by active exercise.

6. **Hip.** Uncomplicated hip dislocations can be immobilized with traction for 5 to 10 days. Range-of-motion exercises (excluding hip flexion) may begin in 2 to 3 days. Gradual weight bearing with crutches can usually begin in 5 to 7 days.

7. **Knee.** After reduction, close observation for neurovascular complications is critical. Ice, elevation, and application of a compressive dressing from thigh to midcalf for the first 3 to 5 days followed by 4 weeks of immobilization with a cast or knee immobilizer are indicated. Since these dislocations are almost always associated with ligamentous injury, surgical repair will often be necessary.

8. **Patella.** After closed reduction of simple patellar dislocations, immobilization with a long leg cast or knee immobilizer for 4 weeks is indicated. While immobilized, the patient should be encouraged to flex the quadriceps repeatedly (quadriceps sitting exercises). The cast or immobilizer can be removed at 4 weeks and active range-of-motion exercises begun.

9. **Ankle.** A large amount of swelling can be expected after reduction of a dislocated ankle; close observation for signs of compartment syndrome of the foot is needed. Bed rest with limb elevation for the first 3 to 5 days can help decrease swelling. Initial immobilization with a bivalved cast to allow extra space is a good idea, with a permanent cast being placed after the swelling subsides. Stable ankles postreduction

require 2 to 3 weeks of immobilization, while those that are unstable should be immobilized for 4 to 6 weeks to allow for ligamentous healing.

C. **Complications**
1. **Ischemic necrosis.** The femoral head, lunate, scaphoid, talus, and humeral head are all at risk for this complication after dislocation. With its vascular supply interrupted, the bone becomes more osteoporotic over time and may collapse on itself. While bone-grafting techniques may be used to promote new bone growth, this condition is notoriously difficult to treat.
2. **Arthritis.** Any joint may develop arthritis after dislocation. However, this complication is especially troublesome after hip dislocations.

V. **Muscle and tendon injuries**
A. **Muscle strains and lacerations.** Most strains can be managed with rest, ice, and anti-inflammatory medication. Gentle stretching and strengthening exercises can begin after pain and swelling have resolved. Muscle lacerations should be immobilized in a position that minimizes muscle stretch for a sufficient period of time to allow adequate healing (usually 4 weeks) before progressive strengthening exercises are begun.
B. **Tendons.** Tendon lacerations should be immobilized in a position of tendon relaxation for long enough to allow sufficient healing (usually 4 to 6 weeks for large tendons). Progressive range-of-motion exercises may then begin. Flexor tendons of the hand are notorious for forming adhesions at the repair site postoperatively. For this reason, many authors advocate early passive range-of-motion exercises as soon as 1 day after surgical repair. For those patients who have limited range of motion due to adhesions despite adequate therapy, tenolysis may be performed after the initial repair has healed.

VI. **Ligamentous injuries.** Most first-degree sprains require only symptomatic treatment with rest, ice, and anti-inflammatory medications. These patients can usually resume their normal activities within a few days. Second-degree sprains require support, with either a cast or a restrictive motion device for 4 to 6 weeks. Gradual resumption of usual activities may then begin. In most active patients, a third-degree sprain requires surgical repair. After repair, immobilization for 4 to 6 weeks is usually needed. Gradual resumption of activity of the involved joint may then proceed. Referral to a physical therapist is frequently helpful, especially with athletes. Patients should be advised that maximum strength of the repaired ligament will not be attained for 12 months; therefore vigorous activity should not resume for many months after repair.

VII. **Replantations.** The primary concern in the immediate postoperative period is maintenance of adequate perfusion in the replanted part. A bulky, nonconstricting dressing should be kept in place with digits exposed to allow for close observation. Continuous monitoring of skin temperature in the replanted part can be used to help assess perfusion. Measures to maximize perfusion include increasing the ambient temperature of the patient's room, cessation of smoking by the patient and all visitors, and peripheral nerve blockades as well as adequate analgesia to prevent vasoconstriction. Anticoagulants are typically used in the postoperative period to help maintain vessel patency. Low-molecular-weight dextran, aspirin, dipyridamole, and sodium warfarin have all been used for this purpose. Heparin has been advocated by some authors for use in replantations at high risk for thrombosis, as after a crush or avulsion injury, or replantations in small children. Replanted limbs and digits should be positioned at the level of the heart. If the replanted part begins to show evidence of hypoperfusion, it can be lowered and, conversely, if signs of venous congestion develop, the part can be elevated. Reoperation for evaluation of all anastomosed vessels is indicated if conservative measures to enhance circulation have failed.

Other complications that may arise in the postoperative period include excessive bleeding due to anticoagulation, skin necrosis caused by nonviable tissue around the amputation site, wound infection, and—in major limb replantations—compartment syndromes. Long-term complications such as nonunion or malunion, tendon adhesions, cold intolerance, joint stiffness, and delay in return of nerve function may present later in the treatment course. The patient is typically kept at bed rest for 3 to 7 days following replantation and usually no movement of the replanted part is attempted for 3 weeks. The patient may then begin a graduated program of stretching and range-of-motion exercises. Most replanted parts now have a greater than 80% chance of long-term viability.

VIII. **Injuries of the spine**
    A. **Cervical spine**
        1. **Stable injuries** are frequently immobilized in a halo vest or other orthotic device such as a SOMI brace. The halo vest is probably the most secure method of immobilization. Serial radiological exams are obtained weekly at first and then with less frequency throughout the treatment course. Most stable injuries of the cervical spine will require 8 to 12 weeks of immobilization.

        The **halo vest** is a commonly used immobilization device that unfortunately has a complication rate as high as 30%. Pin-site pain, infection, and pin loosening as well as vest-induced pressure sores account for the majority of complications. Pins should be routinely retightened 24 to 48 hours after placement. Retightening should be attempted only once and should not progress if no resistance is met during the procedure. Pin sites should be cleaned daily with povidone-iodine or hydrogen peroxide. Pin-site infections should be treated with empiric antibiotics after appropriate wound cultures have been obtained.

2. **Unstable injuries** and other injuries requiring operative intervention can be immobilized postoperatively in a rigid orthotic device for 8 to 12 weeks. Lateral flexion and extension views of the cervical spine should be obtained prior to the removal of the orthotic device to assess fusion and stability.

3. Rehabilitation of patients with cervical cord injuries is a complex issue that requires a multidisciplinary team approach. The common complications that arise in the immediate postinjury period include fluid overload with pulmonary edema during spinal shock, respiratory failure, urinary retention, gastric distention and bleeding, and pressure sores. Ideally, these patients should be cared for in centers equipped to handle their complex needs.

B. **Thoracic and lumbar spine.** Stable fractures can be treated with bed rest until severe pain has resolved (usually 3 to 5 days). Most authors agree that prolonged bed rest or immobilization in an orthotic device will only worsen the patient's condition. Extension exercises to strengthen the paraspinous muscles should be initiated as soon as pain subsides. Operative repair of thoracolumbar injuries may involve the placement of Harrington rods or other hardware and fusion of vertebrae. Bed rest is indicated in the immediate postoperative period, with ambulation being encouraged within the first few days after surgery. The patient may wear a supportive brace until muscle strength improves. Extension exercises should begin as soon as pain subsides. If implanted hardware requires removal, this is usually done 6 to 9 weeks postoperatively.

BIBLIOGRAPHY

Browner BD, Jupiter JB, Levine AM, Trafton PG, eds. *Skeletal trauma.* Philadelphia: WB Saunders, 1992.

Chapman MW, Madison M, eds. *Operative orthopaedics,* 2nd ed. Philadelphia: JB Lippincott, 1993.

Connolly JF, ed. *Fractures and dislocations: closed management.* Philadelphia: WB Saunders, 1995.

Crenshaw AH, ed. *Campbell's operative orthopaedics, 8th ed.* St. Louis: Mosby–Year Book, 1992.

Nickel VL, Bottle MJ, eds. *Orthopaedic rehabilitation,* 2nd ed. New York: Churchill Livingstone, 1992.

II

Upper Extremity Orthopaedics

9

Injuries of the Sternum, Clavicle, and Scapula

Robert W. Wolford

I. **Sternum**
   A. **Anatomy.** The arm is attached to the bony skeleton via the shoulder girdle (scapula, clavicle, and associated joints and ligaments) and its articulation with the sternum. The sternum forms the central portion of the anterior chest and may be injured by blunt trauma. It consists of three main components: **manubrium, body,** and **xiphoid process.** The manubrium articulates with the first rib and clavicle superiorly and with the body of the sternum inferiorly. The costal cartilage of the second rib articulates with the manubrium and body of the sternum at the sternal angle. The sternal angle is easily palpable, lies at the level of the intervertebral disk between the fourth and fifth thoracic vertebrae, and provides a reliable starting point for counting ribs. The costal cartilages of the remaining ribs articulate along the lateral borders of the sternal body. The xiphoid process articulates superiorly with the sternal body and is attached to the linea alba inferiorly. Multiple muscles attach to the sternum, including the pectoralis major, medial head of the sternocleidomastoid, sternohyoid, sternothyroid, transverse thoracic, diaphragm, and rectus abdominis.
   B. **Mechanism of injury.** Fractures of the sternum are most commonly due to blunt trauma, with 70% to 90% due to motor vehicle crashes, 3% to 25% to falls, and the remainder the result of direct blows to the sternum and other causes. In sternal fractures due to motor vehicle crashes, the patients are older, frequently the drivers, and usually seat belt users.

   A minority of patients with sternal fractures will not have a history of direct trauma to the chest. In these patients, spinal fractures, especially of the thoracic spine, must be sought. It is thought that the sternal injury is due to hyperflexion of the anterior chest with buckling of the sternum, resulting in fracture (often displaced) or subluxation/dislocation of the manubriosternal joint (1). A severe kyphotic deformity of the spine may result from a missed vertebral fracture.
   C. **Physical examination.** In most patients, the sternum is superficial and easily palpated. The majority of patients have pain and tenderness over the sternum and 25% have a hematoma overlying the sternum. Dyspnea is a frequent complaint. Physical find-

ings associated with other thoracic injuries must be carefully sought, including rib fractures, pneumothorax, hemothorax, and findings of aortic injury.

D. **Radiography.** Suspected fractures of the sternum may be confirmed radiographically. Approximately one-third of fractures are apparent on the standard trauma anteroposterior (AP) chest roentgenogram, with the remainder visible on the lateral chest film. A sternal view may be obtained but is rarely needed. Occasionally sternal fractures not visible on plain radiographs may be diagnosed by computed tomography (CT) of the chest or by ultrasound.

E. **Diagnosis.** The diagnosis is made by the history of injury and supporting physical and radiographic findings. The majority of sternal fractures (~90%) are of the body, especially the middle portion. A few patients have multiple fractures and may be more likely to have other significant injuries. Some 50% to 80% of sternal fractures are nondisplaced.

F. **Treatment.** Patients are managed with rest, ice, and analgesics. Closed sternal fractures rarely require surgical fixation.

G. **Complications.** It has been suggested that sternal fractures are markers for serious injuries, including myocardial contusion and aortic rupture. Nearly 50% of patients with sternal fractures have other injuries, most commonly other chest injuries. The presence of a sternal fracture, therefore, mandates a search for coexisting injuries. At a minimum, this should include a meticulous physical examination, electrocardiogram, and a chest radiograph (upright posteroanterior and lateral views).

H. **Disposition.** Patients with significant other injuries, severe pain, rib fractures, or electrocardiographic changes should be admitted. Patients with electrocardiographic changes or those 65 years of age or older and meeting any of the above criteria should be admitted to a monitored setting. Patients with an isolated sternal fracture and an otherwise normal chest radiograph, normal electrocardiogram, and adequate pain control may be discharged from the hospital after a short observation period (some suggest 4 to 6 hours) (2–5).

II. **Sternoclavicular joint injuries.** Injuries to the sternoclavicular joint are fortunately rare, as the function of the joint is important in the normal movement of the upper extremity. Grading of injuries to the joint is based on the degree of damage to the supporting ligaments (Table 1). Third-degree injuries frequently result in dislocation of the medial head of the clavicle, with anterior dislocations occurring more commonly than posterior (90% versus 10%, respectively).

A. **Anatomy.** The sternoclavicular joint is a true diarthroidal joint and is stabilized by the capsular, in-

Table 1. Injuries of the sternoclavicular joint

Type	Ligaments
First-degree sprain	Minor stretching or tearing
Second-degree sprain	Rupture of sternoclavicular ligament
	Partial tear of costoclavicular ligament
Third-degree sprain	Complete rupture of both ligaments

terclavicular, sternoclavicular, and costal clavicular ligaments. Normal movements of the scapula and shoulder require rotation of the clavicle, and the majority of this occurs at the sternoclavicular joint. The ossification center of the medial end of the clavicle appears around age 8 and is the last in the body to close, generally in the third decade. "Dislocations" prior to closure may actually be Salter-Harris type I epiphyseal fractures. Structures immediately posterior to the joint include the great vessels, esophagus, trachea, lungs, and vagus nerve (Fig. 1).

B. **Mechanism of injury.** Injuries are commonly due either to a lateral blow to the shoulder or directly to the medial end of the clavicle. The most common etiology is a motor vehicle crash, with sporting activity second. Significant forces are required to cause a sternoclavicular dislocation, mandating a thorough assessment of these patients.

C. **Physical examination.** There is tenderness to palpation directly over the injured joint and patients feel increased discomfort with movement of the shoulder. A bony deformity will be palpable over the joint in those patients with third-degree injuries and anterior dislocations. Hematoma formation, severe pain, and frequent lack of an obvious deformity may interfere in the diagnosis of posterior dislocations. Occasionally, a slight depression of the clavicle, noted while simultaneously palpating the both joints, may identify posterior dislocations. The presence of a posterior dislocation may be suggested by the signs and symptoms of impingement of the clavicular head on adjacent structures, including dysphagia (esophagus), stridor or dyspnea (trachea), and venous congestion of the neck or ipsilateral upper extremity (subclavian vein).

D. **Radiography.** Anteroposterior and lateral radiographs of the joint may be diagnostic. In addition, an anteroposterior radiograph with a 40-degree cephalic tilt may be helpful. Frequently, overlying structures

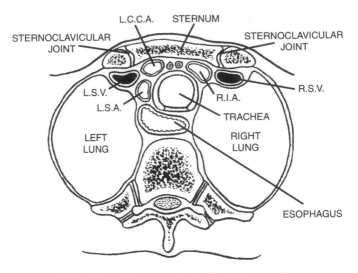

Fig. 1.   Relationship of the sternoclavicular joints to adjacent structures. L. C. C. A., left common carotid artery; L. S. A., left subclavian artery; L. S. V., left subclavian vein; R. I. A., right innominate artery; R. S. V., right subclavian vein.

make plain radiographs difficult to interpret. Particularly in cases of suspected posterior dislocation, CT should be obtained to assess bony as well as pulmonary and vascular structures.

E.   **Treatment**

    a.   **First-degree sprain.** Ice, analgesia, and a simple sling will suffice. Early mobilization should be encouraged, especially for elderly patients.

    b.   **Second-degree sprain.** As in the case of first-degree sprains, ice and analgesia are important. In addition to a sling, a figure-of-eight splint or sling and swathe should be used.

    c.   **Third-degree sprain.** The treatment of this type of injury is controversial, with advocates for both surgical and nonsurgical management. Therefore, early orthopaedic consultation is recommended.

       (1)   **Anterior dislocation.** Closed reduction may be attempted as follows:

          (a)   Position the patient in the supine position with a towel roll between the shoulders.

          (b)   Abduct the ipsilateral arm and apply traction.

(c) Have an assistant apply pressure over the medial clavicular head to push it into position.

After reduction, anterior dislocations are managed similarly to second-degree sprains. These dislocations are unstable and may dislocate after reduction. The patient should be warned of the potential of a cosmetic deformity (lump) at the sternoclavicular joint.

(2) **Posterior dislocation.** Reduction of these injuries often requires general anesthesia. Orthopaedic consultation is recommended prior to attempting reduction. Emergency closed reduction may be attempted if evidence of impingement on the trachea, great vessels, or other structures is present. Reduction is similar to that of anterior dislocations except that upward traction of the medial clavicle is provided by the assistant. This traction may be applied by grasping the clavicle or in some cases using sterile technique and grasping around the clavicle with a towel clip and pulling it into position. Once reduced, these dislocations are typically stable. Management after reduction is the same as that for a second-degree injury.

F. **Complications.** Complications of first- and second-degree sprains are rare. Anterior dislocations may recur and result in a cosmetic deformity. Some 25% or more of posterior dislocations are associated with more serious injuries, including pneumothorax, hemothorax, pulmonary and myocardial contusions, fractures, brachial plexus injuries, tracheal injuries, and injuries to the great vessels.

G. **Disposition.** Patients with first- and second-degree sprains should be referred to their primary care physician in 1 to 2 weeks for evaluation of healing and rehabilitation. Those patients with anterior dislocations should have orthopaedic consultation arranged prior to discharge from the emergency department. Patients with posterior dislocations should generally be admitted to the hospital for observation after other serious injuries are excluded and the dislocation has been reduced.

III. **Clavicle.** The clavicle connects the shoulder to the axial skeleton. It is the first bone to ossify in the fetus and, unlike the other long bones, has an intramembranous origin. This discussion focuses on injuries other than those commonly incurred at birth.

A. **Anatomy.** The clavicle is a greatly curved, horizontally lying tubular bone that articulates with the manubrium medially (sternoclavicular joint). It is firmly attached to the manubrium by the sternoclavicular and costoclavicular ligaments. Laterally, the clavicle articulates with the acromion process of the scapula (acromioclavicular joint) and is anchored to the scapula by the coracoclavicular and acromioclavicular ligaments (Fig. 2). The conoid tubercle is the site of attachment of the conoid portion of the coracoclavicular ligament. The trapezoid portion of the coracoclavicular ligament attaches to the trapezoid line, a bony ridge on the clavicle running lateral to the conoid tubercle. Muscles inserting on the clavicle include the sternocleidomastoid and subclavius. The subclavian vessels and brachial plexus lie directly posterior to the clavicle.

B. **Classification of clavicular fractures.** The clavicle is divided into the medial, middle, and lateral thirds. Mechanically, the weakest portion of the clavicle is the middle third, the most frequent site of fractures. Fractures may be categorized based on the location of the fracture (Table 2).

C. **Mechanism of injury:** Some 87% of patients will have fallen on the ipsilateral shoulder, 7% experience a direct blow, and 6% fall on the ipsilateral outstretched hand (6).

D. **Physical examination.** Patients typically hold the arm adducted against the chest and resist movement. The shoulder of a patient with a group I fracture may appear to slump downward due to loss of support of the clavicle. Palpation over the fracture site reveals swelling and tenderness. The medial portion of the clavicle in group I fractures is frequently elevated by the sternocleidomastoid muscle. A complete vascular and neuromuscular examination of the ipsilateral upper extremity is required to exclude complications involving the brachial plexus or subclavian vessels. A complete examination of the chest is necessary to exclude intrathoracic injuries.

E. **Radiography.** A routine AP radiograph of the clavicle is usually sufficient to detect fractures. To better determine the fracture anatomy or if the AP film is negative and the index of suspicion is high, additional views including lateral, apical lordotic, or apical oblique may be obtained.

F. **Treatment**
   1. **Group I fractures.** Traditionally, commercial clavicular straps (for patients above 10 years of age) or figure-of-eight dressings made from cotton stockinette are recommended. To be effective,
      a. Both shoulders must be pulled backward during the application and tightening of the splint.
      b. The straps must be well padded and careful attention must be paid to preventing inter-

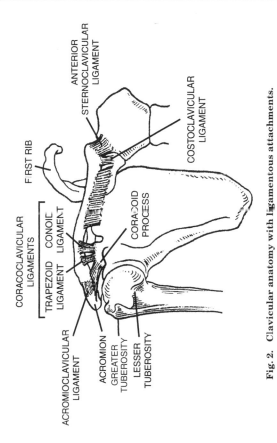

Fig. 2. Clavicular anatomy with ligamentous attachments.

Table 2.   Clavicular fractures

	Fracture site	Frequency
Group I	Middle third Type I—undisplaced Type II—displaced	75%–80%
Group II	Lateral third Type I—lateral to coracoclavicular ligament with intact ligament Type II—disruption of coracoclavicular ligaments Type III—involvement of acromioclavicular joint surface	10%–15%
Group III	Medial third	~5%

ference with normal circulation and neural function.

c. The strap must be worn at all times and kept adjusted. The strap should be worn until the arm may be abducted without pain, usually 3 to 4 weeks in children and 4 to 6 weeks in adults. However, studies comparing outcomes of patients treated with figure-of-eight dressings and simple slings have not demonstrated any difference (7,8), and the use of a sling is usually better tolerated by the patient.

2. **Group II fractures.** In general, uncomplicated fractures of the lateral clavicle may initially be treated symptomatically with analgesia, ice, and a simple sling. Type II fractures, with disruption of the coracoclavicular ligaments, may have nonunion in 20% to 33% of cases. Because of this high rate of nonunion, it is often recommended that surgical fixation be performed. However, a recent review found the majority of patients, even with nonunion, to have a stable shoulder and to be asymptomatic without surgical intervention (9). Type III fractures have been suggested to have a high resorption rate of the distal end, requiring surgical resection, although this was not found in all studies. Owing to the controversy surrounding the management of group II fractures, referral to an orthopaedic surgeon is recommended.

3. **Group III fractures.** Medial fractures are uncommon and generally nondisplaced if the costoclavicular ligament is intact. A simple sling, ice, and analgesia are usually sufficient. If fracture fragments are displaced, orthopaedic referral is recommended.

4. **Surgical management.** Open management of clavicular fracture is rarely required and in fact is associated with significant complications. Indications for surgical management include open fracture, skin compromise, interposition of soft tissue, vascular or neurological injury, or fractures resulting in a "floating" shoulder (ipsilateral fractures of the clavicle and scapular neck).

G. **Complications.** Complications of clavicular fractures are rare: nonunion is most commonly reported. Occasionally, a cosmetically unsatisfactory lump may be seen. Other complications include degenerative arthritis, frozen shoulder, subclavian vessel injury, brachial plexus injury, and pneumothorax. Patients with displaced group I fractures and significant shortening (>15 mm) may be at higher risk for fracture nonunion and persistent pain (10,11).

H. **Disposition.** Patients with uncomplicated group I fractures should be followed by their primary care physician in 1 to 2 weeks for evaluation of fracture healing and to exclude the development of complications. Orthopaedic referral for patients with group II or III fractures should be arranged prior to discharge from the emergency department.

IV. **Scapula.** The scapula is an integral component of the shoulder complex. Injuries to the scapula are uncommon (≤1% of all fractures) and are usually the result of severe blunt force, typically due to a high-speed motor vehicle crash. Owing to the severity of the force required to cause a scapular fracture, associated injuries are common.

A. **Anatomy.** The scapula is a large, triangular bone enveloped by surrounding musculature (supraspinatus, infraspinatus, and subscapularis muscles). It is attached to the clavicle at the acromioclavicular joint and also secured by the coracoclavicular ligaments. It articulates with the humerus at the glenohumeral joint (Figs. 2 and 3). Important landmarks include body, coracoid, acromion, scapular spine, neck, and glenoid fossa. Multiple muscles and ligaments attach to the scapula. Fractures are classified by their location (i.e., body or spine, neck, intraarticular glenoid, acromion, or coracoid process) (Fig. 4).

B. **Specific fractures**
1. **Body or spine.** This is the most common fracture of the scapula, accounting for 40% to 75% of fractures.
   a. **Mechanism of injury.** Scapular fractures are unusual because the scapula is well protected by the surrounding musculature and the thoracic cage. Severe direct trauma is usually required, most commonly associated with a motor vehicle crash. Other etiologies include impact sports, falls, seizures, and electrical injuries. Avulsion fractures associ-

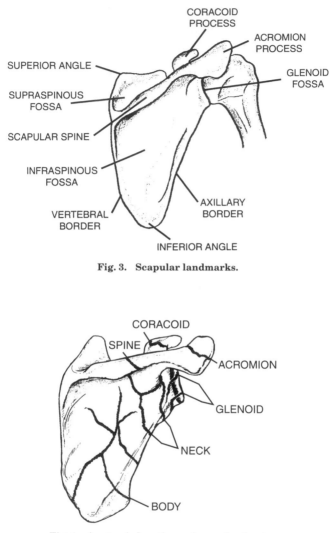

Fig. 3.   Scapular landmarks.

Fig. 4.   Anatomic locations of scapular fracture.

ated with water skiing, "wheelchair racing," etc., may occur, but they are rare.

b. **Physical examination.** Pain and tenderness noted on direct palpation and exacerbated by movement of the shoulder is typical. Swelling and hematoma formation may be found. The patient frequently refuses to abduct the arm because of pain. The injury may be misdiagnosed as a rotator cuff tear.

c. **Radiography.** Fractures are commonly visible on routine chest radiographs but are frequently overlooked. Routine AP and transscapular views are usually sufficient for diagnosis.

d. **Diagnosis.** The diagnosis is made by the history and physical examination and supporting radiographic findings. Fractures are frequently overlooked during the initial evaluation because of severe associated injuries and inadequate attention to the scapula on interpretation of the initial chest film.

e. **Treatment** is directed at patient comfort with sling-and-swathe immobilization, ice, and analgesics. Early mobilization with pendulum exercises initially and limited activity as tolerated after 2 weeks is recommended. The sling should be worn for approximately 2 weeks.

f. **Disposition.** Some 50% or more of patients will have associated injuries, most commonly other thoracic injuries, including rib fractures, clavicular fracture, pulmonary contusions, and hemothorax or pneumothorax. A meticulous physical examination and appropriate diagnostic testing, including a chest radiograph, are mandatory to exclude other injuries. The majority of patients with undisplaced fractures of the scapular body or spine will have good results. Patients should schedule a reevaluation by their primary care physician.

2. **Neck.** Fractures of the scapular neck are the second most common fractures of the scapula and account for 5% to 32% of fractures.

a. **Mechanism of injury.** Usually due to a direct blow to the shoulder, anteriorly or posteriorly, or blunt trauma to the lateral aspect of the shoulder. A fall on the shoulder or on the outstretched hand may also cause fracture of the glenoid neck.

b. **Physical examination.** The patient typically supports the arm in an adducted position. Pressure directed medially over the lateral shoulder exacerbates the pain. If the fracture is displaced, prominence of the acromion may be noted. Associated humeral fractures and dislocations should be sought.

c. **Radiography.** Routine anteroposterior and transscapular views are usually sufficient for diagnosis. The fracture line typically extends from the medial coracoid process to the medial aspect of the subglenoid tubercle. Frequently the fracture is impacted and the fracture line may be difficult to visualize.

d. **Treatment.** Management is similar to that of body fractures with sling or sling and swathe, ice, analgesia, and early mobilization. Operative management may be considered in those patients with displacement, angulation of the glenoid fossa, intraarticular glenoid fractures, or clavicular fracture or ligamentous injuries resulting in a "floating shoulder."

e. **Disposition.** Patients with indications for operative management should have emergent orthopaedic consultation. Those patients with injuries managed on an outpatient basis should have scheduled early orthopaedic follow-up.

3. **Glenoid.** These represent the third most common fracture, accounting for 10% to 25% of all scapular fractures. Glenoid fractures are of two general types, rim fractures and intraarticular fractures of the glenoid.

a. **Mechanism of injury.** Intraarticular glenoid fractures are generally the result of a direct blow to the lateral aspect of the shoulder, driving the head of the humerus medially into the fossa. Glenoid rim fractures may occur with anterior or posterior shoulder dislocations or with forces transmitted along the humerus, driving the humeral head into the rim.

b. **Physical examination.** Swelling and tenderness are usually present, with exacerbation of pain upon movement of the shoulder. In patients with glenoid fractures, pain is increased with medially directed pressure over the humeral head. Shoulder dislocation or subluxation is frequently found in patients with rim fractures.

c. **Radiography.** Standard AP and transscapular views are often sufficient. Small rim fractures may be better visualized on an axillary view. Occasionally, CT may be required.

d. **Treatment.** Small or minimally displaced rim fractures are managed with sling immobilization, ice, and analgesics. Early mobilization is recommended as pain decreases. Large rim fractures or those with displacement may require surgical repair and orthopaedic consultation prior to the patient's discharge from the emergency department.

Intraarticular glenoid fractures are managed similarly to small rim fractures, with sling immobilization, ice, and analgesics. Depressed or displaced fractures may require surgical management.

  e. **Disposition.** All patients with glenoid fractures should have scheduled orthopaedic follow-up prior to discharge from the emergency department.

4. **Coracoid.** Accounting for 3% to 13% of all scapular fractures, these are rare. They may involve either the base or distal coracoid process.

  a. **Mechanism of injury.** A coracoid fracture may be the result of a direct blow or from the humeral head in anterior shoulder dislocations. Avulsion fractures resulting from contraction of the coracobrachialis and biceps brachialis muscles may occur.

  b. **Physical examination.** There is localized pain, tenderness, and swelling in the region of the coracoid process. Pain may be exacerbated by deep inspiration, adduction, and flexion of the shoulder or by flexion and supination of the forearm. There may also be findings of associated acromioclavicular joint injury.

  c. **Radiography.** AP and transscapular views are generally sufficient. An axillary view may be required, particularly to determine displacement. Occasionally special oblique views or CT scans are necessary.

  d. **Treatment.** This consists of sling or sling-and-swathe immobilization, ice, and analgesia. Mobilization is allowed as pain remits. Surgical management may be required in athletes, patients whose occupations involve heavy manual labor, or those with neurovascular complications or other injuries (i.e., acromioclavicular joint injury).

  e. **Disposition.** Orthopaedic follow-up should be scheduled. Associated injuries, such as a clavicular fracture or acromioclavicular joint injury, should be excluded before the patient is discharged from the emergency department.

5. **Acromion.** These fractures are rare, occurring with approximately the same incidence as coracoid fractures, i.e., 8% to 16% of fractures.

  a. **Mechanism of injury.** Fractures of the acromion are usually the result of a direct downward blow to the shoulder. Avulsion and stress fractures may also occur.

b. **Physical examination.** There is localized swelling and pain with abduction of the arm. The weight of the arm may result in downward displacement of the fracture fragment and loss of the normal round contour of the shoulder. Associated brachial plexus injuries should be sought.

c. **Radiography.** The standard AP and transscapular views usually demonstrate the fracture adequately. Os acromiale may be confused with acromion fractures. Radiographs of the uninjured shoulder may be helpful, as os acromiale is bilateral in over 50% of cases. Superior displacement of the acromion suggests a superior shoulder dislocation.

d. **Treatment.** The majority of acromion fractures are undisplaced and are managed with sling-and-swathe immobilization, ice, and analgesia, with mobilization as pain remits. Displaced fractures or fractures with associated injuries of the clavicular or acromioclavicular joint may require surgical management.

e. **Disposition.** Arthritis and bursitis are common complications. Displaced fractures or associated injuries requires orthopaedic consultation. Patients discharged from the emergency department should have scheduled follow-up.

V. **Scapulothoracic disassociation.** This rare entity is associated with a high rate of neurovascular injury and frequently with amputation.

A. **Mechanism of injury.** Typically, a high velocity motor vehicle crash. This results in disruption of the musculature surrounding the scapula (deltoid, pectoralis minor, levator scapulae, trapezius, rhomboids, and latissimus dorsi) and usually injury to the vasculature (generally the subclavian artery but occasionally the axillary artery) and neurologic deficits from avulsion of the brachial plexus.

B. **Physical examination.** Massive soft tissue swelling around the shoulder and chest is typical. Neurological and vascular deficits are usually present as well, although a spectrum of findings, including normal neurovascular examination, have been described. The injury is frequently missed initially due to severe coexisting injuries.

C. **Radiography.** On chest radiographs, the entire scapula is displaced laterally. Associated clavicular fractures or sternoclavicular or acromioclavicular dislocations are frequently present.

D. **Treatment.** Initial treatment is directed toward initial evaluation and resuscitation of the trauma victim. Arteriography is required to assess vascular integrity. Emergent orthopaedic consultation is required.

E. **Complications and associated injuries.** The recognition and treatment of these injuries is often hindered by the severity of coexisting trauma, commonly of the head, chest, and abdomen. A mortality rate of 10% to 20% has been reported (12,13).

Long-term outcome is typically poor, with very few patients (~17%) regaining limited function of the extremity. The severity of the brachial plexus injury often results in an insensate arm. Elective amputation of the involved extremity is common (13).

VI. **Scapular dislocation (locked scapula)**

  A. **Mechanism of injury.** This is an uncommon injury, usually due to low-energy impact (backward fall onto outstretched arm or direct blow to the scapula) in which the tip of the scapula is dislocated into the space between two ribs

  B. **Physical examination** reveals resistance to range of motion of the arm and localized tenderness and swelling over the scapula.

  C. **Radiographs** show lateral displacement of the scapula and the intercostal location of the tip of the scapula (best on oblique views).

  D. **Treatment.** The dislocation may be reduced by traction on the ipsilateral hyperabducted arm with manipulation of the scapula. Following reduction, the arm and scapula are immobilized. The patient must be thoroughly evaluated to exclude coexisting injuries.

REFERENCES

1. Jones HK, McBride GG, Mumby RC. Sternal fractures associated with spine injury. *J Trauma* 1989;29:360–364.
2. Heyes FLP, Vincent R. Sternal fracture: what investigations are indicated? *Injury* 1993;24:113–115.
3. Wright SW. Myth of the dangerous sternal fracture. *Ann Emerg Med* 1993;22:1589–1592.
4. Peek GJ, Firmin RK. Isolated sternal fracture: an audit of 10 years' experience. *Injury* 1995;26:385–388.
5. Chiu WC, D'Amelio LF, Hammond JS. Sternal fractures in blunt chest trauma: a practical algorithm for management. *Am J Emerg Med* 1997;15:252–255.
6. Stanley D, Trowbridge EA, Norris SH. The mechanism of clavicular fracture. *J Bone Joint Surg (Br)* 1988;70B:461–464.
7. Andersen K, Jensen PO, Lauritzen J. Treatment of clavicular fractures: figure-eight bandage versus a simple sling. *Acta Orthop Scand* 1987;57:71–74.
8. Stanley D, Norris SH. Recovery following fractures of the clavicle treated conservatively. *Injury* 1988;19:162–164.
9. Nordqvist A, Petersson C, Redlund-Johnell I. The natural course of lateral clavicle fracture. *Acta Orthop Scand* 1993;64:87–91.
10. Eskola A, Vainionpaa S, Myllynen P, Rokkanen P. Outcome of clavicular fracture in 89 patients. *Arch Orthop Trauma Surg* 1986;105:337–338.

11. Hill JM, McGuire MH, Crosby LA. Closed treatment of displaced middle-third fractures of the clavicle gives poor results. *J Bone Joint Surg (Br)* 1997;79B:537–539.
12. Ebraheim NA, An HS, Jackson WT, et al. Scapulothoracic dissociation. *J Bone Joint Surg (Am)* 1988;70:428–432.
13. Damschen DD, Cogbill TH, Siegel MJ. Scapulothoracic dissociation caused by blunt trauma. *J Trauma* 1997;42:537–540.

Shoulder Injuries

Paul J. Donovan

Shoulder injuries are a common complaint among emergency department patients. The key to accurate diagnosis and treatment is an understanding of shoulder anatomy, with a thorough history, physical exam, and proper radiographic evaluation.

I. **Anatomy.** The shoulder girdle is comprised of four bony articulations: the **glenohumeral, acromioclavicular, sternoclavicular,** and **scapulothoracic.** The soft tissues include the rotator cuff tendons, scapular stabilizing muscles, fibrous capsule, glenohumeral ligaments, and glenoid labrum. These osseous and soft tissue structures provide a stable but flexible unit, allowing the widest range of motion of any joint in the body (Fig. 1).

II. **Mechanism of injury**
    A. **Trauma.** Traumatic shoulder injuries include fractures, dislocations, subluxations, separations, traumatic impingement, and contusions.
    B. **Overuse.** Overuse injuries include bursitis, tendinitis (rotator cuff, biceps), and degenerative or post-traumatic arthritis. The elements of overuse that are frequently implicated are repetitive overhead activities or unaccustomed repetitive strenuous activity (throwing sports, swimming, occupational factors).

III. **Evaluation of the injured shoulder.** With both traumatic and overuse injuries, eliciting the precipitating event is most important. The patient's presenting complaint is most often pain with or without associated weakness. The mechanism of trauma, direction of force or fall, shoulder position at time of injury, patient's age, occupation, hand dominance, and history of previous shoulder disorders should be elicited. When shoulder pain is not preceded by a history of trauma or overuse, a serious underlying cause—such as cardiac disease, systemic arthritis, infection, or neoplasm—should be considered.
    A. **Examination.** Begin with adequate exposure of both shoulders, looking for symmetry, the presence of obvious deformity, swelling, or ecchymosis.
        1. **Range of motion (ROM).** While active and passive ROM and strength testing should be performed, the severity of trauma and degree of pain will often limit this. Limitation of active ROM may be due to pain, weakness, or both. Normal range of shoulder motion is included in Table 1. Partial and complete rotator cuff tears are often accompanied by pain, weakness, or both. In these circumstances, ROM testing should be limited to minimize the risk of further injury. When there is restricted active ROM, passive ROM may help to delineate the cause. In overuse injuries, passive

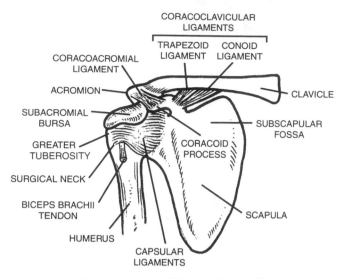

Fig. 1.   Anatomy of the shoulder girdle.

ROM should not be restricted. Restriction of both active and passive ROM suggests a "frozen shoulder" or adhesive capsulitis. In this instance, limitation of external rotation is most dramatic. Specific tests, such as Jobe's and Speed's tests, are used for assessing supraspinatus and biceps tendon integrity respectively. Hawkin's test for impingement is also useful.

2. **Palpation.** On palpation of the injured site, there is often tenderness. The presence of crepitance often indicates a fracture. In overuse injuries, pain and tenderness are more often generalized than with an acute traumatic injury.

Table 1.   Range of normal shoulder motion

Motion	Range (degrees)
Flexion	180
Abduction	180
Adduction	75
Extension	50
External rotation*	65
Internal rotation*	80
External rotation†	90
Internal rotation†	70

*Arm at side.
†Arm abducted 90 degrees.

However, the biceps tendon is readily palpable in its groove, located at the anterior humeral head medial to the greater tuberosity of the humerus. Tenderness on palpation with pain on Speed's test is consistent with bicipital tendinitis. Speed's test elicits pain in the bicipital groove with forward flexion against resistance with the arm abducted and the elbow extended and supinated. Tenderness to palpation over the acromioclavicular joint that worsens with adduction (cross flexion with the arm at 90 degrees) suggests acromioclavicular arthralgia due either to direct trauma with separation or to posttraumatic arthritis. Overuse conditions of the shoulder or glenohumeral instability can often be diagnosed by palpating the humeral head through the deltoid An abnormal finding is when the head can be moved off the glenoid by more than 50% in the anterior, inferior, or posterior direction. When this is done, the patient often exhibits "apprehension" because of a feeling of impending subluxation. Any evidence of instability, a history of the shoulder "popping out," and vague glenohumeral pain support a diagnosis of shoulder subluxation.

3. **Neurovascular examination.** Neurovascular structures should always be evaluated, especially in traumatic shoulder conditions, because injury to the axillary, musculocutaneous and ulnar nerves or to the axillary or brachial artery may be present.

B. **Diagnostic tests**
1. **Plain radiographs** are the first imaging step in the diagnosis of shoulder injuries. Rockwood and Greens recommend that the standard trauma series should include a **true anteroposterior (AP)** or **Grashey** view (x-ray beam perpendicular to the plane of the scapula), **lateral projection in the scapular plane** (Y or transcapular view), and an **axillary** view. However, because of the technical difficulty in proper patient positioning for true AP and axillary views and the patient's pain and limitation of motion, **routine AP (transthoracic)** and **transscapular** views are generally adequate for the vast majority of injuries.

   In cases of shoulder dislocation, postreduction x-rays are always obtained. Additional AP views with internal and external rotation will demonstrate the lesser and greater tuberosities of the humeral head, respectively, and are particularly useful in fractures of the humeral head and proximal humerus. Calcium deposits may be noted on these views as well; these suggest calcific tendinitis or bursitis, given the appropriate clinical scenario.

Special views of the acromioclavicular joint (AP views with cephalad angulation) should be done when injury to the acromioclavicular joint is suspected. These often include the opposite normal side for comparison, with occasional stress views obtained by the patient having a 10-lb weight hung in each hand. In cases of obvious acromioclavicular deformity, stress views are not necessary. To evaluate clavicular trauma, an AP cephalad view is also obtained. Degenerative changes about the glenoid consisting of osteophytic lipping and/or sclerosis may suggest instability or previous subluxation or dislocation. Considerable narrowing of the glenohumeral joint or narrowing of the distance between the acromion and the humeral head in an older person is strongly suggestive of rotator cuff arthropathy. Osteolysis or cyst of the distal clavicle may be evident in someone with a history of acute injury or repeated shoulder stress, such as a manual laborer or a weight lifter.

2. **Computed tomography (CT) and magnetic resonance imaging (MRI)** may be indicated in certain conditions. CT scanning is useful for complicated fractures or dislocations of the shoulder. MRI with contrast is rapidly becoming a diagnostic test of choice for demonstrating soft tissue injuries such as labral or rotator cuff tears.

C. **Treatment.** Most shoulder injuries can be treated by proper immobilization, frequent icing, and nonsteroidal anti-inflammatory drugs (NSAIDs) with or without narcotic medications.

IV. **Specific injuries of the shoulder**

A. **Shoulder dislocation.** The shoulder is the most frequently dislocated major joint of the body. A dislocation may be anterior, inferior, or posterior. Superior and posterior dislocations are rare. Anterior shoulder dislocations are the most common (95%) and can be classified according to the anatomical location of the humeral head: subcoracoid, subclavicular, or subglenoid.

1. **Anterior shoulder dislocation.** The subcoracoid is the most common type of dislocation and usually results from a fall on a flexed, abducted arm.

a. **Examination.** The patient complains of pain about the shoulder. The shoulder and arm are often held in a neutral position with difficulty in flexing at the glenohumeral joint. There is often a prominence of the acromion with loss of the normal deltoid contour laterally. The humeral head can often be palpated anteriorly.

b. **Radiographs.** A routine AP view of the shoulder demonstrates a lack of the normal

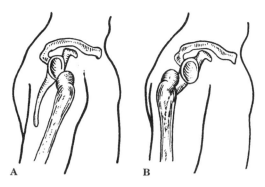

**Fig. 2. Transscapular view of
an anterior shoulder dislocation (A),
and posterior dislocation (B).**

overlap of the humeral head with the glenoid. However, the transscapular view is often most diagnostic, as the humeral head is anterior to the Y of the scapula (formed by the confluence of the acromion, coracoid, and lateral margin of the body of the scapula, centered at the glenoid) (Fig. 2). A posterolateral compression fracture of the humeral head, also called a Hill-Sachs deformity, is present 50% of the time. There may also be an associated fracture, typically of the greater tuberosity, that usually represents an avulsion fracture caused by the external rotators of the rotator cuff tendons (infraspinatus and teres minor muscles).

c. **Treatment.** Various methods of reduction have been described. In general, traction-countertraction techniques are preferred. Leverage techniques, such as Kocher's maneuver, are to be condemned because they are associated with many complications. In general, the least traumatic method that affords the greatest likelihood of success is the one that should be utilized. Ideally the physician should be familiar with at least two methods. Because the patient often has significant pain and the least traumatic reduction method possible is desired, parenteral medications are useful. Analgesics, amnestics, and/or sedative hypnotic agents that are short-acting and reversible should be utilized. Morphine, meperidine (Demerol), fentanyl, midazolam, diazepam, and methohexital are examples. Close monitoring of the cardiorespiratory system is necessary. If

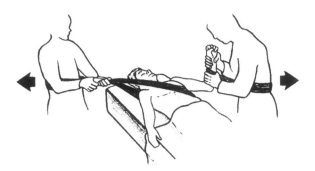

Fig. 3.   Modified Hippocratic technique.

several attempts at reduction are unsuccessful, orthopaedic referral is required. Open dislocations require immediate orthopaedic referral, as do open fracture/dislocations.

(1) **External rotation.** The patient is supine with the arm adducted and the elbow flexed to 90 degrees. The arm is slowly rotated externally with longitudinal traction. This procedure must be performed slowly to allow pain and spasm to resolve. Reduction is usually complete before the coronal plane is reached.

(2) **Modified Hippocratic technique.** The patient is supine with the arm adducted and elbow flexed to 90 degrees. A sheet is wrapped around the patient's chest and held by an assistant. A tied sheet is wrapped around the physician's waist and then around the patient's forearm, with the elbow flexed to 90 degrees. The physician applies gradual traction while the assistant applies countertraction. Gentle internal and external rotation or outward pressure to the proximal humerus may aid reduction (Fig. 3).

(3) **Stimson's scapular manipulation.** The patient is prone on the bed with the affected arm over the side. After complete muscle relaxation, a 10-lb weight is attached to the wrist. Allow approximately 30 minutes for reduction to occur. A modification of Stimson's procedure is to manipulate the scapula by pushing its tip medially with the thumbs while fixing its superior margin with the cephalad hand (Fig. 4).

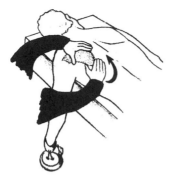

Fig. 4. Stimson's with scapular manipulation.

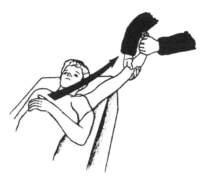

Fig. 5. Milch reduction technique.

(4) **Milch procedure.** With the patient supine, the arm is fully extended, abducted, and then externally rotated to the overhead position. Traction is applied. To aid reduction, an assistant may push the head of the humerus over the lip of the glenoid (Fig. 5).

If adequate reduction is accomplished, the patient is placed in a sling or a shoulder immobilizer to permit adequate capsular healing. The length of immobilization varies with age. In general, the younger the patient, the longer the period of immobilization because the chance of redislocation is greater.

d. **Complications.** Postreduction strength is assessed to rule out a rotator cuff tear. Pre- and postreduction neurovascular exams should also be performed. Axillary neuropraxia can accompany up to 10% of anterior shoulder dislocations. Decreased sensation over the lateral aspect of the shoulder with inability to abduct the shoulder is diagnostic. This usually resolves after relocation. The incidence of vascular complications often increases with age and duration of the dislocation. Any neurovascular compromise requires immediate orthopaedic referral. Persistence of pain or instability may be due to a glenoid labral tear. Recurrent dislocations are common, with a 90% recurrence rate for patients below 20 years of age.

2. **Inferior shoulder dislocation (luxatio erecta).** These are very uncommon but serious injuries. The mechanism is usually a combined hyperadduction and hyperflexion force.

   a. **Examination.** The patient's arm is held in a fixed hyperabducted position, with severe pain and inability to adduct the arm.

   b. **Radiographs.** On the AP view, the entire humeral head and surgical neck of the humerus are inferior to the glenoid fossa. Occasionally fractures of the proximal humerus occur.

   c. **Treatment.** Reduction is sometimes difficult and occasionally requires general anesthesia. Longitudinal traction is applied in the long axis of the humerus and the arm is rotated inferiorly in an outward arc, applying traction throughout (Fig. 6). The presence of a buttonhole deformity at the inferior capsule often makes reduction difficult; therefore open reduction may be required.

   d. **Complications.** Severe soft tissue injury, rotator cuff tears, and neurovascular compromise can often accompany this dislocation. The humeral head is usually forced through the inferior capsule, with accompanying rupture of the rotator cuff tendons. Neurovascular compromise of both the axillary artery and brachial plexus are commonly associated with this injury owing to the proximity of these neurovascular structures to the dislocated inferior head.

3. **Superior shoulder dislocations.** Superior shoulder dislocations are the rarest of shoulder dislocations. The mechanism of injury is usually an extreme upward and forward force on an adducted arm.

   a. **Examination** reveals a superiorly displaced humeral head, often with deformity over the acromion and acromioclavicular joint. This is

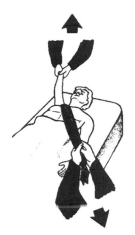

Fig. 6. Longitudinal traction applied in reduction of inferior shoulder dislocation.

an extremely painful condition, and the arm is often shortened and adducted.

b. **Radiographs.** The head of the humerus is displaced superiorly from the glenoid fossa, usually with an associated fracture of the acromion and/or disruption of the acromioclavicular joint.

c. **Treatment.** This involves closed reduction by longitudinal traction directed inferiorly, with slight adduction.

d. **Complications.** Soft tissue damage to the capsule and rotator cuff tendons is common, as is acromioclavicular joint disruption with or without associated acromial fractures. Neurovascular complications can also occur.

4. **Posterior shoulder dislocations** are uncommon and represent approximately 5% or less of shoulder dislocations; however, more than 75% of these are often misdiagnosed as "frozen shoulders." The patient often presents with a history of recent seizure (especially if bilateral) or a posteriorly directed force against the glenohumeral joint.

a. **Examination.** Often the patient presents with the arm held in an internally rotated and flexed position, reporting a great deal of pain on attempted external rotation and abduction.

b. **Radiographs.** With posterior shoulder dislocation, a true AP view of the shoulder demonstrates overlap between the humeral head and the glenoid. On a routine AP view, one can see an "empty glenoid" sign due to loss of a normal elliptical overlap between the humeral head and the glenoid. Also on this view, one may see a "tough line" due to an anteromedial humeral head compression fracture also known as a reverse Hill-Sachs deformity. On a transscapular view, the humeral head is seen posterior to the glenoid. A fracture of the lesser tuberosity of the humerus may be present, which is usually an avulsion fracture that occurs when the strong subscapularis tendon ruptures this bony fragment.

c. **Treatment.** Successful reduction can be accomplished by longitudinal traction in the long axis of the humerus with slight abduction. An assistant gently pushes the humeral head anteriorly in the glenoid fossa. Any difficulty requires orthopaedic consultation.

d. **Complications.** Neurovascular injuries are uncommon with posterior shoulder dislocations because the major neurovascular structures are located anterior, inferior, and medial to the glenohumeral joint.

5. **Chronic shoulder dislocation** is defined as a dislocation that has been present for longer than a week. It is most often seen in nursing home patients, the mentally impaired, and the elderly. These injuries should be approached with caution because of the increased potential for neurovascular injuries. Orthopaedic referral is necessary.

B. **Acromioclavicular (AC) joint injuries.** Injuries of the AC joint can be classified into six types according to the extent of injury sustained at the acromioclavicular and coracoclavicular ligaments (Fig. 7). Often the patient will give a history of a direct blow to the shoulder, either from a fall or particularly in sports such as football during blocking or tackling.

1. **Examination.** There is often swelling and tenderness over the AC joint, with or without ecchymosis.

a. **Type I injury** (Fig. 7A). This type of injury is noted by tenderness over the AC joint with minimal or no ligamentous disruption or instability.

b. **Type II injury** (Fig. 7B). This type implies more tearing of the joint capsule, with complete disruption of the AC ligaments.

c. **Type III injury** (Fig. 7C). In these injuries there is complete tearing of both the AC and the coracoclavicular ligaments. Generally, on physical examination, there is an obvious "step-off" with complete dislocation.

d. **Type IV to VI injuries.** These injuries are rare and are classified according to the associated damage to the surrounding deltoid and trapezius muscles as well as the position

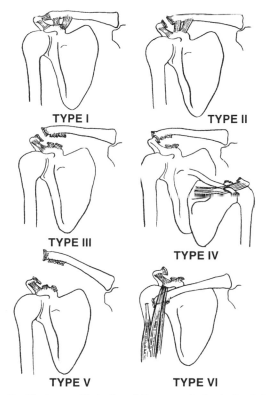

TYPE I

TYPE II

TYPE III

TYPE IV

TYPE V

TYPE VI

Fig. 7. Six types of injuries of the acromioclavicular joint.

of the displaced lateral end of the clavicle. Type IV injuries are type III injuries with posterior displacement of the distal clavicle (Fig. 7D). Often the distal clavicle has penetrated through the body of the trapezius muscle. Type V injuries are type III injuries with superior displacement of the distal clavicle (Fig. 7E). Type VI injuries are type III injuries with inferior displacement of the clavicle, often fixed in the subcoracoid or subacromial space (Fig. 7F).

2. **Radiographs**
    a. **Type I injury** demonstrates a normal x-ray.
    b. **Type II injury** demonstrates a subluxation of the AC joint, usually with less than 1 cm of separation.
    c. **Type III injury** shows greater than 1 cm of AC separation with greater than 50% widening of the coracoclavicular space.

d. **Type IV injury** demonstrates not only AC subluxation but also posterior displacement of the distal end of the clavicle.

e. **Type V injury** illustrates marked superior displacement of the distal clavicle.

f. **Type VI injury** shows the distal clavicle inferiorly displaced.

3. **Treatment.** The mainstay of outpatient treatment is a shoulder immobilizer. The length of immobilization as well as the definitive treatment will depend on the type of injury.

a. **Type I injuries** generally require a minimal amount of immobilization (1 to 2 weeks) followed by early mobilization.

b. **Type II injuries** usually require 2 to 4 weeks of immobilization.

c. **Type III injuries.** Definitive treatment depends on the patient's occupation. These injuries can be treated conservatively and the patient usually returns to normal function. However, the patient must understand that permanent deformity will result. If the patient is an athlete or manual laborer and requires early mobilization or as functional an anatomical repair as possible, surgery provides definitive treatment and has the advantages of offering early mobilization.

d. **Type IV to VI injuries** require surgical intervention definitively because they involve significant injury to the deltoid and trapezius muscles and/or significant displacement of the distal end of the clavicle.

4. **Complications.** Neurovascular complications and rotator cuff tears are rare.

C. **Traumatic impingement.** The impingement syndrome is defined as the impingement of the periarticular soft tissues between the greater tuberosity of the humerus and the corocoacromial arch. This usually results from a fall on an outstretched hand or a lateral blow to the proximal humerus. It is often misdiagnosed as "shoulder contusion" and is often a source of chronic shoulder pain and weakness because of underlying rotator cuff injury.

1. **Examination.** The patient often presents with pain, swelling, and ecchymosis and demonstrates limitation of active ROM. Weakness may be present because of pain or injury to the accompanying rotator cuff tendons.

2. **Radiographs.** The radiographs are usually normal.

3. **Treatment.** Immobilization with a sling for comfort for 1 to 2 weeks. Proper evaluation of the integrity of the rotator cuff tendons is often difficult because of the patient's concomitant pain. There-

fore orthopaedic referral is mandatory. Follow-up radiographic assessment methods include CT, arthrography, ultrasound, and MRI. Persistence of pain or weakness after shoulder injury indicates a rotator cuff or labral tear until proven otherwise.

4. **Complications.** Chronic pain can often accompany this injury, owing to undetected rotator cuff or labral injury.

D. **Rotator cuff tears.** Rotator cuff tears often go unrecognized because of failure to consider them as a complication of significant trauma and/or because a precise detailed history and physical exam are omitted. Rotator cuff tears can be acute or chronic and involve a partial or full thickness. Acute rotator cuff tears are usually a complication of severe trauma, such as shoulder dislocation or traumatic impingement. Chronic tears are usually present in the patient with a long-standing history of shoulder pain or weakness and are usually the result of underlying degenerative disease or long-standing tendinitis and impingement. Functionally, the supraspinatus is involved in abduction, the infraspinatus and teres minor in external rotation, and the subscapularis in internal rotation. While all four of the rotator cuff tendons—supraspinatus, infraspinatus, teres minor, and subscapularis—can be involved, the supraspinatus is most frequently torn.

1. **Examination.** The presenting complaint is often pain with or without associated weakness. Pain is often the predominant symptom in the acute injury that results from trauma. This is in contrast to the situation with chronic symptoms, where weakness predominates. Generally, greater than 30% of the involved rotator cuff tendon must be torn to demonstrate weakness. Several tests can be performed to assess the integrity of the rotator cuff tendons. Jobe's test for supraspinatus function is performed with the arm at 90 degrees of abduction and 30 degrees of forward flexion with internal rotation against resistance. Pain and weakness are consistent with a supraspinatus tear. The presence of pain generally implies a minor tear or an inflammatory condition (tendinitis). The drop-arm test is also useful. The arm is passively abducted to 90 degrees and the patient attempts to lower it slowly. If pain develops or the patient is unable to lower the arm slowly, the presence of a rotator cuff tear should be suspected.

Often these tests are difficult to perform in the patient with acute trauma, as pain often limits the patient's ability to perform them. Therefore a patient should be specifically instructed that the presence of continued pain with associated weakness after a shoulder injury should be closely followed up to rule out a rotator cuff tear.

2. **Radiographs.** Radiographic clues to the presence of a rotator cuff tear in acute trauma are often subtle. In the young patient with acute shoulder dislocation, an avulsion of the greater or the lesser tuberosity (insertion sites for the supraspinatus, infraspinatus, teres minor, and subscapularis tendons, respectively) instead of an in-substance rotator cuff tear can occur. In the individual above 40 years of age, there is a 40% to 50% chance of a concomitant rotator cuff tear with a shoulder dislocation, and this percentage increases with increasing age.

   In the patient with chronic shoulder symptoms, some periarticular calcification may be seen radiographically consistent with degenerative changes within the tendons and associated subacromial bursa. Also, elevation of the humeral head on the AP view such that the acromiohumeral interspace is less than 5 mm is strong evidence of a chronic rotator cuff tear with resulting superior displacement of the humeral head. MRI and CT arthrography can confirm the diagnosis. Ultrasound, which may be used as well, is an underused modality for the diagnosis of rotator cuff tears.

3. **Treatment.** The presence of a displaced greater tuberosity or lesser tuberosity avulsion (greater than 1 cm) with a shoulder dislocation often requires surgical repair to optimize the patient's functional outcome. If a rotator cuff tear secondary to an acute traumatic episode is suspected, immobilization in a sling for comfort for 1 to 3 weeks is recommended. The length of immobilization depends on the patient's age. Close follow-up is necessary, as a full-thickness tear due to an acute traumatic event usually requires surgical repair. In the individual with chronic underlying rotator cuff disease, conservative treatment by immobilization is often useful. The persistence of pain and/or weakness with failure to respond to conservative rehabilitation may be an indication for surgery.

4. **Complications.** Unrecognized rotator cuff tears can lead to long-standing pain, weakness, and glenohumeral arthropathy. The longer the tear remains undetected, the poorer the prognosis for both conservative and surgical interventions.

E. **Overuse injuries.** Overuse injuries such as rotator cuff tendinitis, subacromial bursitis, bicipital tendinitis, and degenerative or posttraumatic conditions of the shoulder can occur. A history of previous trauma or repetitive or overhead types of activity is an important historical clue.

1. **Examination.** Pain is often generalized. Active ROM is often limited secondary to pain or significant rotator cuff pathology. Passive ROM is often intact. Specific tests such as Jobe's, as already described for supraspinatus pathology, are useful. Speed's test for bicipital tendinitis elicits pain in the bicipital groove with forward flexion against resistance with the arm abducted and elbow extended and resupinated. Often this represents not only an acute inflammatory condition but also some underlying biomechanical instability.

2. **Radiographs.** These are often normal. The presence of periarticular calcification, such as that seen adjacent laterally or superior to the humeral head, is helpful in diagnosing calcific tendinitis or bursitis but is not pathognomonic.

3. **Treatment.** In general the treatment of inflammatory conditions of the shoulder involves NSAIDs, ice, and a brief period (1 week) of immobilization. Subacromial injection utilizing aseptic techniques with a local anesthetic such as lidocaine and a steroid preparation (e.g., triamcinolone, dexamethasone) is appropriate in the emergency department provided that there is no suspicion of a septic joint and the patient's history, physical exam, and radiographic findings are consistent with an overuse inflammatory condition. The preferred approaches for subacromial bursal injection into the shoulder are the posterolateral and lateral. It is often recommended that if there is acute calcific bursitis, aspiration of the calcium should be attempted with a large-bore needle (18 to 20 gauge). However, this rarely succeeds and will probably only worsen the patient's pain.

   If the patient has tendinitis of the long head of the biceps, infiltration of the medial lateral edge of the long head of the biceps at the level of the bicipital groove can also be accomplished with a local anesthetic and dexamethasone. Orthopaedic referral is recommended. Treatment for acute rupture of the long head of the biceps tendon is immediate sling immobilization. Close orthopaedic referral is required because surgical reattachment may be necessary in the most active patients. In the sedentary or older individual, surgical repair may not be indicated, since the loss in overall biceps strength is usually less than 15% to 20%.

4. **Complications.** Adhesive capsulitis (frozen shoulder) can result from chronic inflammation or prolonged periods of immobilization, with resulting limitation of active and passive ROM.

BIBLIOGRAPHY

Donovan PJ, Paulos LE. Common injuries of the shoulder—diagnosis and treatment. *West J Med* 1995;163:351–359.

Bigliani LV, Craig EV, Butters KP. Fractures of the shoulder. In: Rockwood CA, Green DP, Buscholz RW, eds. *Fractures in adults;* 3rd. ed. Philadelphia: JB Lippincott, 1991:871–1020.

Rockwood CA, Thomas SC, Matsen FA. Subluxations and dislocations about the glenohumeral joint. In: Rockwood CA, Green DP, Buscholz RW, eds. *Fractures in adults;* 3rd. ed. Philadelphia: JB Lippincott, 1991:1021–1179.

Quaday KA. The shoulder. In: Ruiz E, Cicero JJ, eds. *Emergency management of skeletal injuries.* St. Louis: Mosby, 1995:179–210.

Simon RR, Koenigshnecht SJ. The shoulder and upper arm. In: *Emergency orthopedics—the extremities,* 3rd ed. Appleton & Lange, 1996:385–412.

Proximal and Midshaft Humeral Injuries

Brian Aldred

I. **Fractures of the proximal humerus**
   A. **Introduction.** Shoulder injuries frequently present to the emergency department with fractures of the proximal humerus. A fall is the usual mechanism of injury, with osteoporosis a likely contributing factor. Intricate movements of the shoulder are necessary for optimal function of this extremity. The shoulder complex involves an intricate anatomy and biomechanics to allow for these elaborate movements. Included in the shoulder complex are four major joints; the glenohumeral, acromioclavicular, sternoclavicular, and scapulothoracic. The glenohumeral joint is a focus in our discussion of proximal humeral fractures. The physician must understand its anatomy and mechanics for proper diagnosis and treatment. A thorough assessment entails history, including mechanism of injury, physical examination, and adequate radiographic studies. Although various treatments exist, the majority of patients are best suited for conservative therapy with sling and swath or shoulder immobilizer. Close orthopaedic follow-up and appropriate rehabilitation helps to ensure a successful outcome.

   The first documentation of a fracture of the proximal humerus was made in 460 B.C. by Hippocrates. Many other reports discuss treatment of most fractures by immobilization in a sling followed by range-of-motion exercises. Many well-known orthopaedists attempted classification schemes to aid in diagnosis and treatment. In 1970, Neer developed a comprehensive system based on an earlier anatomical classification. It involves fracture type, anatomy, biomechanics, and displacement, providing uniformity of diagnosis and treatment. It is currently the most commonly used classification system (1).
   B. **Anatomy and mechanics.** The glenohumeral joint includes the glenoid cavity, which has enough surface area for only one-fourth to one-third the size of the humeral head. This property aids in the joint's vast range of motion but relies on capsule, ligaments, and muscles for stability. The proximal humerus consists of the head, lesser tuberosity, greater tuberosity, and shaft (Fig. 1). These four fragments form anatomical landmarks that can help to define treatment and prognosis (1,2).

   The anatomical neck is at the junction of the head and tuberosities, just distal to the articular surface of the humerus. It is differentiated from the surgical

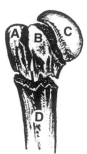

Fig. 1. Codman's four fragments of the proximal humerus. A: Greater tuberosity. B: Lesser tuberosity. C: Head. D: Shaft.

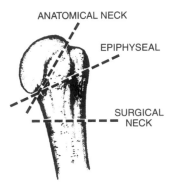

Fig. 2. Anatomical levels of proximal humeral fractures: anatomical neck, epiphysis and tuberosities, and surgical neck.

neck, which is distal to the greater and lesser tuberosities (Fig. 2). Fractures through the anatomical neck, although rare, have a poor prognosis. Such a fracture disrupts the blood supply to the humeral head from the arcuate artery, an ascending branch of the anterior humeral circumflex artery (1).

The proximal humerus is unstable in the glenoid fossa with its bony articulation, but is secured by numerous muscular attachments. The major muscles to be considered are the rotator cuff muscles (supraspinatus, infraspinatus, teres minor, and subscapularis), the deltoid and pectoralis major. The tendon insertions of these muscles influence displacement of fracture fragments (Fig. 3).

1. **The supraspinatus, infraspinatus, and teres minor** cause superior and posterior displacement via their insertion on the greater tuberosity.
2. **The deltoid and pectoralis muscles** insert distal to the surgical neck and cause proximal and medial displacement.

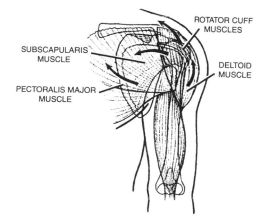

Fig. 3. Bony and muscular structure of the shoulder, showing displacing forces. Fractures are displaced according to the pull of muscular attachments upon the proximal humeral fragments.

3. **The subscapularis** inserts on the lesser tuberosity and causes medial and anterior displacement (1).

   The anterior humeral circumflex artery provides the major blood supply to the proximal humerus. An ascending branch, the arcuate artery, is the principal supplier to the humeral head. The brachial plexus and axillary artery can be injured with trauma to the proximal humerus. Isolated injuries can also occur to three important nerves of the shoulder: the axillary, suprascapular, and musculocutaneous nerves. These all arise from fibers from the fifth and sixth cervical roots. The axillary nerve supplies the deltoid and teres minor muscles and the suprascapular nerve innervates the supraspinatus and infraspinatus muscles. The musculocutaneous nerve supplies the coracobrachialis, biceps, and brachialis muscles. These nerves are usually injured by traction at points of fixation.

C. **History.** Proximal humeral fractures account for 4% to 5% of all fractures and occur at nearly 70% of the reported rate of proximal femur fractures. The proximal humerus is the most common site of humeral fractures, and women outnumber men almost 2 to 1. Osteoporosis is the most common risk factor, although there is also an increased incidence of alcoholism and prior gastric resection in individuals who sustain proximal humeral fractures (2–5).

   Most commonly, a fall on the outstretched hand from standing height or lower is the mechanism of injury.

Besides falls, direct blows, either blunt or penetrating, can result in proximal humeral fractures. Pathological fractures due to metastatic disease commonly affect the proximal humerus and can result from relatively minor trauma. Less commonly, electric shock and seizures have been etiological factors.

D. **Assessment.** As with all patients, a primary survey of the general status, including the airway, breathing, and circulation (ABCs), must precede any localized assessment of the extremity. The clinical presentation of most proximal humeral fractures will be acutely after a fall. Pain, swelling, and arm deformity are common complaints. Physical examination will usually confirm tenderness and edema. Crepitation and ecchymosis may also be present. Arm deformity is common and can be manifest as shortening or angulation, depending on the location of injury. The patient commonly has a very limited range of motion and holds the arm closely against the torso. The definitive diagnosis is made radiographically.

Neurovascular status is assessed initially and again after manipulation of the arm. The brachial plexus and axillary artery lie in close proximity to the proximal humerus. A high index of suspicion for neurovascular injuries is needed in a patient with complaints of paresthesias or sensory deficits. Intact lateral sensation to the arm is indicative of preserved deltoid neurological function via the axillary nerve. This is important, since motor examination is likely to be limited because of pain. Distal neurovascular status should be tested and documented. Head, eye, ear, nose, and throat (HEENT) and chest examination are also important. Rare complications of proximal humeral injuries include thoracic penetration and pneumothorax (1,2,6).

Fracture/dislocations need special mention owing to the diagnostic difficulties they pose. Posterior fracture/dislocations are commonly missed by the initial treating physician (7). Observation of shoulder contour, including palpation of the anterior and posterior joint for bulging or depression, can aid in diagnosis. A high index of suspicion is necessary, especially in patients with multiple trauma, altered mental status, or those who are postictal or have a history of electric shock. Ultimately the diagnosis must be made with the appropriate radiographs.

E. **Radiography.** The essential views necessary for proper assessment are included in the shoulder series. These consist of anteroposterior and lateral (Y-view) radiographs in the scapular plane and, if possible, an axillary view. With these three views, the joint is viewed in three separate perpendicular planes. The axillary view is best for visualizing the glenoid surface. The Y view is most helpful in the diagnosis of anterior and posterior dislocations. If the diagnosis is yet unclear, further imaging can include tomograms or computed tomography (CT).

F. **Diagnosis.** The Neer four-part classification of proximal humeral fractures is based on the relationship of the four major fragments: the lesser tuberosity, greater tuberosity, humeral head, and humeral shaft. Proper x-rays can identify these anatomical fragments. This classification is not a memorization scheme but is based on the anatomical relations of the fracture segments to each other. This scheme provides uniformity for describing proximal humeral fractures (Fig. 4). The focus is on recognition of more complex *displaced* fractures that more likely will disrupt the vascular integrity to the humeral head. Thus, with proper identification, avascular necrosis and its long-term sequelae can be minimized. Displacement is defined as a separation from a neighboring segment of more than 1 cm or angulation of more than 45 degrees. Multiple fracture lines may be present, but if these criteria are not met, the lesion is classified as a minimally displaced fracture. Surrounding soft tissue will keep the fragments in close proximity. Fortunately, the majority, over 80%, of proximal humeral injuries are minimally displaced (1,2,4,7,8).

Multiple-part fractures are more difficult to treat. Complications are more common, including avascular necrosis, nonunion, and neurovascular compromise. Recognition of displacement is essential to minimize these pitfalls (1,4,9). In a two-part fracture, one fragment is displaced in relation to the other three fragments. If the anatomical neck is involved, vascular integrity to the head may be impaired. Displacement of the surgical neck may damage the brachial plexus and axillary artery. Three-part fractures have two fragments displaced in reference to each other and the other two fragments, but the humeral head is within the glenoid. Four-part fractures have all fragments displaced and the head out of the glenoid. A fracture/dislocation is described by Neer as either anterior or posterior and according to the number of fracture fragments. By definition, a fracture/dislocation must have a humeral fracture and the head must be outside the joint space. Fractures of the greater tuberosity are more likely seen with anterior dislocations and are commonly associated with rotator cuff tears. Impression and head-splitting fractures are special fractures that Neer described as involving injuries to the articular surface (1,4,7). An orthopaedic surgeon should be consulted early after recognition of displaced fractures. These fractures are illustrated in the Neer classification in Fig. 4.

G. **Treatment.** A simple sling with or without swath will usually suffice during transport in the prehospital setting prior to definitive diagnosis and therapy. The optimal positioning of the patient is upright, if possible,

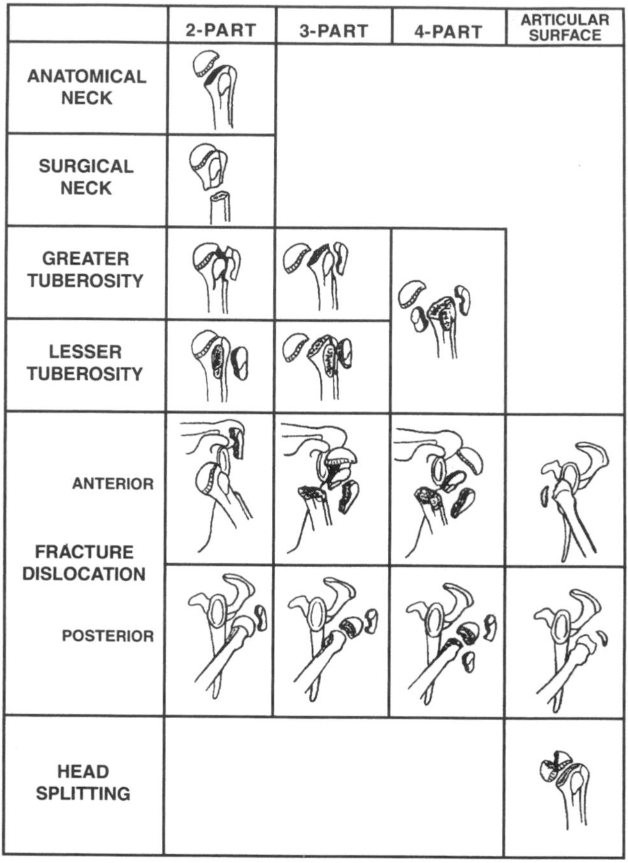

	2-PART	3-PART	4-PART	ARTICULAR SURFACE
ANATOMICAL NECK				
SURGICAL NECK				
GREATER TUBEROSITY				
LESSER TUBEROSITY				
FRACTURE DISLOCATION — ANTERIOR				
FRACTURE DISLOCATION — POSTERIOR				
HEAD SPLITTING				

Fig. 4.   Neer classification. This is a four-part scheme based on the displacement of the four major fragments and their relation to each other. Displacement is defined as separation of more than 1 cm or angulation of more than 45 degrees. Minimally displaced fractures, even with multiple fracture lines, are not included in this classification. With proper diagnosis of displaced fractures, optimal treatment can be applied, minimizing such complications as avascular necrosis.

allowing mild gravity distraction to the injury. The arm should be against the torso in full adduction with the elbow flexed 90 degrees.

Fortunately, conservative treatment is ideal for the majority of patients, since most fractures of the proximal humerus are minimally displaced. Furthermore, more severe fractures may occur in patients with limited functionality who are poor surgical candidates. Therefore, more conservative therapy may be adequate and preferred in these situations.

Successful outcomes are usually obtained with a simple sling of the extremity and early range-of-motion exercises. Minimally displaced fractures of the proximal humerus should be immobilized in a sling at the side or in the Velpeau position. A swath or shoulder immobilizer helps optimize initial immobilization and thus increases patient comfort. Outpatient treatment and orthopaedic referral are recommended provided that there is adequate pain control and there are no complicating concomitant injuries. If the fracture segment is clinically stable and moves as a unit, gentle range-of-motion exercises may be initiated by 7 to 10 days postinjury. Pain and muscular spasm will have decreased. Aggressive exercising should be avoided to prevent distraction of the fracture segments, which may lead to malunion or nonunion. Within 4 to 8 weeks, range of motion usually increases vastly, but patients should be followed closely for improvement through a rehabilitation program.

Displaced fractures commonly require more complex treatment. Closed reduction may be attempted for displaced fractures, although an understanding of the deformity and displacing forces is necessary. It is important to provide adequate analgesia and sedation to allow muscular relaxation. One should always obtain premanipulation and postreduction radiographs as well as documentation of neurovascular status after any manipulation of the fracture. Many displaced fractures are infrequently amenable to closed reduction.

Closed reduction can be attempted for a two-part fracture of the surgical neck. Success may be limited owing to the interposition of soft tissue, usually the long head of the biceps. On the other hand, a two-part fracture involving the anatomical neck will usually require open reduction and internal fixation (ORIF), since adequate alignment and reduction of fragments are difficult to achieve by closed techniques. Two-part fractures of the greater tuberosity and lesser tuberosity may sometimes be treated closed but more likely will require inpatient treatment for ORIF. If a two-part fracture of the greater tuberosity is associated with an anterior dislocation, closed reduction of the humeral head dislocation can reduce the fracture. The

Neer classification shown in Fig. 4 illustrates these fractures. Again, the basis of this classification and treatment recommendations are to optimize the vascular integrity of the humeral head. By adequate reduction of the fracture with open or closed techniques, complications and especially avascular necrosis of the humeral head can be decreased. Patients treated with closed reduction may be followed as outpatients by an orthopaedist.

Inpatient treatment with ORIF is probably necessary for best results in three- and four-part fractures. There is a greatly increased incidence of avascular necrosis, especially in four-part fractures treated with closed reduction (1,6,7). Most fracture/dislocations and comminuted fractures as well as significantly displaced fractures must be treated with operative techniques. The Neer classification can act as a guide for optimal therapy and outcome. After proper identification of the type of displaced fracture of the proximal humerus, this classification scheme helps categorize fractures that are best suited for closed or open techniques.

ORIF has been a popular operative treatment for various fractures. Numerous other treatments have useful roles in fracture care including percutaneous techniques, external fixation and humeral head replacement. These decisions will be made in close consultation with an orthopaedic specialist. Fracture type, bone quality, the patient's underlying health status, as well as patient compliance will help the orthopaedist to choose the definitive treatment (1).

H. **Complications.** Fortunately, most proximal humeral fractures are minimally displaced, with infrequent complications. Many complications have, however, been reported. These include early problems, such as rotator cuff or biceps tendon rupture, neurovascular injuries, and thoracic injuries. The source of these is usually the initial trauma. Late complications may become evident on follow-up examination or during rehabilitation; they include avascular necrosis, nonunion, malunion, infection, hardware failure, and frozen shoulder (1,6,7).

Vascular injury, usually to the axillary artery, has been reported in nearly 5% of displaced fractures (6). The key to successful treatment is early diagnosis and repair. It is important to check the radial pulse even in seemingly trivial trauma. Paresthesias should raise the physician's index of suspicion of vascular injury. Angiography can confirm the diagnosis and repair should be done on an emergent basis to prevent limb-threatening sequelae.

Brachial plexus injuries can occur in up to 6% of proximal humeral fractures (6). Axillary nerve injury is the most common isolated injury. Thorough neurological examination, including sensory and motor power, is required. Pain and muscular spasm make assessment of motor strength in the acutely injured patient difficult. Intact sensation over the deltoid indicates good axillary nerve function. With minor brachial plexus injuries, nerve dysfunction may not be apparent until the rehabilitation period. Any neurological impairment should trigger emergent orthopaedic consultation. Nevertheless, neuropraxia of the axillary nerve is often given a 2- to 3-month trial of conservative therapy prior to surgical exploration.

Late complications vary and may result from the initial injury or the subsequent treatment. A frozen shoulder or adhesive capsulitis occurs secondary to inadequate rehabilitation, prolonged immobilization, or, rarely, impinging mechanical hardware. This is the most common complication of proximal humeral fractures. Operative release of adhesions is sometimes necessary to alleviate stiffness and pain. This should occur only after an adequate program of physical therapy fails. **Malunion** describes a healed fracture after inadequate reduction or fixation and often requires surgical repair. **Nonunions** are rare and occur more often in older, osteoporotic patients. Occasionally, overaggressive rehabilitation or inadequate immobilization via hanging cast methods is responsible. Nonunion due to infection, poor bone quality, or failed fixation is a known complication of operative interventions.

Avascular necrosis has occurred in up to 34% of patients, especially in the more complex three- and four-part fractures (9). To relieve the stiff, painful joint, treatment entails the use of a humeral head prosthesis or even total shoulder replacement if the glenoid is affected.

I. **Disposition.** Most patients will have minimally displaced fractures and can be treated as outpatients with shoulder immobilization, analgesics, and early mobilization. Early follow-up with an orthopaedist and the importance of beginning passive motion within 7 to 10 days should be stressed to these patients. More complex fractures—including displaced, comminuted and unstable fractures as well as fracture/dislocations—require emergent orthopaedic referral for definitive care. A high index of suspicion is needed for any signs or symptoms of neurovascular compromise even in the case of seemingly trivial injuries. Emergent referral for further diagnostic studies and definitive therapy should be made in any patient with neurovascular impairment.

J. **Rehabilitation.** Proper rehabilitation will optimize patient outcome and can prevent some complications. A well-organized regimen involving the surgeon, therapist, and patient is essential. Early passive motion has been shown to be a key to success in fractures of the proximal humeral. To allow this, the fracture must be stable and pain and muscular spasm must be controlled. Early in the course of nondisplaced proximal humeral fractures, elbow and wrist range-of-motion exercises should be performed while the sling and swath is in place. Most authors recommend a three-phase rehabilitation program. This consists of passive assistance exercises initially, then stretching exercises and active and early resistive training, and finally maintenance therapy and strengthening (1,7).

K.   **Summary.** Proximal humeral fractures are relatively common; therefore the physician should understand the complex anatomy of the shoulder as well as the appropriate diagnostic and treatment options. Assessment must include mechanism of injury, physical examination, and adequate radiographs. A thorough examination for associated injuries and neurovascular compromise is essential for proper assessment and therapy. The definitive diagnosis is made radiographically. The Neer classification can act as a diagnostic guide to optimize treatment and outcome. Fortunately, most shoulder fractures are minimally displaced and treated easily with closed techniques, usually with a shoulder immobilizer. Operative treatment is probably necessary for more complex displaced fractures. Also, close orthopaedic referral and adequate rehabilitation will ensure a successful outcome.

II.   **Fractures of the humeral shaft**

A.   **Introduction.** Fractures of the humeral shaft represent approximately 1% to 2% of all fractures. Closed treatment options are numerous and usually successful. Because the glenohumeral joint has the greatest mobility of any joint in the body, shortening and angulation of the humerus is well tolerated. With special attention given to injuries of the radial nerve, complications rarely occur. Proper rehabilitation and follow-up can help optimize results (10–12).

B.   **Anatomy and mechanics.** The humeral shaft extends from the upper border of the insertion of the pectoralis major muscle to the supracondylar ridges proximal to the elbow. The arm is divided into two soft tissue compartments, anterior and posterior. The humerus is not designed anatomically for weight bearing, which is the main mechanism of injury from falls on an outstretched hand. Because of the muscular attachments, the humeral fragments displace differently according to the level of injury. A thorough understanding of the anatomy and distracting forces involved will greatly aid the physician in reduction and treatment.

In fractures proximal to the attachment of the pectoralis major muscle, the proximal fragment is pulled laterally and superiorly by the rotator cuff. In a fracture proximal to the deltoid insertion, the distal fragment is displaced laterally and the proximal fragment is pulled medially. A fracture line distal to the deltoid

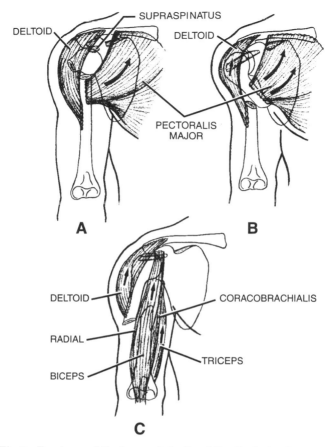

Fig. 5. Fractures of the humeral shaft and the displacing forces. Above the pectoralis insertion, the proximal fragment is pulled laterally and superiorly by the rotator cuff. Proximal to the deltoid insertion, the proximal humerus is displaced medially by the pectoralis. A fracture below the deltoid causes shortening.

insertion causes shortening of the extremity, with the proximal portion pulled laterally and anteriorly and the distal portion pulled upward by the biceps and triceps muscles (Fig. 5).

C. **History.** The most frequent mechanism of injury to the humeral shaft is a fall. There is a bimodal distribution, with younger males (between the ages of 16 and 24) involved in more motor vehicle accidents and with penetrating wounds. Rarely, stress from vigorous activity has been implicated. A suspicion for a pathological process should be sought in fractures due to less severe trauma in younger patients. In older women (aged 56 to 65), falls are the most frequent cause. Osteoporosis and metastatic disease are common contributing factors. Bending mechanisms usually affect the shaft, whereas compression forces tend to injure either end of the humerus. The patient with a humeral fracture usually presents with pain, swelling, and occasionally deformity. Complaints of distal weakness or paresthesias should heighten suspicion for neurovascular injury (12–14).

D.   Physical examination. Always assess the patient for life-threatening problems prior to focusing on examination of the extremity. A fracture of the humeral shaft is associated with tenderness, edema, and sometimes deformity. Crepitation and instability may be present at the fracture site. Palpation of the anterior and posterior arm should be performed for any signs of compartment syndrome. This complication is rare, since the compartments are relatively spacious. Vascular integrity can be ascertained by palpation of brachial, radial, and ulnar pulses and by assessment of distal capillary refill. Evaluation of neurological function includes examination of the distal motor and sensory function of the radial, ulnar, and median nerves. Special attention should be given to the radial nerve as it traverses the humeral shaft from posterior to anterior. Radial nerve injury is the most common complication associated with fractures of the humeral shaft. A wrist drop may make the diagnosis obvious. Neurovascular status should be documented prior to and following any manipulation. This is best illustrated with radial nerve palsy. If this palsy is associated with the original injury, the treatment is usually conservative. The usual cause is a stretching injury to the nerve, which usually heals well without invasive treatment. Contrarily, treatment is often surgical if radial nerve dysfunction occurs after reduction techniques due to impingement of the nerve between fracture fragments. Untreated, this will more likely result in long-term neurological dysfunction. Finally, skin integrity should be observed.

E.   Radiography. Proper radiographs should include at least two views of the entire shaft of the humerus. Also, the shoulder and elbow joints should be visualized. Other diagnostic tests such as angiography may be performed, although this would be done after emergent referral to a surgeon.

F.   Diagnosis. The fracture may be classified initially as open or closed. The fracture fragments will be displaced according to muscular attachments. Bending mechanisms usually produce transverse fractures. Falls with axial loading and torsion forces cause oblique or spiral fractures. Comminution should be documented. Associated injuries with special attention given to neurovascular status should be sought.

Also, the integrity of bone can influence treatment and outcomes. The humerus is a common site of metastasis with such intrinsic conditions as osteoporosis and neoplasms susceptible to fractures.

G. **Treatment.** Many treatment options are available for fractures of the humeral shaft. Primary goals of treatment are reduction of fracture fragments, immobilization to allow callus formation, and early mobilization to maintain range of motion. As always, initial assessment of the ABCs is necessary prior to treatment of non-life-threatening conditions. In the prehospital setting, immobilization is usually best accomplished by positioning the arm against the chest in an upright patient. This may be difficult and is unacceptable in a patient with multiple trauma. After proper assessment and diagnosis, a fracture of the humeral shaft is usually best treated by distraction to help align fracture fragments and reduce angulation. Adequate analgesia and muscular relaxation are necessary for success.

Treatment can be divided into open and closed techniques. In most patients, closed treatment is preferred. Indications for operative intervention are as follows:

1. Open fractures, which are almost always treated with open reduction and internal fixation (ORIF)
2. Missile injuries such as gunshot wounds
3. Pathological fractures
4. Vascular injuries
5. Shaft fractures associated with elbow injuries
6. Severely comminuted fractures with poor alignment
7. Certain underlying disease states or other associated injuries
8. Multiple trauma, to allow early mobilization and help reduce later complications (10,12–15)

Interestingly, an associated isolated radial nerve palsy is not an absolute indication for ORIF. Most such palsies will resolve spontaneously within weeks to months. Conversely, any radial nerve injury occurring after reduction may require open treatment to reduce entrapment of the radial nerve. ORIF is usually accomplished via primary plate or intramedullary fixation.

Most fractures of the humeral shaft are appropriately treated closed. In the emergent treatment of fractures, swelling can be a complicating factor and circumferential casts should be avoided. Commonly, a coaptation or U-shaped splint is the best initial immobilizer. Also known as a sugar-tong splint, it is a plaster or fiberglass splint placed from high in the axilla in a U shape, down and under the elbow, extending up the lateral arm to the top of the shoulder. The arm is held in approximately 90 degrees of flexion with a sling or collar and cuff. Advantages include ease of application, adequate immobilization, and slight gravity traction to the fracture site. It also allows exercising of the elbow, hand, wrist, and shoulder. It is not a circumferential cast, thus allowing for swelling. Sugartong splints may be used exclusively throughout the course of healing of humeral shaft fractures.

Another frequently used treatment is the hanging cast. Circumferential casting is placed from at least 1 in. proximal to the fracture to the wrist, with the elbow flexed at 90 degrees and the forearm neutral. A sling is affixed to the distal cast via a loop of cast material. The arm must always be dependent to allow traction to the fracture. Thus, the patient must sleep sitting upright. Angulation may be corrected by adjustments to the loop location. The cast must not be made too heavy, as this may cause overdistraction and possibly nonunion. Since 1933, after having been made popular by Caldwell, the hanging cast has been the standard closed treatment (10). More recently, the sugar-tong splint has come into more common use. Criticism of the hanging cast has grown, claiming it to be inconvenient and uncomfortable. Also, the circumferential immobilization can cause a hinging effect at the fracture site and possibly delayed union. Obviously, a compliant and cooperative patient is required for its success.

Other methods used are sling and swath, shoulder spica casting, abduction humeral splinting, skeletal traction, and functional bracing. External fixation has also been used in some cases. Indications include markedly comminuted fractures, bone loss, extensive skin and soft tissue injuries including burns, and multiple limb fractures in which early mobilization is indicated (10).

H. Complications. Both early and late complications may occur after a fracture of the humeral shaft. The most common early complication is radial nerve injury. An estimated 5% to 10% of patients will experience radial nerve problems (10,13,14,16,17). Over 70% of radial nerve injuries occur with fractures to the middle third of the humeral shaft (15). Often, a benign neurapraxia results, which resolves spontaneously in 80% of patients. This may take up to 6 months; but if palsy does not resolve within 3 to 4 months, operative nerve reconstruction may be necessary (15,17). The mechanism of radial nerve injury is usually a stretching or bruising, but even complete lesions have been shown to resolve better with delayed repair versus early operative intervention. Penetrating or open fractures with complicating radial nerve injuries may not resolve; therefore early open techniques may be justified. Radial nerve injuries that occur after reduction or fracture manipulation should be emergently referred to an orthopaedist, who may opt for operative treatment.

Vascular complications are uncommon, but injuries to the brachial artery have been reported in a small portion of humeral shaft fractures (14). Severe sequelae may result, including reflex sympathetic dystrophy, gangrene, infection, and limb loss. Immediate referral and repair are warranted with any vascular injury. Angiography is a good diagnostic test, although emergent evaluation by a surgeon is of utmost importance. In obtaining diagnostic tests, long ischemic times (over 4 to 6 hours) and thus delay in providing definitive therapy should be avoided. Compartment syndromes are rare owing to the fairly roomy compartments of the arm.

Late complications can occur with both open and closed treatments. Nonunion of the bony fragments occurs after at least 4 to 6 months of unsuccessful therapy. Contributing causes are overdistraction of the fracture fragments and interposition of soft tissue. Transverse fractures are more susceptible secondary to minimal contact of the bone surfaces. Union of uncomplicated fractures normally occurs by 10 weeks. Postoperative complications can include infection, radial nerve injury, and unsuccessful repair (10). Without adequate rehabilitation, decreased joint mobility and strength can be seen.

I. **Disposition.** Initially, the physician must assess all injured patients for life-threatening injuries. After a fracture to the humeral shaft has been diagnosed, a decision for open or closed repair must be made. Most fractures can be treated with closed techniques, as by using a coaptation (sugar-tong) splint. Pre- and posttreatment radiographs must be documented and neurovascular status ascertained. Close outpatient orthopaedic referral for an isolated humeral shaft fracture is adequate. If a hanging cast is applied, reexamination by the orthopaedist should take place within 24 to 48 hours to check alignment. Immediate referral to a surgeon is required with radial nerve injury, vascular injury, or fracture requiring ORIF. ORIF is usually indicated for open fractures, severely displaced or comminuted fractures, or fractures with multiple associated injuries.

J. **Rehabilitation.** Long-term care and successful rehabilitation are dependent on many factors. Fracture type, location, complications, associated injuries, and treatment modalities all affect outcomes. More importantly, patient cooperation will greatly influence functionality. A directed treatment plan should be individualized for maximal success. Rehabilitation begins immediately, so that attaining premorbid function is possible. Shoulder, wrist, and hand motions may be started within 1 to 2 days of injury. After stability of the fracture fragments has been established, a well-organized exercise routine should begin. Close supervision by the treating surgeon is an integral part of this rehabilitation.

K.   Summary. After assessing for other injuries, the emergency physician can effectively treat most humeral shaft fractures. Closed techniques such as sugar-tong splinting are adequate for most injuries. Careful examination of the neurovascular status is important. Emergent referral must be made for complicated fractures, including those with neurovascular compromise or requiring ORIF. With proper treatment and disposition, excellent functional outcomes can be attained.

REFERENCES

1. Bigliani LU, Craig EV, Butters KP. Fractures of the shoulder. In: Rockwood CA Jr, Green DP, eds. *Fractures in adults.* Philadelphia: JB Lippincott, 1991:871–927.
2. Basti JJ et al. Management of proximal humeral fractures. *J Hand Ther* 1994;7(2):111–121.
3. Lind T, Kroner TK, Jensen J. The epidemiology of fractures of the proximal humerus. *Arch Orthop Trauma Surg* 1989;108:285–287.
4. Neer CS. Displaced proximal humeral fractures: Part I. Classification and evaluation. *J Bone Joint Surg* 1970;52A:1077–1089.
5. Rose SH, Melton LJ, Moorey BF, et al. Epidemiologic features of humeral fractures. *Clin Orthop* 1982;168:24–30.
6. Stableforth PG. Four-part fractures of the neck of the humerus. *J Bone Joint Surg* 1984;66B:104–108.
7. Neer CS. Four-segment classification of displaced proximal humeral fractures. *AAOS Instr Course Lect* 1975;24:160–168.
8. Neer CS, Rockwood CA Jr. Fractures and dislocations of the shoulder. In: Rockwood CA, Green DP, eds. *Fractures.* Philadelphia: JB Lippincott, 1984:675–707.
9. Hagg O, Lundberg B. Aspects of prognostic factors in comminuted and dislocated proximal humeral fractures. In: Bateman JE, Welsh RP, eds. *Surgery of the shoulder.* Philadelphia: BC Decker, 1984:51–59.
10. Epps CH Jr, Grant RE. Fractures of the shaft of the humerus. In: Rockwood CA Jr, Green DP, eds. *Fractures in adults.* Philadelphia: JB Lippincott, 1991:843–868.
11. Foulk DA, Szabo RM. Diaphyseal humerus fractures: natural history and occurrence of nonunion. *Orthopaedics* 1985;18:3333–3335.
12. Sterner S. Fractures of the humeral shaft. In: Ruiz E, Cicero JJ, eds. *Emergency management of skeletal injuries.* St. Louis: Mosby, 1995:211–219.
13. Bleeker WA, Nijsten MW, ten Duis HJ. Treatment of humeral shaft fractures related to associated injuries. *Acta Orthop Scand* 1991;62:148–153.
14. Mast JW, Spiegel PG, Harvey JP, et al. Fractures of the humeral shaft: a retrospective study of 240 adult fractures. *Clin Orthop* 1975;112:254–262.
15. Moda SK, Chadha NS, Sangwan SS, et al. Open reduction and fixation of proximal humeral fractures and fracture-dislocations. *J Bone Joint Surg* 1990;72B:1050–1052.

16. Samardizic M, Grujiac D, Milinkovic ZB. Radial nerve lesions associated with fractures of the humeral shaft. *Injury* 1990;21: 220–222.
17. Holm CL. Management of humeral shaft fractures: fundamental nonoperative techniques. *Clin Orthop* 1970;71:132–139.
18. Salter RB. *Textbook of disorders and injuries of the musculoskeletal system,* 2nd ed. Baltimore: Williams & Wilkins, 1983: 332–333.

Elbow Injuries

Alok C. Saxena and Jefferson D. Bracey

I. **Anatomy.** The elbow is a synovial hinge joint formed by articulations between the humerus, radius, and ulna. The humerus widens distally to form the medial and lateral condyles. The capitellum of the lateral condyle articulates with the radial head and the trochlea articulates with the ulna. The head of the radius also articulates with the lateral ulna and is held in position by the orbicular ligament. Medial and lateral collateral ligaments provide additional stability. The flexor-pronator muscle group originates from a common tendon that attaches to the medial epicondyle. The extensor-supinator muscle group similarly originates from the lateral epicondyle. The triceps attaches to the olecranon posteriorly and the biceps and brachialis muscles attach to the radius and ulna, respectively. The median nerve passes deep in the antecubital fossa medial to the biceps and brachialis, while the radial nerve passes lateral to the same group of muscles. The ulnar nerve passes posteriorly in a groove between the medial epicondyle and the olecranon process. The brachial artery is palpable medial to the biceps tendon in the antecubital fossa. The olecranon bursa lies over the olecranon process just below the skin. The radiohumeral bursa allows for smooth movement over the radial head with supination and pronation. A third bursa protects the biceps tendon from the radius during flexion of the elbow.

II. **History and physical examination.** Evaluation of an elbow injury in the emergency department begins with obtaining a history and doing a physical examination. A detailed history of the mechanism of injury, description of the location and duration of pain, aggravating factors, and presence of paresthesias or loss of movement should be obtained. Patients most commonly complain of pain, restriction of movement, and swelling. Pain in the elbow may be referred from injuries to the shoulder, forearm, or wrist. Occupational history is especially relevant in the patient presenting with chronic pain. The extremity should be examined for presence of swelling, open wounds, deformities, effusions, and discoloration. Brachial, radial, and ulnar pulses should be palpated and capillary refill assessed. The brachioradialis, biceps, and triceps reflexes should be tested. The radial nerve is responsible for wrist and finger extension. Wrist drop results from a radial nerve injury. Flexion of the wrist and digits, abduction of the thumb, and pronation of the forearm is the function of the median nerve. The ulnar nerve provides adduction of the thumb and motor strength to the interosseus muscles. The radial nerve provides sensation to the dorsum of the hand and is best tested in the web space between the thumb and index finger. The median nerve provides sen-

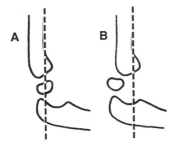

Fig. 1. A: The anterior humeral line should intersect the anterior portion of the middle third of the capitellum. B: With supracondylar fractures, this line passes more anteriorly.

sation over the palmar aspect of the thumb, the index and middle fingers, and the radial half of the ring finger. Sensation to the little finger and the ulnar half of the ring finger is the function of the ulnar nerve. A neurovascular examination should be done initially and then repeated after any manipulation of the injured extremity.

III. **Radiography.** The radiographic examination of the elbow consists of anteroposterior and lateral views. Oblique and specialized views such as the radial head–capitellum view are indicated when specific injuries are suspected. The anterior humeral line is seen on the lateral radiograph and is parallel to the anterior border of the humerus; it should intersect the anterior portion of the middle third of the capitellum. The anterior humeral line is displaced anteriorly in supracondylar fractures such that it passes through the anterior third of the capitellum or is entirely anterior to it (Fig. 1). The radial-capitellar line extends from the center of the radius and should intersect the middle third of the capitellum on the lateral view. Disruption of this line should raise suspicion for a radial head dislocation or fracture and is also useful in evaluating subtle fractures in children.

Fat-pad signs are helpful in diagnosing occult fractures. The anterior fat pad appears as a "ship's sail." The posterior fat pad is associated with a fracture in greater than 90% of patients in the setting of trauma. An effusion in the joint capsule displaces the fat pads. The fat-pad sign is not pathognomonic for fracture, as it is also seen in arthritis, gout, pseudogout, infection, neoplasm, and other disease processes causing an intraarticular fluid collections.

IV. **Fractures of the elbow**

A. **Supracondylar fractures**

1. **Mechanism of injury.** Supracondylar fractures are most commonly seen in children. The mechanism is a fall on an outstretched hand with the elbow in extension. The strength of the collateral ligaments and joint capsule of the elbow is greater than that of bone in children. A similar mechanism of injury in adults may result in an elbow dislocation.

2. **Physical examination.** The child will present holding the upper extremity immobilized with the elbow flexed at 90 degrees and localized swelling and tenderness. A neurovascular examination is important to exclude brachial artery and median nerve injury as a result of anterior angulation of the sharp, distal end of the proximal fragment into the antecubital fossa. Some 25% of supracondylar fractures in children are of the greenstick variety.

3. **Treatment**
   a. **Nondisplaced or minimally displaced fractures.** Treatment is a posterior splint from axilla to palm with the elbow flexed to 90 degrees and referral to an orthopaedic surgeon. Because of the possibility of **occult fracture,** a child with localized tenderness and swelling should be splinted even in the absence of a definite radiographic fracture.
   b. **Displaced fractures**
      (1) **Closed reduction.** In displaced fractures, the distal fragment is usually displaced posteriorly (extension type). Anterior displacement of the distal fragment is caused by a direct blow to the posterior aspect of the flexed elbow (flexion type). An arteriogram should be obtained if an arterial injury is suspected. Closed reduction of a displaced fracture should be attempted by the emergency physician if neurovascular compromise is present. After appropriate parenteral anesthesia, the patient's wrist is grasped and firm traction in line with the longitudinal axis of the arm is applied. The forearm is kept in neutral position (thumb up). Medial or lateral displacement is corrected while traction is maintained. After correction of angular deformity and restoration of length, the elbow is gently flexed to just beyond 90 degrees. Angulation is corrected to a normal carrying angle of 12 to 15 degrees (Fig. 2).
      (2) Displaced fractures require **internal fixation** or **percutaneous pinning** if closed reduction is not successful. Flexion-type fractures may also require surgical treatment and should be splinted in extension. Range-of-motion exercises should be started 1 to 2 weeks after internal fixation.

      Patients with displaced supracondylar fractures should be admitted because of the risk of delayed swelling and neu-

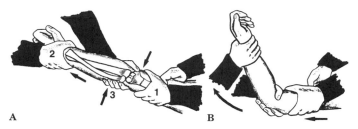

Fig. 2. Technique for reduction of supracondylar fractures. A: Firm traction (2) countertraction (1) is applied while medial or lateral displacement is corrected (3). B: The elbow is flexed just beyond 90°.

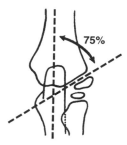

Fig. 3. Baumann's angle as measured on an anteroposterior film.

rovascular compromise, including development of Volkman ischemic contractures. Delayed swelling may also lead to transient loss of the radial pulse in 10% of patients.

4. **Complications.** Some 25% to 60% of patients experience a loss of the normal carrying angle of 10 to 15 degrees valgus. Baumann's angle is formed by the intersection of a line on the anteroposterior (AP) film through the midshaft of the humerus and growth plate of the capitellum. This normally measures 75 degrees and is abnormally increased with medial tilting of the distal fragment. Measurement of Baumann's angle is predictive of an acceptable carrying angle (Fig. 3).

B. **Intercondylar fractures** are rare; they are seen in older patients with brittle bones.

1. **Mechanism of injury** is a direct blow to the flexed elbow.

2. **Physical examination.** Patients present to the emergency department with a complaint of elbow pain. Tenderness to palpation is found on examination; neurovascular compromise is uncommon.

3. **Radiographs.** Intercondylar fractures are described by their radiographic appearance as T- or Y-shaped fractures.
4. **Treatment** is based on the degree of separation of the condyles from each other and from the proximal humeral fragment. Treatment rarely requires manipulation by the emergency physician. Referral is made to orthopaedic surgery.
    a. **Nondisplaced fractures** should be placed in a posterior splint for 3 weeks followed by an active range-of-motion program.
    b. **Displaced fractures** require internal fixation and range-of-motion exercises in 1 week. Severely comminuted fractures are treated with olecranon traction for 3 to 4 weeks if operative repair is not possible. Traction across the elbow with the arm extended may relieve neurovascular compromise. Admission may be recommended by the orthopaedic surgeon.

C. **Medial condylar fracture**
1. **Mechanism of injury.** Medial condylar fractures are less common than lateral condylar fractures; they result from a fall on an outstretched hand, a direct blow to the elbow applied medially through the olecranon, or forced abduction with elbow in extension.
2. **Physical examination.** Patients present with pain in the medial aspect of the elbow and pain with flexion of the wrist.
3. **Radiographically** the fracture involves the articular surface and nonarticular epicondylar portion of the distal humerus. The distal fragments may be displaced anteriorly and inferiorly by the pull of forearm flexors.
4. **Treatment**
    a. The treatment of a **nondisplaced** or **minimally displaced condylar fracture** is immobilization of the flexed elbow in a long arm posterior splint with forearm pronated and wrist flexed. Range-of-motion exercises should be started as early as 2 to 3 weeks postinjury.
    b. Fractures with **displacement greater than 3 mm** require surgical intervention.
5. **Complications.** A high rate of complications (valgus/varus deformity, lateral transposition of forearm, posttraumatic arthritis, delayed ulnar nerve palsy, and avascular necrosis of the trochlea) necessitates orthopaedic consultation.

D. **Lateral condylar fractures**
1. **Mechanism of injury.** Lateral condylar fractures are the result of a fall on an outstretched hand, a direct blow to the lateral aspect of the flexed elbow, or a force that causes adduction and hyperextension with avulsion of the lateral condyle.

2. **Physical examination.** Patients present with pain and tenderness over the lateral elbow.
3. **Radiographs** may show widening of the intercondylar distance with the distal fragment displaced posterior and inferior to its normal position.
4. **Treatment**
   a. Treatment of a **nondisplaced** or **minimally displaced condylar fracture** is immobilization of the flexed elbow in a long arm posterior splint with forearm supinated and wrist extended to relieve tension on the extensor muscle attachments. Active range-of-motion exercises should begin 2 to 3 weeks postinjury.
   b. Surgery is indicated in cases of **displaced fracture**
5. **Complications** are similar to those seen with medial condylar fractures.

E. **Epicondylar fractures**
   1. **Mechanism of injury.** Epicondylar fractures are more common in children and often involve the apophyses. The medial epicondyle is more commonly involved than the lateral. These fractures are caused by direct blows to the medial epicondyle or a posterior elbow dislocation in children. A third mechanism results in avulsion of the medial epicondyle or a compression fracture of the subchondral bone of the lateral condyle or or radial head ("Little Leaguer's elbow") and occurs from a repetitive valgus stress (as in throwing a ball).
   2. **Physical examination.** Patients present with the elbow held in flexion, a prominent olecranon if associated with a dislocation, and tenderness to palpation over the medial epicondyle. Flexion of the forearm increases pain. The young, athletic patient will present with pain in the medial epicondyle or radial head in the absence of an acute injury. Paresthesias or decreased sensation over the palmar aspect of the fifth digit and hypothenar eminence or motor weakness in the interossei suggests ulnar nerve injury.
   3. **Radiographs** should be carefully examined to identify presence of intraarticular fragments.
   4. **Treatment** of a nondisplaced or minimally displaced fracture is immobilization with a posterior splint, with the elbow and wrist flexed and forearm pronated. Orthopaedic consultation is indicated with displaced fractures or interarticular fragments.
   5. **Complications.** The most common complication is ulnar nerve palsy, seen in 60% of patients.

F. **Capitellum fractures**
   1. **Mechanism of injury.** Fractures of the capitellum are the result of a fall on an outstretched

hand or a posterior elbow dislocation and may be associated with a radial head fracture. The capitellum has no muscular attachments; therefore the fragment may remain nondisplaced.

2. **Physical examination.** Patients may not experience pain or tenderness until there is significant swelling within the capsule. Flexion of the elbow will increase pain.

3. **Treatment** includes immobilization in a posterior splint, use of ice packs, elevation, compression, and analgesia. Surgery may be indicated in fractures with displaced fragments or if perfect anatomical alignment is not seen on radiographs.

4. **Complications** include posttraumatic arthritis, avascular necrosis of fracture fragments, nonunion, and restricted range of motion.

G. **Trochlear fractures**

1. **Mechanism of injury.** Fractures of the trochlea are extremely rare. They are highly unusual as isolated injuries and are more often the result of posterior elbow dislocation.

2. **Physical examination.** Although joint stability is maintained by the condyles, motion may be impeded by fracture fragments.

3. **Treatment.** Nondisplaced fractures may be treated with immobilization, whereas more complicated fractures may require internal fixation.

4. **Complications** are similar to those seen with fractures of the capitellum.

H. **Radial head fractures** are the most common elbow injuries in adults.

1. **The mechanism of injury** is a fall on an outstretched hand that drives the radial head into the capitellum. There is usually associated damage to the articular surface of the capitellum and collateral ligaments; in cases of radial head displacement, there is significant soft tissue injury.

2. **Physical examination.** Patients present with pain and tenderness over the radial head and pain with pronation and supination of the forearm.

3. **Radiographs** demonstrate fad-pad signs even in the absence of a visible fracture. A radial head–capitellum view may aid in identification of the fracture.

4. **Treatment.** Radial head fractures are classified as **nondisplaced, displaced,** or **comminuted.**

   a. Treatment of a **nondisplaced** or **minimally displaced fracture** is a sling support or posterior splint and range-of-motion exercises within 24 to 48 hours. Aspiration of the hemarthrosis and injection of 0.5% bupivacaine (Marcaine) into the joint space in the emergency department may provide dramatic pain relief and expedite mobilization of the extremity. Limited range of motion after joint anesthesia may identify entrapped fragments.

b. **Fractures displaced more than 3 mm or involving more than one-third of the joint surface** should be treated surgically with the insertion of small screws.

c. **Comminuted fractures** are treated with a sling and range-of-motion exercises in 1 to 2 weeks. The treatment of **severely comminuted and displaced fractures** is controversial; options include excision of fragments or complete radial head excision with or without Silastic implants. Examination of the wrist for tenderness is important to identify the **Essex-Lopresti lesion**—a radial head fracture with disruption of the distal radioulnar joint ligaments and forearm interosseous membrane. For best results, treatment calls for early internal fixation.

I. **Olecranon fractures**

1. **The mechanism of injury** is a direct blow or fall on an outstretched hand. These fractures are usually intraarticular. The pull of the triceps displaces the proximal olecranon proximally.

2. **Physical examination** reveals tenderness over the olecranon, a palpable separation at the fracture site, and inability to extend the elbow against resistance. The ulnar nerve is particularly susceptible to injury. Loss of sensation over the palmar aspect of the fifth digit and hypothenar eminence or motor weakness of the interosseus ligament confirms ulnar nerve injury.

3. **Treatment** varies with the amount of displacement and requires orthopaedic consultation.

a. **Nondisplaced fractures** should be treated with rest, ice, compression, elevation of the extremity, and analgesia, with immobilization of the elbow in a posterior splint and range-of-motion exercises in 2 to 3 weeks.

b. **Displacement of more than 2 mm** on a lateral radiograph is an indication for open reduction and internal fixation.

4. **Complications** may include an associated ulnar nerve injury in 10% of cases.

J. **Radial head subluxation** or **"nursemaid's elbow"** represents 20% of upper extremity pediatric injuries and is most commonly seen in children 1 to 3 years of age.

1. **The mechanism of injury** is a sudden longitudinal pull on the forearm. The child presents with the arm in passive pronation and slight flexion at the elbow. Supination of the forearm is difficult owing to the presence of fibers of the annular ligament that are stuck between the capitellum and head of the radius.

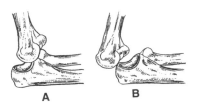

Fig. 4.   Posterior (A) and anterior (B) elbow dislocations.

2. **Physical examination.** The child is unable and unwilling to move the arm; direct tenderness is palpated over the head of radius, with resistance to supination noted.
3. **Radiographs** are required only if the child will not resume use of the arm after reduction and in the presence of swelling, deformity, or an uncharacteristic history.
4. **Treatment** is reduction by supination of the forearm while the examiner's thumb places slight pressure on the radial head. In one continuous motion, the elbow is supinated and flexed. A click may be felt as the radial head reduces. The patient should be asymptomatic within several minutes unless the subluxation has been present for several hours.

K. **Elbow dislocation** accounts for 20% of all dislocations; it is second in frequency only to dislocations of the shoulder and fingers.
   1. **Posterior dislocations**
      a. **Mechanism of injury.** Posterior dislocation accounts for 80% to 90% of elbow dislocations and is the result of a fall on an outstretched arm. The olecranon is displaced posteriorly in relation to the distal humerus (Fig. 4).
      b. **Physical examination.** Patients present to the emergency department with the elbow held in 45 degrees of flexion with prominence of the olecranon posteriorly and moderate swelling and deformity at the joint.
      c. **Radiographs** are necessary to exclude fractures of adjacent bony structures. Early reduction is important to prevent damage to the articular cartilage and excessive swelling or circulatory compromise. Neuropraxia involving the ulnar and median nerves occurs in 20% of patients. Brachial artery injury is commonly associated with open dislocations and dislocations with associated fractures.
      d. **Treatment.** The technique for reduction of posterior, medial, and lateral dislocations is the same. The patient lies supine with the in-

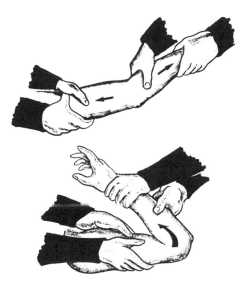

Fig. 5. Technique for reduction of posterior elbow dislocation.

jured elbow in the position of most comfort. The area of the wrist and distal forearm is grasped and traction is applied along the long axis of the forearm. The other hand applies downward pressure over the proximal forearm to disengage the coronoid from the olecranon fossa. An assistant provides countertraction to the upper arm. Any medial or lateral displacement is corrected. While forearm traction is continued, the elbow is flexed and a palpable "clunk" should be noted as the elbow is reduced (Fig. 5). Neurovascular examination should be repeated postreduction and radiographs should be done to confirm proper reduction. The elbow should be flexed to 90 degrees and immobilized in a posterior splint. All patients require prompt orthopaedic follow-up. Range-of-motion exercises may begin within 1 week. Indications for open reduction include associated fractures, open dislocation, neurovascular injury, or inability to accomplish a closed reduction.

    c. Complications. Long-term complications include contractures, neurovascular injury, heterotropic bone formation, and ankylosis.

2. Anterior elbow dislocations are rare.

    a. Mechanism of injury is a blow from behind to the olecranon while the elbow is flexed.

    b. **Physical examination.** The upper arm appears shortened and the forearm elongated. The patient presents with the elbow fully extended and forearm supinated. The olecranon fossa is palpable posteriorly. Associated injuries to vessels and nerves around the joint are much more common with anterior dislocations.

    c. **Treatment.** Reduction is accomplished with distal traction of the wrist and backward pressure on the forearm. Many of these dislocations are open and complete avulsion of the triceps mechanism is a commonly associated soft tissue injury.

BIBLIOGRAPHY

Greenspan A, Norman A. The radial head, capitellum view: useful technique in elbow trauma. *AJR* 1982;138:1186–1188.

Harwood-Nuss AL, Shepard SM. *The clinical practice of emergency medicine.* Philadelphia: Lippincott-Raven, 1996.

Horne JG, Tanzer TL. Olecranon fractures: a review of 100 cases. *J Trauma* 1981;21:469–472.

Hurley JA. Complicated elbow fractures in athletes. *Clin Sports Med* 1990;9:39–57.

Karasick D, Burk DL. Trauma to the elbow and forearm. *Semin Roentgenol* 1991;26:318–330.

Linscheid RL, Wheeler DK. Elbow dislocations. *JAMA* 1965;194: 113–118.

Murphy WA, Siegel MJ. Elbow fat pads with new signs and extended differential diagnosis. *Radiology* 1977;124:659–665.

Norell HG. Roentgenologic visualization of the extracapsular fat: its importance in the diagnosis of traumatic injury of the elbow. *Acta Radiol* 1954;42:205.

Pitt MJ, Speer DP. Imaging of the elbow with an emphasis on trauma. *Radiol Clin North Am* 1990;28:293–305.

Rosen P, Baker FJ II, Barkin RM, et al. *Emergency medicine: concepts and clinical practice,* 2nd ed. St Louis, CV Mosby, 1988.

Simon RR, Koenigsknecht SJ. *Orthopedics in emergency medicine.* New York: Appleton-Century-Crofts, 1982.

13

Injuries of the Wrist

Harold Chin

Injuries to the wrist are common but can present diagnostic problems because of the complexity of the joint. The most common error is the diagnosis of a sprained wrist because of the mere absence of an obvious fracture on the radiograph. Even subtle injuries can lead to significant impairment if not properly diagnosed and treated. Knowledge of the anatomical relationships between these various bones and carpal dynamics is essential for understanding the various types of injuries that can occur.

I. **General anatomy.** The wrist includes the distal radius and ulna and the carpal bones. The distal radius is the only forearm bone that articulates directly with the carpal bones (scaphoid and lunate). The distal ulna is separated from the carpals, lunate, and triquetrum by the triangular fibrocartilage complex, which is the main stabilizer to the distal radioulnar joint.

The carpal bones are held together by intrinsic ligaments between one another and extrinsic ligaments that bind the carpals to the radius and ulna. The carpal bones are arranged in two rows. Beginning on the radial side, the trapezium, trapezoid, capitate, and hamate form the distal carpal row. These bones are joined rather tightly with the adjoining distal metacarpals and move together as a unit in the wrist. The proximal carpal row, however, is a mobile unit. In fact, wrist movement is equally divided between the midcarpal joints (i.e., between the proximal and distal carpal rows) and the radiocarpal joint. The proximal carpal row functions as a mobile middle link in this system, which explains its propensity for injury and instability. The proximal carpal row includes the scaphoid, lunate, triquetrum, and pisiform. The scaphoid also holds a key position by serving as a bridge between the proximal and distal carpal rows along their radial side. This explains why trauma to the scaphoid and scapholunate joint is the most common carpal injury in the wrist.

II. **Physical examination.** Examination of the injured wrist is aided by the use of topographical anatomy. Pinpointing areas of tenderness and correlating them to visible anatomical landmarks on the wrist can assist in determining what potential injury may have occurred, so that appropriate radiographic studies can be obtained to confirm the diagnosis.

A. **Dorsal surface.** The "anatomic snuffbox" is the most visible feature on the radial aspect of the wrist. The scaphoid is palpable within this triangle; the bony prominence that forms the base of this triangle is the radial styloid. The ulnar border of this triangle is

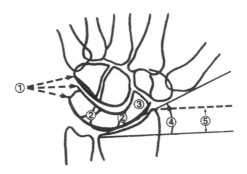

Fig. 1.   PA radiograph. Notable radiographic features are *(1)* three smooth arcs, *(2)* carpal space of 1 to 2 mm, *(3)* elongated shape of scaphoid, *(4)* radial inclination of 22 degrees, and (5) radial length of 13 mm.

formed by the extensor pollicis longus, which crosses around Lister's tubercle, a small bony prominence on the distal radius. The area immediately distal to Lister's tubercle marks the junction of the scapholunate joint. Just ulnar to Lister's tubercle, the lunate and capitate are palpable in the shallow indentation that is present in the middle of the wrist. The bony prominence on the ulnar aspect of the wrist is the ulnar styloid. The area immediately distal to this is the location of the triquetrum.

B.   **Volar surface.** The proximal flexor crease identifies the location of the proximal carpal row. The small bony prominence at the base of the hypothenar eminence is the pisiform. The hook of the hamate is palpable 1 cm away, at a 45-degree angle radial to the pisiform. The bony prominence at the base of the thenar eminence is the scaphotrapezial junction.

III.   **Radiography.** The clinical evaluation should dictate which radiographic views will assist in supporting a diagnosis. Proper positioning must be assured, since skewed views may create misleading artifacts. The standard posteroanterior, lateral, and oblique views are sufficient in the vast majority of cases. Motion studies and other specialized views are useful in profiling specific carpal injuries.

A.   **Posteroanterior (PA) view.** On a properly positioned PA view, the axis of the third metacarpal should be parallel to the axis of the radius. There should be no overlap between the radius and ulna at its distal articulation. Besides disruption of the bony cortex, other major items to examine on a PA view are as follows (see Fig. 1):

1.   The carpals form three smooth arcs. The proximal and distal articular surfaces of the scaphoid, lu-

nate, and triquetrum form two arcs. A third arc is formed by the proximal surface of the capitate and hamate.

2. The carpal bones are separated by a 1- to 2-mm space. Obliteration or an increase in the joint space occurs with torn ligaments, carpal instability patterns, fracture/dislocations, or improper positioning when the radiograph was taken.

3. The scaphoid has a relatively elongated shape. It is an oblong bone which normally lies flexed toward the palm. Scaphoid fractures or tears of the scapholunate ligament may cause the scaphoid to rotate further in the direction of the palm, making it appear shortened in a frontal PA view.

4. Radial inclination of 13 to 30 degrees (average, 22) and radial length of 8 to 18 mm (average, 13 mm). The radial styloid normally projects 13 mm past the radioulnar joint, creating a radial slope or inclination of 22 degrees. Fractures of the distal radius may change these measurements.

5. At least half the lunate makes contact with the radius. The slope of the radial articular surface would cause the carpals to shift toward the ulnar (ulnar translocation) if it were not for the support of radial ligaments and the triangular fibrocartilage complex, which prevents this. Injuries to either supporting structure can cause this ulnar shift. This can also produce shear stress and fracture of the lunate.

B. **Lateral radiograph.** On a properly positioned radiograph, the hand should be in a neutral position, the radius and ulna should overlap completely, and the radial styloid should be centered over the radial articular surface. The lateral radiograph is the single most important view. The degree of fracture angulation or displacement and carpal alignment are best seen on this view. Key elements on this view are as follows (Fig. 2):

1. **Three C's sign.** The axis of the radius, lunate, and capitate should be in a straight line. If their concave and convex articular surfaces were highlighted, they would appear as three consecutive letter C's in a row. A disruption in this arrangement occurs with torn ligaments and dislocations of the carpals.

2. The **capitolunate angle** is less than 10 to 20 degrees; the scapholunate angle is between 30 and 60 degrees. This goes one step further than noting the three C's sign. The axis of the lunate runs through the center of the concave and convex surfaces of the lunate. The axis of the capitate and scaphoid run lengthwise through each bone. The angle formed by the intersection of the axis of the lunate and capitate should measure less than 20 degrees; i.e., the two should nearly overlap. The

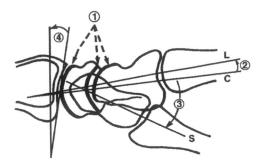

Fig. 2. Lateral radiograph. Key elements are *(1)* **three C's sign,** *(2)* **capitolunate angle <20 degrees,** *(3)* **scapholunate angle of 30 to 60 degrees, and** *(4)* **volar tilt of radius of 1 to 23 degrees (average, 14 degrees).**

scaphoid lies flexed in the direction of the palm and forms an angle of 30 to 60 degrees with the lunate. A change in these angles occurs with torn ligaments and carpal instability patterns or with improper positioning.

3. The radius has a **volar tilt** of 1 to 23 degrees (average, 14). The distal articular surface of the radius normally tilts slightly toward the palm. Angulated radial fractures will alter this measurement. A goal of fracture reduction is to restore this angle to normal.

C. **Oblique view.** These views are done in partial pronation or supination and project the scaphotrapezial joint or the pisiform, respectively, away from the overlapping patterns of the other carpals.

D. **Scaphoid view.** This is a coned down PA view of the wrist in ulnar deviation. Ulnar deviation causes the scaphoid to shift from its palmarflexed position into a more upright position. This radiographic view therefore profiles more of the scaphoid along its long axis, which may assist in revealing subtle fractures of the bone.

E. **Motion studies.** These are dynamic views in flexion, extension, and radial and ulnar deviation. They demonstrate carpal movement at the midcarpal and radiocarpal joint and change the orientation of the bones to one another.

F. **Grip compression, fist view.** This is a stress view of the wrist in the PA projection with the hand held in a tightly clenched fist, which pushes the capitate into the proximal carpal row and may force the carpals apart if torn ligaments are present.

G. **Carpal tunnel view.** A tangential view through the carpal tunnel is used to visualize the pisiform and hook of the hamate for injuries.

IV. Ligamentous injuries. Many of the ligamentous injuries are centered around the lunate and occur sequentially from varying degrees of force. The mechanism of injury is often similar: forced dorsiflexion of the wrist. The injuries range from an isolated tear to perilunate and lunate dislocations.

  A. Scapholunate ligamentous instability. This is the most common ligament injured.

   1. **Anatomy.** Each carpal row has intraarticular or intrinsic ligaments that hold them together as a unit. The intrinsic ligaments of the proximal carpal row, scapholunate, and triquetrolunate are particularly important, since they, along with the extrinsic ligaments of the radius and ulna, are the main supports in the wrist. These intrinsic ligaments hold the lunate tightly between the scaphoid and triquetrum in a delicate balance of opposing forces of flexion and extension.

   2. **Mechanism of injury.** This injury results most often from a fall on the outstretched hand in slight ulnar deviation.

   3. **Physical examination.** There will be pain and swelling on the radial side of the wrist. The patient may complain of a clicking sensation when moving the wrist. Palpation reveals point tenderness on the dorsum of the wrist just distal to Lister's tubercle. Ballottement of the scaphoid may also produce pain in this area.

   4. **Radiography.** This injury is frequently cross-referenced after the various radiographic appearances it may produce. The injury may manifest in any combination of three radiographic patterns (Fig. 3):

      a. **Scapholunate dissociation.** On the PA view, an increase in the joint space between the scaphoid and lunate of 3 mm or more may be present. Partial tears in the ligament may not be revealed unless a grip compression stress view or motion study is obtained. The grip compression stress view pushes the capitate into the proximal carpal row and forces the bones apart if the ligament is torn.

      b. **Rotatory subluxation of the scaphoid.** This is best seen on the lateral projection. The scaphoid tilts further into the palm and the scapholunate angle is greater than 60 degrees (the normal angle is 30 to 60 degrees). On the PA view, the scaphoid's axis rotates further toward the observer. Therefore the scaphoid appears shorter, with a dense cortical ring around its center, from being viewed down its axis (ring sign). Scapholunate dissociation often accompanies this picture.

      c. **Dorsal intercalary segment instability (DISI).** When viewed from the side, the

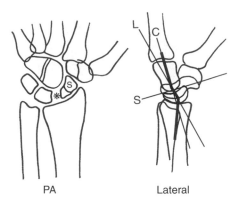

Fig. 3.   Scapholunate ligamentous instability (all three radiographic patterns are illustrated). PA view: scapholunate dissociation with a wide gap between the bones *(asterisk)*. **The scaphoid (S) appears shorter from notatory subluxation. Lateral view: dorsal intercalary segment instability (DISI) pattern is present. Note the zigzag appearance of the radial, lunate, and capitate axes. The capitolunate and scapholunate angles are increased and the scaphoid tilts more volarly (rotatory subluxation).**

scaphoid sits in a flexed posture. This imparts a flexion torque on the lunate that is counterbalanced by an extension torque from the triquetrum. When the scapholunate ligament is disrupted, so is the balance between the scaphoid and the triquetrum. The lunate then rotates dorsally from the unopposed force of the triquetrum. The proximal carpal row is also the middle link or intercalated segment of this three-link system in the wrist, hence the name DISI. The pathology is illustrated best in the lateral radiographic view, in which the lunate has a dorsal tilt and the capitolunate and scapholunate angles are increased. The normal linear arrangement of the axis through the radius, lunate, and capitate takes on a skewed zig-zag pattern (Fig. 4).

5. **Treatment.** Application of a radial gutter or posterior mold splint is adequate initial treatment until the patient can be seen by the orthopaedist. This injury can be treated with closed reduction and percutaneous pinning but more often requires open reduction and repair of the ligament.

6. **Complications.** Failure to recognize this condition can lead to the development of early degenerative arthritis and a chronically painful wrist.

B. **Triquetrolunate ligamentous instability.** This is the ulnar counterpart to the scapholunate injury on the radial side, but it occurs less often.

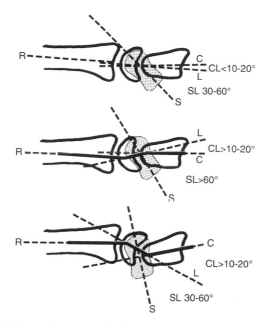

Fig. 4. **A:** Normal wrist, sagittal view. The axes of the radius (R), capitate (C), and lunate (L) are nearly colinear. The capitolunate angle (C) is less than 10 to 20 degrees. The scapholunate (SL) angle is 30 to 60 degrees. **B:** DISI: lunate tilts dorsally and slides toward the palm. Capitate shifts slightly to the posterior. Scaphoid flexes toward the palm. Capitolunate and scapholunate angles both increase. **C:** volar intercalary segment instability (VISI). Lunate tilts volarly. Capitolunate angle increased. Scapholunate angle normal. The axes take on a zig-zag pattern *(dark lines)* with both DISI and VISI.

1. **Anatomy.** This is the intrinsic ligament that holds the lunate and triquetrum together (see Sec. IV.A, on the scapholunate ligament).
2. **Mechanism of injury.** A fall on the outstretched hand with the wrist in dorsiflexion and impact on the hypothenar eminence is the most common cause of this injury.
3. **Physical examination.** There will be localized tenderness just distal to the ulnar styloid on the dorsum of the wrist. In severe injuries, when the triquetrum is moved back and forth between the examiner's fingers, a painful click can be palpated.
4. **Radiography.** A pattern of volar intercalary segment instability (VISI) is present on the lateral radiograph. Rupture of the triquetrolunate liga-

ment causes the lunate to tilt volarly from the unopposed action of the scaphoid. The capitolunate angle is increased but the scapholunate angle is unchanged. A line through the axis of the radius, lunate, and capitate forms a zig-zag pattern in the opposite direction from that seen in scapholunate tears.

5. **Treatment.** Application of an ulnar gutter or posterior mold is adequate initial treatment until the patient can be seen by the orthopaedist. Cast immobilization for 6 to 8 weeks followed by a protective splint for an additional 6 to 8 weeks produces satisfactory results in most cases. Chronic injuries often require open reduction and internal fixation and fusion.

6. **Complications.** Failure to recognize this condition can lead to the development of early degenerative arthritis and a chronically painful wrist.

C. **Perilunate and lunate dislocation.** With the application of enough force, the ligamentous disruptions continue around the lunate and culminate into these dislocations.

1. **Anatomy.** In addition to the intrinsic ligaments that hold the individual carpal bones together, the carpals are also held to the radius and ulna by extrinsic ligaments that form three arcs stretching across the wrist. There are two volar arcs and one dorsal arc. The two volar arcs attach at the radial styloid and distal ulna. They form two slings; one travels across and holds the lunate while the other one reaches up to hold the capitate. An inherently weak area adjacent to the capitolunate joint is present between these two volar arcs (space of Poirer). This space closes with a flexed wrist but widens when the wrist is extended. This explains why forced dorsiflexion of the wrist is responsible for this injury.

2. **Mechanism of injury.** A fall on the outstretched hand with very forceful dorsiflexion of the wrist is the most common cause of this injury. Perilunate instability is a progressive injury that most often begins with rupture of the scapholunate ligament, followed by the peeling away from the lunate of the capitate and triquetrum. This displaces the capitate posterior to the lunate, creating a perilunate dislocation. The capitate can also push the lunate off the radius and into the palm as it rebounds back and creates a lunate dislocation. The injury pattern just described is also capable of fracturing any number of the carpals that surround the lunate in the semicircular pattern.

3. **Physical examination.** There is often diffuse swelling, pain, and tenderness to palpation. Contrary to what one might expect with a "wrist dis-

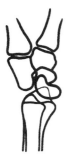

Fig. 5. Perilunate dislocation, lateral view. The lunate maintains its contact with the radius while the capitate is pushed posterior to the lunate.

location," a highly visible gross deformity of the wrist is often absent. Except for diffuse swelling, the wrist may appear misleadingly normal.

4. **Radiography**
   a. **Perilunate dislocation.** On the PA view, the joint space between the lunate and the capitate is obliterated. The scaphoid may appear shortened or fractured. Fractures of the capitate and triquetrum are also possible. The lateral view shows more specific findings of the capitate positioned posterior to the lunate, while the lunate maintains contact with the radius (Fig. 5).
   b. **Lunate dislocation.** On the PA view, the lunate has a triangular shape that is pathognomonic for lunate dislocation ("piece-of-pie" sign). The lateral view shows the lunate pushed off the radius and into the palm by the capitate ("spilled teacup" sign). As with perilunate dislocations, fractures to the surrounding carpal bones are possible (Fig. 6).
5. **Treatment.** If possible, closed reduction and casting in a long arm splint is done. Open reduction, internal fixation, and repair is the more likely scenario.
6. **Complications.** Carpal instability patterns, early degenerative arthritis, and any of the complications associated with carpal fractures such as delayed union, nonunion, malunion, and avascular necrosis are possible. Lunate dislocation can also compress the median nerve in the carpal tunnel.

V. **Carpal fractures.** These fractures can be subtle and elude early detection. Unfortunately, this can produce early degenerative arthritis and a chronically painful wrist. The various carpal fractures are discussed below in decreasing order of frequency.
   A. **Scaphoid fractures.** The scaphoid fracture is the most common carpal bone fracture and among all

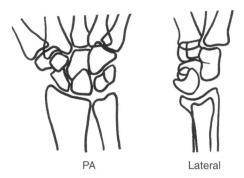

PA   Lateral

Fig. 6. Lunate dislocation. PA view: the lunate has a triangular appearance ("piece-of-pie" sign). The scaphoid is also fractured. Lateral view: the lunate is pushed off the radius ("spilled teacup" sign), and the capitate is positioned posterior to the lunate.

wrist fractures, is second only to fractures of the distal radius.

1. **Anatomy.** The scaphoid is an irregular, oblong-shaped bone that articulates with five other bones. Two-thirds of its external surface is articular to accommodate these numerous connections. In general, articular fractures are more difficult to heal, which adds to the scaphoid's problems. The scaphoid lies in a volarflexed position in the wrist and functions as a strut between the two carpal rows. The scaphoid's unique role of linking and forming the radial border of the proximal and distal carpal rows exposes it to potential injury.

    The vascular supply to the scaphoid comes from branches off the radial artery and the palmar and superficial palmar arteries that enter on the distal portion of the bone. This explains the increased risk of avascular necrosis of the proximal portion in proximal fractures.

2. **Mechanism of injury.** A fall on the outstretched, dorsiflexed hand or by an axial force directed along the thumb's metacarpal produces a compression and tension load across the scaphoid, making various fracture patterns possible.

3. **Physical examination.** These individuals present with pain on the radial side of the wrist. There is well-localized tenderness in the anatomical snuffbox. Ulnar deviation of the wrist exposes more of the scaphoid in the snuffbox and may assist the exam. Eliciting pain in this same area when the patient is asked to resist any attempt to supinate or pronate the wrist or when a longitudinal force is directed along the thumb metacarpal is also very suggestive of injury.

4. **Radiography.** Standard and scaphoid views should be obtained. The scaphoid view straightens out the normally flexed posture of the scaphoid. This may help to delineate more subtle nondisplaced fractures. Distortion or loss of a soft tissue fat stripe that lies along the radial side of the bone is also suggestive of injury. Approximately two-thirds of the fractures occur in the waist or midportion of the scaphoid, 16% to 28% in the proximal third, and 10% in the distal third. Some 12% of individuals will also have accompanying injuries that include fractures of the radius, ulna, or neighboring carpals, carpal instability patterns, or dislocations.

5. **Treatment.** As many as 10% of initial radiographs may fail to demonstrate a fracture when one is present; therefore treatment should be dictated by clinical suspicion as well. Nondisplaced fractures and those that are only clinically suspected may be treated with a thumb spica cast or splint.

   Signs of an unstable fracture are (a) as little as 1 mm of displacement; (b) rotation, angulation, or shortening of the bone; or (c) the presence of a carpal instability pattern. Prognosis for healing is also influenced by the site and orientation of the fracture. Proximal, oblique, and displaced fractures pose a greater risk of avascular necrosis of the proximal segment because the blood supply enters in the distal part of the scaphoid. Unstable fractures should be evaluated promptly by the orthopaedic surgeon and immobilized in a long arm thumb spica cast or splint.

6. **Complications.** The risk of the development of avascular necrosis, delayed union, nonunion, or malunion is the greatest concern.

B. **Triquetrum fractures**

1. **Anatomy.** The triquetrum is encased by strong ligamentous attachments. It is supported proximally by the triangular fibrocartilage and it helps to stabilize the neighboring lunate through the triquetrolunate ligament.

2. **Mechanism of injury.** Triquetral fractures are of two basic types: avulsion fractures and fractures through the body. The mechanism of injury is a twisting motion that is resisted, shear forces from impaction with the ulnar styloid, or wrist hyperextension that pushes the hamate against the triquetrum. Fractures through the body may also be seen in combination with the arc fractures that occur with perilunate dislocations.

3. **Physical examination.** There is localized tenderness over the dorsum of the wrist just distal to the ulnar styloid.

4. **Radiography.** An avulsion fracture is usually dorsal and is best visualized on the lateral and

oblique views as a flake of bone dorsal to the body of the triquetrum. The fractures through the body are usually nondisplaced and are seen on the PA view.

5. **Treatment.** Dorsal avulsion fractures are treated with a simple splint or cast immobilization for 6 weeks. These do extremely well. Fractures through the body are treated with cast immobilization for 6 weeks. Those associated with perilunate dislocations require internal fixation.

6. **Complications.** Nonunion may occur with body fractures. Fortunately, avascular necrosis has not been reported.

C. **Lunate fractures**
1. **Anatomy.** The lunate is relatively well protected in the lunate fossa of the radius and supported by the triangular fibrocartilage on the ulnar aspect, so that an isolated injury is rare. Nevertheless, the lunate is under the influence of the other carpal bones, and fractures in association with them may occur. The lunate's blood supply enters on its volar and dorsal surfaces at the distal end. An osteochondral fracture can compromise the blood supply to the proximal segment and produce avascular necrosis.

2. **Mechanism of injury.** Injury most often occurs from a fall on the dorsiflexed hand.

3. **Physical examination.** There is localized pain in the shallow indentation over the middorsum of the wrist. When the wrist is flexed, the lunate moves closer to the examiner's palpating digit. Pain in this area when axial compression is applied along the middle finger ray is also suggestive of injury.

4. **Radiography.** These injuries are difficult to visualize on standard radiographs. Tomography, bone scan, or magnetic resonance imaging (MRI) may be necessary to determine whether an injury is present.

5. **Treatment.** Since these fractures may not be detectable with standard radiographic techniques, treatment is dictated by clinical suspicion. A thumb spica cast or splint will provide sufficient immobilization until the patient can be evaluated by the orthopaedist.

6. **Complications.** Like the scaphoid, the blood supply enters on the distal end and the potential for avascular necrosis exists. The lunate can also undergo osteonecrosis (Kienbock's disease), lunate collapse, osteoarthritis, chronic pain, and decreased grip strength. Kienbock's disease is avascular necrosis of the lunate resulting from repetitive trauma to the lunate and produces microfractures of the bone.

D. Trapezial fractures

1. **Anatomy.** The trapezium is a saddle-shaped bone that is attached to the thumb metacarpal, scaphoid, and trapezoid.

2. **Mechanism of injury.** Injury occurs from a direct blow to the thumb or from a dorsiflexion and radial deviation force.

3. **Physical examination.** Movement of the thumb will be painful. There is palpable tenderness at the base of the thenar eminence and at the apex of the anatomical snuffbox.

4. **Radiology.** The fracture is best seen on a 20-degree pronated oblique view.

5. **Treatment.** Nondisplaced fractures are treated in a thumb spica cast for 6 weeks. Displaced fractures require reduction and internal fixation.

6. **Complications.** Nonunion.

E. Pisiform fractures

1. **Anatomy.** The pisiform is a sesamoid bone enveloped in the tendon of the flexor carpi ulnaris. It sits against the volar surface of the triquetrum. The pisiform and hook of the hamate form the side walls of Guyon's canal. The ulnar nerve and artery course through this canal.

2. **Mechanism of injury.** A fall on the outstretched hand with the point of impact on the hypothenar eminence is the most common mechanism of injury.

3. **Physical examination.** There may be mild swelling, but generally there is no deformity. There is point tenderness over the bony prominence at the base of the hypothenar eminence. With the wrist held in passive flexion, the pisiform can be palpated between the examiner's fingers.

4. **Radiography.** These fractures are best visualized in a partial supination or carpal tunnel view. The presence of multiple ossification centers within the pisiform, a normal variant, is a potential source of confusion.

5. **Treatment.** A compression dressing or short arm splint in 30 degrees of flexion and ulnar deviation is sufficient. These fractures do extremely well.

6. **Complications.** Ulnar nerve injury in Guyon's canal is remotely possible.

F. Hamate fractures. Fractures generally involve the hook of the hamate. Body fractures are rare and are generally associated with a fracture or dislocation of the fourth or fifth metacarpal or axial ulnar carpometacarpal dislocations.

1. **Anatomy.** The hamate is a triangular bone with a palmar bony process or hook. The hook of the hamate and the pisiform form the walls of Guyon's canal, which contains the ulnar nerve and artery.

2. **Mechanism of injury.** The classic mechanism is an interrupted swing with a racquet, club, or bat that compresses against the hypothenar eminence.

3. **Physical examination.** There is point tenderness over the base of the hypothenar eminence. The hamate hook is located approximately 1 to 2 cm away from the pisiform in a radial direction at a 45-degree angle.

4. **Radiography.** The fracture may be seen on the PA view but is best visualized on the carpal tunnel view.

5. **Treatment.** Initial treatment with a compression dressing or wrist splint is sufficient, but nonunion is common and requires excision of the bone fragment.

6. **Complications.** Nonunion of the hook is common. Compression of the ulnar nerve and intrinsic muscle weakness is possible.

G. **Capitate fractures**

1. **Anatomy.** The capitate is the largest carpal bone. It is centrally located and connected to the third metacarpal. The large proximal articular expansion is called the **head,** the midportion is the **neck,** and the distal end is the **body.** The blood supply of the capitate enters through its distal end; therefore fractures of the neck may result in avascular necrosis of the head. Fracture of the capitate most frequently occurs in combination with that of the scaphoid; this condition is called the **scaphocapitate syndrome.** Isolated fractures are rare.

2. **Mechanism of injury.** Isolated fractures result from direct trauma. The scaphocapitate syndrome occurs from forceful dorsiflexion of the wrist in radial deviation, usually from a fall on the outstretched hand. The scaphoid fractures first, followed by a fracture usually through the neck of the capitate. If the force is sufficient, displacement of the capitate posteriorly creates a perilunate dislocation with associated "arc fractures" around the lunate.

3. **Physical examination.** There will be diffuse swelling and tenderness over the wrist.

4. **Radiography.** PA, lateral, and scaphoid views should be obtained. The lateral view best reveals the fractures that most often occur in the neck. The head of the capitate and proximal scaphoid may rotate together in the scaphocapitate syndrome. The head is capable of rotating as much as 180 degrees. Fractures of the capitate are often missed, being overshadowed by the more obvious scaphoid fracture or perilunate dislocation.

5. **Treatment.** The rare isolated fracture is treated with splint or cast immobilization. Displaced

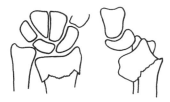

Fig. 7. Colles' fracture. PA view: the distal radius is fractured and shortened. Lateral view: the distal fragment is dorsally displaced and angulated. Comminution is common on the dorsal surface.

fractures require closed or open reduction with internal fixation and immobilization.

6. **Complications.** Nonunion, malunion, avascular necrosis of the proximal portion, and the complications associated with scaphoid fractures and perilunate dislocations are possible.

H. **Trapezoidal fracture**

1. **Anatomy.** The trapezoid is a wedge-shaped bone that articulates with the second metacarpal distally. Trapezoidal fractures account for only 1% of carpal fractures.

2. **Mechanism of injury.** This injury is produced by an axial load along the second metacarpal.

3. **Physical examination.** There is tenderness on the radial aspect of the wrist. Pain with compression along the index finger ray is suggestive of injury.

4. **Radiography.** This injury is extremely difficult to detect with standard radiographs because it is rare, and the difficulty is compounded by the overlap of adjacent carpal bones. CT may be necessary to visualize it.

5. **Treatment.** A thumb spica splint is adequate immobilization until the patient can be seen by the orthopaedist.

VI. **Distal radial and ulnar fractures.** Fractures of the distal radius and ulna are common and account for as many as 15% of all fractures. The peak occurrence is in the elderly 60-to 70-year age group.

A. **Colles' fracture.** This is the most common fracture of the wrist. It is a fracture of the distal radial metaphysis with dorsal displacement and angulation (Fig. 7).

1. **Anatomy.** The distal radial articular surface has two shallow concave surfaces to accommodate the scaphoid and lunate and a small notch on its ulnar aspect that articulates with the distal ulna. The radius is attached to the ulna by volar and dorsal ligaments that attach to the sides of the lunate fossa. So-called die-punch injuries to the lunate fossa will affect these attachments. The distal articular surface of the radius has an alignment to the long axis of the radius of 22 degrees of radial inclination and 14 degrees of volar tilt.

2. **Mechanism of injury.** This fracture most often occurs from a fall on the outstretched hand with the wrist in dorsiflexion. This mechanism creates a sharp break on the volar surface of the distal radius. As the distal radius is displaced dorsally, the dorsal surface is bent and compressed, producing comminution there. The individual's age can influence the type of fracture produced. In general, extraarticular fractures occur in the elderly because they have a thinner metaphyseal cortex, whereas young adults are prone to sustain complicated intraarticular fractures because of their propensity to be involved in high-impact athletic activities.

3. **Physical examination.** There is localized pain and swelling over the distal radius. The dorsal angulation produces the so-called silver-fork deformity. The median nerve may be compressed in the carpal tunnel and produce paresthesias on the palmar radial aspect of the hand and weakness of the thenar muscles. The elbow and shoulder should also be examined for any associated injuries.

4. **Radiography.** On the PA view, the cortex of the distal radius is disrupted in the metaphyseal region and the radius may appear shortened. Comminuted fractures may extend into the radioulnar joint or distal radiocarpal joint. These intraarticular fractures are variants of the Colles' fracture. They typically have an "inverted T"-shaped appearance on the PA view. Fractures through the lunate fossa have been referred to as die-punch fractures, after the visible step-off and depression on the articular surface. These fractures are often comminuted and involve the distal radioulnar joint. The lateral view reveals the extent of dorsal angulation and comminution of the dorsal cortex.

5. **Treatment.** These fractures are often divided into stable and unstable fractures, depending on their radiographic appearance. In general, unstable fractures have more than 20 degrees of angulation, shortening of 10 mm or more, and comminution or intraarticular involvement. Stable fractures are treated either with a splint or with closed reduction and immobilization until the patient can be evaluated by an orthopaedist. Closed reduction and immobilization can be attempted with unstable fractures, but the reduction is difficult to maintain; therefore open reduction and internal fixation may be required. Closed reduction is achieved with the use of finger traps and a counterweight applied to the arm. The fracture fragment is manipulated by applying pressure on its dorsal aspect and then immobilization with

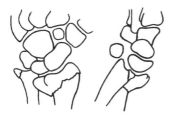

Fig. 8. Dorsal Barton's fracture. PA view: the distal radius is fractured and shortened. Lateral view: the carpus is dislocated posteriorly. The posterior dorsal rim of the radius is fractured.

the hand in slight flexion and ulnar deviation. The goal is to restore the normal length and volar tilt to the radius. Intraarticular involvement requires perfect alignment, which often calls for open reduction and internal fixation. Die-punch fractures are often irreducible by traction and closed reduction, requiring open reduction and repair.

6. **Complications.** Loss of reduction, malunion, nonunion, median nerve compression, and delayed carpal instability patterns with degenerative arthritis are possible complications.

B. **Smith's fracture**
   1. **Anatomy (see Sec. IV. A, Colles' fracture).**
   2. **Mechanism of injury.** Smith's fracture results from a direct blow or fall on the dorsum of the hand or from a fall on the hand initially in supination and then turning in pronation.
   3. **Physical examination.** There is local swelling and tenderness over the distal radius and a characteristic "garden spade" deformity with volar displacement of the hand. The elbow and shoulder should be examined carefully for an accompanying injury.
   4. **Radiography.** On the PA view, the radius has a metaphyseal fracture and appears shortened. The lateral view shows the opposite of a Colles' fracture, hence the name *reverse Colles'* is also given to this fracture. The distal radius fracture is displaced volarly and angulated dorsally. The fracture may be either extraarticular or intraarticular.
   5. **Treatment.** The treatment is identical to that for Colles' fracture except that the reduction maneuver is in the opposite direction.
   6. **Complications (see Colles' fracture, Sec. VI.A)**

C. **Barton's fracture.** This is an intraarticular fracture involving the volar or dorsal rim of the radius. Dislocation or subluxation of the carpus in the direction of the fracture segment produces a fracture/dislocation or subluxation (Fig. 8).
   1. **Anatomy (see Colles' fracture, Sec. VI.A).**

2. **Mechanism of injury.** Volar and dorsal Barton's fractures are actually intraarticular variants of Smith's and Colles' fractures, respectively. The dorsal Barton's fracture or intraarticular Colles' is the more common of the two. The mechanism of injury is similar to the respective Smith's or Colles' fracture counterpart.

3. **Physical examination.** There will be an obvious deformity of the wrist with either volar or dorsal displacement of the hand. Injury of the median nerve is also possible.

4. **Radiography.** On the PA view, the carpus overlaps the distal radius, and the radius appears shortened with a metaphyseal fracture. On the lateral view, the subluxation or dislocation of the carpus overshadows the radial injury, which involves either the volar or dorsal lip of the articular surface.

5. **Treatment.** Stable fractures can be treated with a splint until the patient can be evaluated by an orthopaedist. Fractures involving more than 50% of the articular surface or with carpal subluxation or dislocation are unstable and require reduction with either external fixation or open reduction and plating.

6. **Complications.** Malunion, nonunion, posttraumatic arthritis, carpal instability, and median nerve injury are possible.

D. **Radial styloid fractures (chauffeur's fracture)**

1. **Anatomy.** The radial styloid is a key point for the attachment of the extrinsic carpal ligaments; these ligaments hold the carpals to the forearm.

2. **Mechanism of injury.** These injuries classically occurred when the old hand-crank automobiles would backfire while being started and torque the operator's wrist back, hence the name *chauffeur's fracture.*

3. **Physical examination.** There is point tenderness and mild swelling immediately over the visible bony prominence of the radial styloid.

4. **Radiography.** The PA view shows a thin lucent line crossing the base of the radial styloid.

5. **Treatment.** A radial gutter splint is sufficient until the patient can be evaluated by an orthopaedist. Closed reduction or percutaneous pinning may be necessary for displaced fractures. Definitive treatment for nondisplaced fractures is cast immobilization for 4 to 6 weeks.

6. **Complications.** Carpal instability and posttraumatic arthritis.

E. **Ulnar styloid fractures**

1. **Anatomy.** The ulnar styloid is attached to the triangular fibrocartilage complex, which is the

main stabilizer to the distal radioulnar joint. It supports the extrinsic ligaments and carpus, acting as a shock absorber between the carpals and the ulna.

2. **Mechanism of injury.** Injuries occur through forced dorsiflexion (it frequently accompanies a Colles' fracture), radial deviation, or rotation of the wrist.

3. **Physical examination.** Local tenderness is present over the ulnar styloid. A torn triangular fibrocartilage complex may produce pain or clicking with wrist rotation.

4. **Radiography.** The PA view shows a lucent line or displacement of the ulnar styloid. A fracture of the ulnar styloid is rather innocent-appearing, but it should suggest the possibility for tears of the triangular fibrocartilage complex.

5. **Treatment.** Splint immobilization in neutral or ulnar deviation is adequate initial and definitive treatment for isolated ulnar styloid fractures. Those associated with fractures of the distal radius or tears of the triangular fibrocartilage complex may require open reduction and repair. Painful nonunions may require excision of the fragment.

6. **Complications.** Nonunion and distal radioulnar instability.

F. **Radioulnar disruption**
1. **Anatomy.** The distal radioulnar joint is a trochlear joint that assists forearm rotational movement. It is supported by dorsal and volar radioulnar ligaments that attach at the sides of the lunate fossa. The triangular fibrocartilage also supports the distal end.

2. **Mechanism of injury.** Injury to the radioulnar joint accompanies intraarticular fractures of the distal radius, e.g., intraarticular Colles', Smith's, and Galeazzi fracture/dislocation. Isolated injury most commonly occurs from falls in hyperpronation.

3. **Physical examination.** There is pain on the ulnar aspect of the wrist with prominence of the ulna on the dorsum of the wrist (volar dislocation is rare). Patients may complain of pain and a snapping or clicking sensation with wrist movement. Laxity of the joint can be detected by grasping the distal radius and ulna separately and moving them in opposite directions like piano keys ("piano keys" sign).

4. **Radiography.** On the PA view, one may see the radius and ulna overlap at the distal radioulnar joint instead of seeing the normal space in this area. The lateral view will show dorsal displacement of the ulna.

AQ3:
Au:
Ok?

5. **Treatment.** The dislocation is easily reduced and the wrist is splinted in supination for 4 weeks. This is the treatment of choice. Open reduction is necessary for late cases or if closed reduction is unsuccessful.
6. **Complications.** Dorsal dislocation has a high recurrence rate. Reconstruction may be necessary in these cases.

BIBLIOGRAPHY

Altissimi M, Antenucci R, Fiacca C, Mancini GB. Long-term result of conservative treatment of fractures of the distal radius. *Clin Orthop* 1986;206:202–210.

Bradway JK, Amadio PC, Cooney WP. Open reduction and internal fixation of displaced, comminuted intra-articular fractures of the distal end of the radius. *J Bone Joint Surg* 1989;71A:839–847.

Breckenbaugh RD. Accurate evaluation and management of the painful wrist following injury. *Orthop Clin North Am* 1984;15: 289.

Bryan RS, Dobyns JH. Fractures of the carpal bones other than the navicular. *Clin Orthop* 1980;149:107.

Carter PR. *Common hand injuries and infections: a practical approach to early treatment.* Philadelphia: WB Saunders, 1983.

Chernin MM, Pitt MJ. Radiologic disease patterns at the carpus. *Clin Orthop* 1984;187:72.

Chin HW, Propp DA, Orban DJ. Forearm and wrist. In: Rosen P, Barkin RM, eds. *Emergency medicine: concepts and clinical practice,* ed 3, vol 1. St. Louis: Mosby–Year Book, 1992.

Cooney WP, Bussey R, Dobyns JH. Difficult wrist fractures. *Clin Orthop* 1987;214:136.

Cooney WP, Dobyns JH, Linscheid RL. Fractures of the scaphoid: a rational approach to management. *Clin Orthop* 1980;149:90.

Cooney WP, Linscheid RL, Dobyns JH. Fractures and dislocations of the wrist. In: Rockwood CA, Green DP eds. *Fractures in adults,* ed 3, vol. 1. Philadelphia: JB Lippincott, 1991.

Dunn AW. Fractures and dislocations of the carpus. *Surg Clin North Am* 1972;52:1513.

Frykman G. Fractures of the distal radius: a clinical and experimental study. *Acta Orthop Scand* 1967;108:1.

Green DP. The sprained wrist. *Am J Fam Pract* 1979;19:114–122.

Green DP, O'Brien ET. Classification and management of carpal dislocations. *Clin Orthop* 1980;149:55.

Johnson R. The acutely injured wrist and its residuals. *Clin Orthop* 1980;149:33.

Linscheid RL. Kinematic considerations of the wrist. *Clin Orthop* 1986;202:27–39.

Linscheid RL, Dobyns JH, Beabout JW. Traumatic instability of the wrist. *J Bone Joint Surg* 1972;54:1612.

Malone CP. Open treatment for displaced articular fractures of the distal radius. *Clin Orthop* 1986;202:104.

Mayfield JK. Wrist ligamentous anatomy and pathogenesis of carpal instability. *Orthop Clin North Am* 1984;15:209.

O'Brien ET. Acute fractures and dislocations of the carpus. *Orthop Clin North Am* 1984;15:237.

Rand JA, Linscheid RL, Dobyns JH. Capitate fractures. *Clin Orthop Rel Res* 1982;165:205–216.

Wiessman BN, Sledge CB. *Orthopedic radiology.* Philadelphia: WB Saunders, 1986.

Waeckerle JF. A prospective study identifying the sensitivity of radiographic findings and the clinical efficacy of clinical findings in carpal navicular fractures. *Ann Emerg Med* 1987;16:733.

14

Forearm Injuries

John L. Zautcke

I. **Anatomy.** The **radius** and **ulna** make up the bony structure of the forearm. They are approximately parallel,
touching only at the ends. The ulna is a relatively straight
bone and the radius has an outward bow. During pronation and supination, the radius rotates around the relatively fixed ulna. Proximally, the bones are bound by the
capsule of the elbow joint and by the annular ligament.
Distally they are bound by the capsule of the wrist joint,
the anterior and posterior radioulnar ligaments, and the
fibrocartilaginous articular disk. The distal radioulnar
joint supports articulations with the scaphoid, lunate,
and the ulna itself. The triangular fibrocartilaginous ligament separates the ulna from the carpal bones and is the
main stabilizer of the distal radioulnar joint. Between the
shafts of both bones is the strong interconnecting interosseous membrane, whose fibers originate on the radius and run obliquely to insert on the ulna. Owing to
their proximity and strong interconnections, both bones
and their ligamentous attachments are often disrupted by
serious injuries.

   A. **Muscles of the forearm.** The forearm is divided
   into two compartments, anterior and posterior, separated by the antebrachial fascia. A total of 19 muscles
   of the forearm are responsible for motion of the hand
   and wrist, including pronation and supination. Fracture fragments are displaced primarily by the actions
   of the **supinator, pronator teres,** and **pronator
   quadratus** muscles. As their name implies, these
   muscles are responsible for pronation and supination. Supination is controlled by the supinator and biceps brachii, which insert on the proximal radius. The
   pronator teres inserts distal to these attachments on
   the radius and is responsible for pronation. Because
   of the opposing forces between these muscle groups,
   proximal radial fractures result in marked displacement (Fig. 1A). For middle-third radial fractures
   distal to these muscle groups, the opposing forces are
   neutralized and there is less displacement (Fig. 1B).

   B. **Nerves of the forearm.** The nerves of the forearm
   consist of the **median, ulnar,** and **radial.**

      1. The **median nerve** controls basic motions of the
      wrist and finger flexion. It is responsible for sen-
      sation of the volar surface of the thumb, index,
      and middle fingers and the radial half of the ring
      finger. The nerve is evaluated by testing its three
      distal branches. Motor function is evaluated by
      the ability to both abduct the thumb and oppose
      it to the little finger. Sensation is evaluated by

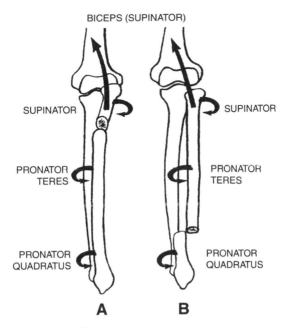

BICEPS (SUPINATOR)

SUPINATOR

SUPINATOR

PRONATOR
TERES

PRONATOR
TERES

PRONATOR
QUADRATUS

PRONATOR
QUADRATUS

A   **B**

Fig. 1. **Displacement of radial fractures in relation to forearm muscles.**

two-point discrimination of the thumb, index, and middle fingers, normal is 2-5 millimeters.

2. The **ulnar nerve** supplies only the flexor carpi ulnaris muscle and the ulnar portions of the flexor digitorum profundus. It provides sensation to the little finger and ulnar half of the ring finger. It is evaluated by the ability to abduct the index finger against resistance and by two-point discrimination of the little finger.

3. The **radial nerve** innervates all the muscles of the posterior compartment, controlling wrist, finger, and thumb extension. The sensory portion innervates the posterior aspect of the hand from the thumb to the radial half of the ring finger. The nerve is evaluated by testing sensation of the dorsum of the hand and the ability to extend the wrist and fingers against resistance.

C. **Vascularture of the forearm.** Blood is supplied to the forearm by the **radial** and **ulnar arteries.** Both are branches of the **brachial artery,** which bifurcates at the level of the radial neck.

1. The **radial artery** passes distally along the radial aspect of the forearm to the wrist. In the hand it crosses the metacarpals to the ulnar bor-

der, where it forms an anastomosis with the ulnar artery to give the deep palmar arch.

2.   The **ulnar artery** is the larger of the two terminal branches of the brachial artery. It runs along the ulnar border of the forearm to the wrist and into the hand. The deep branch of the ulnar artery joins the radial artery to form the deep palmar arch.

II.   Fractures of the forearm

A.   **General principles.** Because of the close relationship of the radius and ulna, solitary fractures of the forearm are unusual. Fractures usually occur at two or more sites or involve a fracture of one bone along with a ligamentous injury, with or without an associated joint dislocation. The accompanying injury often involves the wrist or elbow joint, so these areas need to be routinely examined. When shortening is present, there is a very high likelihood of associated injuries.

Successful treatment of forearm fractures involves healing of the fracture site, restoration of length, and maintaining function of the wrist, elbow, and forearm itself. In order to achieve these goals, surgeons often prefer open reduction and internal fixation (ORIF) as the treatment of choice for most adults with forearm fractures. Surgery is usually performed within 24 hours of the injury. Problems associated with closed reduction include malunion, nonunion, and loss of function. Standard radiographs of the forearm include anteroposterior and lateral views. Both the wrist and elbow must be visualized to identify occult fractures or dislocations in these areas. Standard views of the wrist and elbow should be obtained if these areas are not seen well on the forearm views and suspicion for injury is high.

B.   **Fractures of the radius**
1.   **Proximal and middle thirds**
a.   **Mechanism.** A direct blow to the radius. These injuries are uncommon because the surrounding musculature provides abundant protection in this area. Most injuries severe enough to fracture the radius will also fracture the ulna.
b.   **Physical examination.** Tenderness will be present over the fracture site. The amount of tenderness and deformity may be masked by the soft tissue surrounding this area.
c.   **Radiography.** Routine views of the forearm are usually adequate. If there is suspicion of an injury to the elbow or wrist, these joints should be radiographed as well.
d.   **Treatment.** The rare undisplaced fracture should be immobilized in a standard long arm cast or posterior mold. The location of the ra-

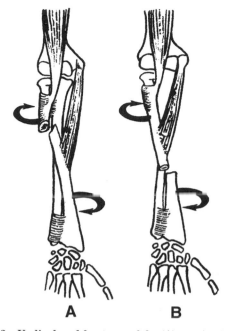

Fig. 2. Undisplaced fractures of the (A) proximal radius and (B) middle or lower shaft radius.

dial fracture determines the degree of supination of the distal fragment needed to correct the rotational alignment. In fractures of the proximal radius between the insertion of the supinator and pronator teres, an unopposed supinating force is exerted on the proximal fragment (Fig. 2A). The forearm is therefore placed in full supination. In a fracture of the middle or lower shaft of the radius below the insertions of the pronator teres, the proximal fragment is in a more neutral position (Fig. 2B). The forearm is then placed in mild supination.

Displaced fractures of the proximal and middle third of the radius are treated with ORIF. The only exception is a displaced fracture of the proximal fifth of the radius. This is best treated closed with the forearm in full supination.

e. **Complications.** Compartment syndrome is rare with these fractures. Most complications involve malunion or nonunion because of inadequate or lost reduction.

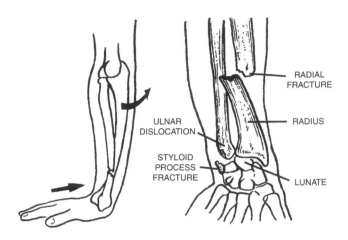

Fig. 3.   Galeazzi fracture of the distal radius.

    f.   Disposition. Close follow-up is required. For fractures treated by closed reduction, weekly radiographs should be done to ensure that the reduction is maintained. Even with adequate immobilization, the reduction is often lost because of the strong deforming forces present in the forearm.

    g.   Pediatrics. Treatment is the same as in adults. Children often obtain better results than adults when treated with closed reduction and immobilization.

2.   Distal third fractures

    a.   Mechanism. A direct blow or fall on an outstretched hand is the most common mechanism for fractures of the distal radius. Solitary injuries, however, are rare. More commonly, fractures occur at the junction of the middle and distal thirds and have an associated dislocation or subluxation of the distal radioulnar joint **(Galeazzi fracture, Fig. 3).**

    b.   Physical examination. Swelling and tenderness are present at the fracture site. A prominent distal ulna and tenderness are present with injuries to the radioulnar joint.

    c.   Radiography. The fracture may be transverse or oblique and is seen on standard forearm views. The injury to the radioulnar joint may be subtle. Moore described **four radiographic signs of injury** to the distal radioulnar joint:

        (1)   Fracture of the ulnar styloid

        (2)   Widening of the radioulnar joint space on anteroposterior views

(3) Dislocation of the distal radius relative to the ulna on lateral views

(4) Shortening of the radius more than 5 mm on anteroposterior views

d. **Treatment.** ORIF is the treatment of choice for the Galeazzi fracture. Prior to surgery, the patient should be placed in a long arm cast or posterior mold with the elbow flexed to 90 degrees and the forearm in pronation.

e. **Complications.** Complications include infection, nonunion, and malunion. Injuries to the ulnar nerve and anterior interosseous branch of the median nerve have been reported. These usually recover spontaneously. Radioulnar subluxation is a result of shortening of the radius and rotational deformity. When the radius heals with a rotational deformity, there is pain at the distal radioulnar joint with extreme pronation and supination.

f. **Disposition.** These patients are usually admitted to an orthopaedist for surgery.

g. **Pediatrics.** Galeazzi fractures are rare in children. When they occur, treatment is the same as in adults.

D. **Fractures of the ulna**
1. **Proximal third.** Fractures of the proximal third of the ulna can either be solitary or associated with dislocation of the radial head (**Monteggia fracture**).

a. **Mechanism.** Solitary fractures are caused by a direct blow, sometimes called a **nightstick fracture** (arm held above the head in a defensive position to guard against a head injury). The mechanism of injury of Monteggia fractures is controversial, and up to five types of injuries have been described. Each type of injury has a different mechanism and a different combination of ulnar fracture and dislocation of the radial head. The most common mechanisms and fracture/dislocation patterns are falls backward, which force the forearm into supination and hyperextension of the elbow, or direct blows over the posterior ulna (Fig. 4). These result both in a fracture of the proximal third of the ulna with anterior angulation and a dislocation of the anterior radial head. In general the radial head dislocates in the same direction as the angulation of the ulnar fracture.

b. **Physical examination.** Pain and tenderness are present at the fracture site. The forearm is shortened and the radial head is prominent and may be palpated. If the radial nerve is involved, weakness of hand and wrist extensors will be present.

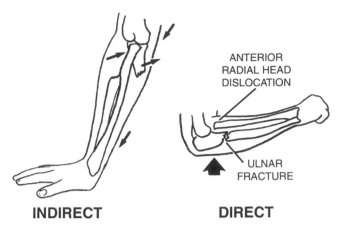

ANTERIOR
RADIAL HEAD
DISLOCATION

ULNAR
FRACTURE

INDIRECT   **DIRECT**

**Fig. 4.   Diagrams of injury mechanisms
related to Monteggia fractures.**

c. **Radiography.** The ulna fracture is easily
seen on standard views of the forearm. The
dislocation of the radial head, however, is often overlooked and may result in ankylosis
and myositis ossificans. Additional views of
the elbow joint are often necessary. On all
views of the elbow, a line drawn through the
middle of the long axis of the proximal radius
should extend through the middle of the
capitellum.

d. **Treatment.** Successful treatment includes
early diagnosis, rigid internal fixation of the
fractured ulna, and reduction of the radial
head. When the radial head can be reduced
by closed means, open reduction is not necessary. The arm should be immobilized in a long
arm posterior mold prior to surgery. The elbow should be flexed 90 degrees and the forearm placed in a neutral position.

e. **Complications.** As many as one-third of
these injuries are initially missed. Complications include infection and nonunion. Recurrent or persistent dislocation of the radial
head is the usual feature of a missed dislocation and is secondary to an unrepaired tear of
the annular ligament. The deep branch of the
radial nerve may be impinged or contused by
the radial head. This usually resolves spontaneously in 6 to 8 weeks.

f. **Disposition.** Adults with Monteggia fractures are usually admitted for ORIF. Close

follow-up is required to ensure maintenance of the reduction.

g. **Pediatrics.** Monteggia fractures are rare in children. Unlike adults, they are treated with closed reduction and plaster immobilization, usually performed under general anesthesia. The arm is immobilized with the elbow in moderate flexion (15 to 20 degrees past 90 degrees) and the forearm in supination.

2. **Middle and distal thirds**

a. **Mechanism.** Fractures of the middle and distal thirds are usually caused by a direct blow. As in proximal ulnar fractures, these solitary lesions are called **nightstick fractures.** Falls associated with pronounced pronation or supination can cause these fractures as well.

b. **Physical examination.** Pain and swelling are present at the fracture site. Significant deformities will also be easily seen.

c. **Radiography.** Standard forearm views are adequate to visualize these fractures. If pain or tenderness is present in the wrist or elbow or displacement of the fracture is more than a few millimeters, these joints should be radiographed as well.

d. **Treatment.** For these fractures, a long arm cast or posterior mold is adequate if there is less than 50% or 5 mm of displacement or less than 10 degrees of angulation. The elbow is flexed to 90 degrees and the forearm is placed in neutral position. For fractures with displacement or angulation exceeding these measurements, ORIF is required.

e. **Complications.** Associated injuries are rare; they include vascular injuries, compartment syndrome, infection, and nonunion. Occasionally, the deep branch of the radial nerve is injured, manifested by a wrist drop. This usually resolves spontaneously.

f. **Disposition.** Undisplaced and minimally displaced nightstick fractures are treated on an outpatient basis. Repeat radiographs are done to ensure maintenance of the reduction.

g. **Pediatrics.** Nightstick fractures in children are treated the same as in adults. Displacement is usually minimal, so ORIF is rarely required.

E. **Radius and ulnar ("both bone") fractures**

1. **Mechanism.** Significant force is required to fracture both the radius and ulna; therefore the fractures are often displaced. The most common mechanisms are motor vehicle accidents, direct blows, falls from significant heights, and injuries

sustained during sports activities. The fractures are often open.

2. **Physical examination.** Pain and swelling are evident at the fracture site. In addition, deformities are usually present. Although neurological injury is rare, injuries to the median, ulnar, and radial nerves can occur and must be identified by careful examination. Nerve injuries are more likely with open fractures. With some more serious injuries, forces are exerted along the interosseous membrane and result in subluxations or dislocations of the wrist or elbow. Therefore it is important to closely examine these joints as well. Finally, the vascular status of the forearm should be evaluated, as well as the amount of swelling. Vascular compromise is usually not a problem because of the excellent collateral circulation. If the forearm is tense, compartment pressures should be measured to rule out compartment syndrome.

3. **Radiography.** The fractures are obvious on standard views of the forearm. The amount and degree of angulation, displacement, rotation, and shortening should be noted. Comminuted fractures are common. It is important to include the wrist and elbow because of the high likelihood of an associated dislocation or articular fracture.

4. **Treatment.** Treatment depends on the location of the fracture and the amount of angulation and displacement. For the rare fracture that is neither angulated nor displaced, a long arm cast or posterior mold will suffice. The elbow should be placed at 90 degrees with the forearm in a neutral position. Casts should be bivalved to avoid vascular compromise. For the most common fractures with angulation and displacement, ORIF is necessary to maintain the reduction.

5. **Complications.** Neurological injuries are rare, but compartment syndrome is not unusual. In addition, because of the instability of these fractures, loss of reduction and nonunion are common. Other complications include osteomyelitis and loss of ability to supinate and pronate.

6. **Disposition.** For fractures treated with immobilization alone, close follow-up is necessary owing to frequent loss of reduction. This usually occurs when the swelling from the fracture subsides and the cast loosens.

7. **Pediatrics.** Torus and greenstick fractures with less than 15 degrees of angulation are treated with immobilization in a long arm cast. For greenstick fractures with more than 15 degrees of angulation, completion of the fracture and immo-

bilization are sometimes performed. King et al. disagree, believing that completing the fracture makes it more difficult to maintain the reduction. They recommended closed reduction under general anesthesia with immobilization in a long arm cast.

For complete fractures in children less than 10 to 12 years old, closed reduction and immobilization in a long arm cast is indicated. For children over the age of 12, the treatment is controversial. Permanent loss of rotation can be expected from treatment with closed reduction. Some argue that ORIF is required, depending on the amount of residual deformity after closed reduction.

III. Compartment syndrome

A. Mechanism. Although it is much more common in the lower extremity, compartment syndrome may occur in the forearm. The forearm is divided into compartments by fascial planes. Closed fractures, especially of the shafts of the radius and/or ulna, can cause elevation of the compartmental pressures due to bleeding, swelling, or pressure from a tight cast, splint, or bandage. The resulting high pressure leads to neurovascular damage and muscle necrosis.

B. Physical examination. Patients often present with pain that is out of proportion to the degree of their injury. The forearm feels tense to palpation, and there is pain on passive flexion or extension of the wrist and fingers. Although pulses usually remain intact, the pressures are great enough to compromise capillary blood flow to the affected muscles and nerves. The individual nerves themselves should be tested by light touch and/or two-point discrimination rather than pinprick. Paresthesias are often present and can progress to total anesthesia and paralysis.

C. Diagnosis. The diagnosis is primarily clinical, but it should be confirmed by measurement of compartmental pressures. Various devices are available to support the diagnosis. Pressures greater than 25 to 30 mm Hg are considered diagnostic. Normal compartmental pressure is 0 to 8 mm Hg.

D. Treatment. Once the diagnosis is made, urgent fasciotomy is required. Ideally, this should be carried out within 8 hours of the onset of symptoms.

E. Complications. Failure to recognize and treat this condition promptly leads to myonecrosis and the formation of **Volkmann's contractures.** These contractures are the end result of the ischemic process involving the affected muscles and nerves. They are classically associated with supracondylar fractures of the humerus but may occur with fractures of the forearm as well. The resulting contractures are frequently debilitating and often leave the arm nonfunctional.

BIBLIOGRAPHY

Bado JL. The Monteggia lesion. *Clin Orthop* 1976;50:71–86.

Dormans JP, Rang M. The problems of Monteggia lesions in children. *Orthop Clin North Am* 1990;21:251–256.

Fowles JV, Slinman N, Kassab MT. The Monteggia lesion in children. *J Bone Joint Surg* 1983;65A:1276–1283.

King RE. Fractures of the shafts of the radius and ulna. In: Rockwood CA, Wilkens KE, King RE, eds. *Fractures in children,* 3rd ed. Philadelphia: JB Lippincott, 1991.

Moore EM, Klein JP, Patzakin MJ, et al. Results of compression plating of closed Galeazzi fractures. *J Bone Joint Surg* 1985;67: 1015–1021.

Rockwood CA, Green DP, Bucholz RW. *Rockwood and Green's fractures in adults.* Lewis B. Anderson and Frederick N. Meyer, eds. Philadelphia: JB Lippincott, 1991.

Ruiz E, Cicero JJ. *Emergency management of skeletal injuries.* Mosby, St. Louis, MO:1995.

Simon RR, Koenigsknecht SJ. *Emergency orthopedics: the extremities* 3rd ed. Norwalk, Connecticut: Appleton and Lange, 1995.

15

Fractures of the Metacarpals

Thomas S. Pannke

Fractures of the hand are common owing to its unprotected position and the forces to which it is exposed. Fractures involving the metacarpals are among the most commonly seen and can usually be managed easily in the emergency department. Mechanisms of injury can include crushing, penetrating, shearing, avulsing, and lacerating forces as well as direct blows. Most metacarpal fractures seen in the emergency department are due to direct blows, and several fracture types are seen frequently. Because of different treatments and outcomes, the thumb metacarpal is considered separately from the metacarpals of the rest of the hand.

I. **Anatomy.** The bones of the hand are specialized in their function. The metacarpals form a strong, stable base that allows the fingers to perform multiple complex tasks. The metacarpals of the index and middle fingers have limited movement and, with the fixed distal carpal bones, form the stabilizing structure from which the rest of the hand functions. They are fixed in place by strong ligamentous attachments. The thumb metacarpal is freely mobile, as are the bases of the ring and little finger metacarpals. Metacarpals are divided anatomically into a head, neck, shaft, and base. The tendons of several muscles attach to the metacarpals, including the flexor carpi radialis, extensor carpi radialis longus and brevis, extensor carpi ulnaris, abductor pollicis longus, and the interossei. There are strong ligaments at the distal ends of the second through fifth metacarpals that hold these bones closely together. This transverse metacarpal ligament is essential to the function of the hand, and disruption of the bony attachments or of the ligament itself will cause a dysfunctional grip and affect other hand movements.

II. **Mechanism of injury.** Fractures of the metacarpals can occur from direct blows, torque forces, axial loads, and crushing injuries. It is important to understand the mechanism of injury, as this helps to predict the type of fracture, the severity of the fracture, and associated injuries.

III. **Physical examination**

A. **Function.** In general, injuries to the hand should be examined with attention to function. A thorough neurovascular exam is important. Flexion and extension of the carpometacarpal (CMC) joints, the metacarpophalangeal joints (MCP), and the proximal and distal interphalangeal joints (PIP and DIP respectively) are crucial. Function can be difficult to evaluate at times because of the injury and its associated pain. Describing the point of maximal tenderness and noting any deformity will help to direct the x-ray studies and aid in their interpretation. A low threshold for obtaining radiologic studies should be maintained when hand injuries are encountered.

B. **Rotational deformities** resulting from fractures require early detection and correction. An undetected rotational deformity of 5 degrees that is allowed to heal can lead to 1 cm of finger overlap in flexion. Rotation can be detected in three ways:

1. Inspection of the fingers flexed at 90 degrees at the MCP and PIP joints, with the DIP joints extended. The fingers should point to approximately the same spot on the scaphoid.

2. Viewing the slightly flexed fingers from the tips. The planes of the nails should be level and, when compared with those of the uninjured hand, should look the same.

3. Noting any discrepancy of the widths of the fracture fragments on the x-ray.

IV. **Fractures of metacarpals 2 to 5.** These metacarpals are more often fractured than the thumb. Anatomically, the second and third metacarpals are firmly fixed and immobile. This immobility provides a firm base from which the rest of the hand can function. The fourth and fifth metacarpals have greater mobility, allowing the hand to better grasp and move. Because of this anatomical relationship, the second and third metacarpals are poorly tolerant of angulation deformities, while the fourth and fifth are much more tolerant without functional impairment.

A. **Head of the metacarpals**

1. **Mechanism of injury.** These fractures are unusual. They result from direct, often crushing blows to the hand and most frequently involve the second metacarpal. These fractures are usually comminuted and always intraarticular.

2. **Diagnosis.** Look for associated soft tissue and extensor tendon injuries.

3. **Treatment** depends on the amount of joint space involved, with attention to restoring the articular surface. Minimally comminuted fractures are often treated with open reduction and internal fixation (ORIF), while more comminuted fractures are treated by closed manipulation, with molding of the fragments and plaster immobilization. Emergency treatment includes a soft, bulky dressing with the hand in the "position of function." Conservative management often produces adequate functional results, with residual bony defects filling in with fibrocartilage.

4. **Complications** include degenerative arthritis, interosseous muscle scarring from the crush injury, and extensor tendon injuries.

B. **Neck of the fourth and fifth metacarpals**

1. **Mechanism of injury.** These fractures are common and usually result from direct blows, as by punching a solid object.

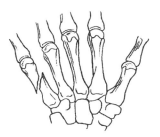

Fig. 1. Oblique and spiral fractures tend to shorten and rotate.

2. **Diagnosis.** Routine hand x-rays are usually diagnostic. These fractures tend to present with an gulation deformities with the apex dorsal; rotational deformities also occur. The interosseus muscles, which flex the MCP joints, are responsible for the angulation deformities. Angulation is well tolerated from a functional standpoint owing to the mobility of the CMC joints. The "boxer's fracture" results when a clenched fist strikes a solid object, causing a fracture of the fifth metacarpal neck.

3. **Treatment.** Treatment is controversial. There have been many series that report good function and quicker return to work with no reduction of angulation. Others argue that residual angulation of greater than 40 degrees should be avoided by proper reduction. Once a fracture is reduced, maintenance of reduction is difficult or impossible. A more devastating deformity is rotation, which must be sought and reduced. Even small rotational deformities can cause significant functional impairment. A similar fracture of the fourth metacarpal requires reduction for angulation greater than 20 degrees. Reduction may be attempted for lesser angulation, although these fractures tend to lose reduction even with splinting. They can be reduced and splinted in the emergency department as follows:

   a. Obtain adequate anesthesia by hematoma or ulnar nerve anesthetic injection.

   b. Hang the affected finger in a "finger trap" for 10 minutes.

   c. Flex the PIP and the MCP joints to 90 degrees.

   d. Apply a volar force over the metacarpal head while applying an axially directed dorsal force through the proximal phalanx of the finger. Rotation can be corrected by using the proximal phalangeal shaft as a crank to reduce the deformity.

Once reduced, these fractures should be splinted to the fingertips in an ulnar gutter splint or an anterior or posterior splint. The MCP joint is flexed 70 to 90 degrees, the IP joints extended, and the wrist extended 30 degrees, in a position that is similar to that of holding a tennis ball. As previously noted it is extremely difficult to hold the reduction in this manner. Close follow-up within several days is needed to assure that the reduction continues to be adequate. The patient can expect about 2 weeks of splinting, followed by range-of-motion exercises. Most patients can be back to work in 2 to 4 weeks.

4. **Complications** in up to 75% of patients can include deformity, painful grip, and loss of power. Very few patients, however, have any noticeable disability from these complications.

C. **Angulated neck fractures of the second and third metacarpals**

1. **Treatment.** These fractures require anatomical reduction because of the lack of compensatory motion at the CMC joints. This is accomplished outside of the emergency department setting. In the emergency setting, treatment includes immobilization in a short arm volar splint and elevation.

2. **Complications** of all metacarpal neck fractures include collateral ligament dysfunction, extensor tendon injuries, nonunion due to inadequate immobilization (relatively uncommon), residual rotation, and excessive angulation with compromise of grip and function of the hand.

D. **Nonangulated fractures of the metacarpal neck** are less common. The treatment of these includes splinting and elevation. Close follow-up is necessary within several days to make sure that the fracture did not angulate after splinting.

E. **Shaft fractures of metacarpals 2 through 5** occur as a result of either a direct blow to the hand or a twisting force applied to the corresponding finger. These fractures are either transverse, oblique, spiral, or comminuted.

1. **Transverse**
   a. **Mechanism of injury.** Direct blows cause these fractures. Because of the pull of the interossei and long flexor muscles, these are angulated with the apex dorsal (Fig. 2). The more proximal the fracture, the more noticeable the deformity, with "clawing" of the hand resulting in a weakened grip. Similar to fractures of the neck, angulation is less well tolerated for the second and third metacarpals than the fourth and fifth. Residual angula-

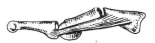

Fig. 2. Transverse fractures of the metacarpals generally angulate apex dorsal because of the pull of the interosseus muscles.

tion of greater than 10° is not acceptable for the second and third metacarpals, and patients may not tolerate the visible bump on the dorsum of the hand seen with residual angulation deformities; reduction may be necessary for this reason.

Residual angulation can be hard to control owing to excessive swelling from the fracture hematoma. Any residual rotation is unacceptable and requires correction.

b. **Treatment.** Emergency reduction may be attempted in a manner similar to that described above (fractures of the fifth metacarpal neck). Splinting of nonangulated or reduced transverse fractures utilizes a gutter splint that extends from the elbow to the fingertips with the joints in the position of function. These tend to lose reduction, and close follow-up is recommended for possible wire or screw fixation. Multiple transverse fractures may require surgical treatment and are best splinted with rapid follow-up.

2. **Spiral and oblique fractures**
   a. **Mechanism of injury.** These occur secondary to twisting of the associated finger.
   b. **Diagnosis.** In addition to standard AP and lateral x-ray views, an oblique view is often helpful in defining this fracture. These fractures tend to shorten and rotate due to the proximal pull of the intrinsic muscles. Residual shortening of more than 3 mm or any rotation is unacceptable.
   c. **Treatment.** These fractures are often easy to reduce but rarely remain reduced with splinting; therefore close orthopaedic follow-up is needed. Both spiral and oblique fractures may exhibit rotational deformities. In general, these fractures should be reduced anatomically. Residual angulation is less well tolerated in the fourth and fifth metacarpals. The more proximal the fracture, the less angulation may be tolerated by the patient after healing.

3. **Comminuted fractures**
   a. **Mechanism of injury.** These fractures are due to direct blows and crush injuries and may have significant overlying soft tissue injury.

      b. Treatment. Because of the comminution and loss of integrity of the shaft, the affected bones can shorten and rotate. These fractures frequently require operative repair, occasionally with bone grafting, so close follow-up is needed. Splinting with bulky dressing is appropriate in the emergency department.

      c. Complications include chronic pain from excessive angulation, weak grip from shortening or rotation, scarring of the associated interossei muscles, and nonunion, which is relatively uncommon.

F. Fractures of the base of the metacarpals

    1. Mechanism of injury. These are uncommon and can result from falls on the outstretched hand, punching with axial loads to the metacarpal, or direct blows.

    2. Diagnosis. Routine x-rays of the hand are usually sufficient for diagnosis, although these lesions can easily be missed on x-ray. Be suspicious if the point of tenderness is at the base of the metacarpal, with an appropriate mechanism. CMC joint dislocation may occur as well, which can be difficult to discern on x-ray but can lead to significant functional impairment if not corrected. An intraarticular fracture of the fifth metacarpal may act like a Bennett's fracture owing to the pull of the extensor carpi ulnaris muscle.

    3. Treatment. Depending on which bone is fractured, tendon pull may preclude closed reduction. Intraarticular fractures frequently require operative reduction. Extraarticular fractures are usually stable because of the CMC and interosseous ligaments. The initial management of these fractures consists of a bulky dressing and close follow-up.

    4. Complications can include damage to one of the tendons that attaches to the fracture site, nonunion (uncommon), and stiffness of the carpometacarpal joint.

V. Fractures of the thumb

  A. Thumb metacarpal. The mobility of this bone at the CMC joint affords significant resistance to fracture. It also allows the healing fracture to better tolerate residual angulation deformities. Standard x-rays of the thumb and hand usually suffice to visualize these fractures.

  B. Fractures of the shaft and nonintraarticular base are more commonly seen than intraarticular fractures. Most of these fractures occur as a result of direct blows to the hand or axial loading, as is seen when the hand strikes a solid object. These fractures can be transverse (the most common) or oblique. Inspect oblique fractures carefully to rule out intraarticular extension. Extraarticular fractures are often oblique and comminuted. These tend to shorten and

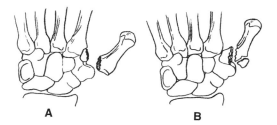

Fig. 3. A: Bennett's fracture/dislocation. The distal fragment is displaced proximally by the pull of the abductor pollicis lengus. B: Rolando's fracture. This is a comminuted intraarticular fracture.

rotate because of the forces imposed by the tendons on the fragments. Residual angulation of up to 30 degrees is well tolerated. Rotational deformity must be sought and corrected; if this is not done early, permanent functional impairment will result. These fractures are treated with attention to immobilization, elevation, and follow-up. The emergency physician may attempt reduction of angulation for most of these fractures; however, it is not mandatory. Close follow-up for ongoing care is important. Oblique and comminuted fractures often do not remain reduced in a splint; therefore operative fixation may be necessary. A short arm splint with the fingers in the position of function (as in holding an apple) will usually be sufficient for initial treatment. Other options include a soft, bulky dressing. Indications for operative reduction include persistent rotation, shortening, and angulation of greater than 30 degrees.

C. **Intraarticular fractures at the base of the thumb metacarpal** are relatively uncommon. These can cause significant long-term problems, including painful grip, weak grip, and loss of normal opposition function.

   1. **Bennett's fracture/dislocation**
      a. **Mechanism of injury.** This involves an oblique fracture into the joint space of the first CMC joint (Fig. 3A). These fractures are often caused by an axial load on the partially flexed metacarpal, as is seen in a fist-fight. Anatomically, this fracture is unstable because of the tendon forces exerted on the distal metacarpal fragment, which contains most of the joint surface. The proximal fragment maintains contact with the trapezium because of its strong ligamentous attachments. The distal fragment is pulled by the tendon of the abductor pollicis longus and is displaced proximally.

b. **Treatment.** This injury can be treated surgically by percutaneous K-wire fixation if displacement is minimal. If there is greater displacement open reduction and fixation will be necessary. In the emergency department, the digit can be held immobile with a thumb spica splint pending anatomical reduction.

2. **Rolando's fracture**

   a. **Mechanism of injury.** This is a comminuted intraarticular fracture of the thumb metacarpal (Fig. 3B). It is relatively rare and is caused by the same mechanism as a Bennett's fracture. In addition to the proximal fixed fragment, also with Bennett's fracture, Rolando's fracture has at least a second dorsal fragment and often multiple fragments.

   b. **Treatment.** Anatomical reduction is required. The prognosis can be poor even with expert management. Depending on the size of the fragments involved, management may consist of open reduction, attempts at molding the comminuted fragments in a thumb spica cast, or traction to align the fragments, with ROM exercises after 4 weeks. The more comminution of the fragments, the worse the prognosis will be. Emergency department treatment is directed at immobilization in plaster and rapid follow-up.

   c. **Complications** consist mainly of chronic pain from arthritic degeneration of the joint surface, with loss of grip strength and decreased function of the hand.

BIBLIOGRAPHY

Bodell LS, Martin ML. Hand and wrist fractures in occupational medicine. *Occup Med* 1989;4:497–524.

Bowman SH, Simon RR. Metacarpal and phalangeal fractures. *Emerg Med Clin North Am* 1993;11:671–702.

Green DP. Complications of phalangeal and metacarpal fractures. *Hand Clin* 1986;2:307–328.

Lowden IMR. Fractures of the metacarpal neck of the little finger. *Injury* 1986;17:189–192.

Ruiz E, Cicero JJ. *Emergency management of skeletal injuries.* St Louis: Mosby, 1995.

Rockwood CA, Green DP. *Fractures in adults.* Philadelphia: JB Lippincott, 1991.

Simon RR, Koenigsknecht SJ. *Emergency orthopedics,* 2nd ed. Norwalk, CT: Appleton and Lange, 1987.

Phalangeal Fractures

Todd H. Chaffin

The digit's architecture permits soft tissue and the skeletal structures to perform a wide range of motor and sensory functions. Most digit injuries can be definitively treated upon initial presentation. It is vital that clinicians be able to take a methodical and detailed history and perform a careful physical examination. For injuries that require referral, adherence to a comprehensive evaluation will ensure an intelligent discussion with a consultant and assist the patient toward functional recovery. Additionally, most well-managed digit injuries will heal satisfactorily with minimal morbidity. With the advent of microsurgical techniques and orthopaedic fixation devices, many digits that were once deemed unsalvageable are now repairable. Replantation of amputated digits, bone grafting, and newer immobilization devices allow useful, early functional recovery of the once mangled digit. Initial management—such as pain relief, wound cleansing, immunization, antibiotics when indicated, and preservation of the amputated part—can reduce morbidity and improve surgical outcomes.

I. **Anatomy.** The digits are indicated by name: thumb index, long, ring, and little fingers. The thumb has two phalanges, proximal and distal, and, at its base, two sesamoid bones. The remaining digits are comprised of three bones each: proximal, middle and distal phalanges. The associated joints are the metacarpophalangeal (MCP), proximal interphalangeal (PIP), and distal interphalangeal (DIP). The exception is the thumb interphalangeal joint (IP).

II. **Examination**
   A. **History.** The age of the patient, hand dominance, occupation (job description and how it is performed), time and location of injury, immunization status, allergies, and medications require documentation. The mechanism of injury, symptomatology, perceived loss of function and digit's position at the time of injury (extension, flexion, clenched) should be determined. Chemical exposure, environmental contaminants, use of protective garments, and observation of proper machine safety should be sought when evaluating occupational injuries along with any prehospital care received, such as wound cleansing, irrigation, or manipulation. The patient's past medical history should be checked for immunosuppression, diabetes, circulatory or rheumatological disorders, prior injuries, or other factors influencing healing such as smoking, alcohol, or impaired lymphatics (mastectomy, lymph node dissection, or radiation therapy). Last, hobbies or activities important to the patient should be determined.

B. **Physical.** A systematic exam under proper lighting, with an outstretched extremity on an arm board, provides for optimal physical examination. Often adequate examination cannot be performed without first providing a bloodless field by digit or forearm tourniquet and digital, common digital, or wrist block anesthesia. First, however, neurovascular function must be documented and, when indicated, a specialist consulted.

1. **Inspection**

    a. The digit's **position** should be documented relative to its normal position of function, along with **deformity, deviation,** or **rotation** (metacarpal or phalangeal fractures can result in rotational deformities that must be corrected). Rotational deformity is noted if the planes of the nails are not relatively parallel or if the fingers fail to point toward the scaphoid when alternately flexed.

    b. **Make note of soiling, swelling, ecchymosis, color, foreign bodies, or gross wound contamination.**

    c. **Soft tissue loss or penetration** (loss may indicate the need for skin grafting or flaps), exposed tendon or bone, fingernail condition and extent of subungual hematoma must be documented (adding a drawing is useful).

2. **Circulation** is checked by noting temperature, capillary refill, and results of Allen's test of the digits or hand.

3. **Nerve function** is assessed by light touch and two-point discrimination (normal <2 to 6 mm).

4. **Tendon function** is revealed by simple observation. The hand at rest forms a cascade of increasing flexion from the index through little fingers. A complete tendon laceration disrupts this normal cascade. Range-of-motion testing is as follows:

    a. Radial and ulnar deviation at the MCP joint.

    b. Thumb adduction, abduction, and opposition.

    c. Flexion by immobilizing the PIP and MCP joints and asking the patient to flex the DIP or thumb IP joint (profundus test). Then, with the examiner holding the adjacent digits, the patient is asked to flex the PIP joint (superficialis test).

    d. Extension by fully extending all digit joints, especially the DIP.

    e. Strength testing against resistance (but not to the extent that a partial injury is made into a complete one).

5. Joint injuries are found by locating pain and swelling and stress-testing the collateral, volar, and dorsal capsular structures after the digit has been x-rayed and—usually—anesthetized.

6. **Bone injury** may be detected when there is gross deviation, protrusion of bony fragments, rotation, or limited joint motion.

7. **Wound exploration** (after x-ray and anesthesia) is required if skin disruption exists. All wound recesses are explored in a bloodless field to ensure that deep vital, structure lacerations or foreign bodies are not missed. Tendon injury is eliminated only after moving the digit through its entire excursion under direct visualization.

C, **Radiography.** Many injuries require an x-ray, as physical examination is often unreliable in detecting fractures, subluxations, dislocations, or radiopaque foreign bodies. Additionally, swelling and ecchymosis may be minimal or nonexistent shortly after the injury or in the pediatric patient. Large subungual hematomas, nail-plate disruption, restricted motion, or significant mechanisms of injury are indications for radiographs, as these indications imply substantial trauma. On occasion a distal phalangeal fracture presents as a posttraumatic paronychia, this may be an additional indication for radiographs. At least three images are needed, including posteroanterior (PA), true lateral, and 45-degree externally rotated oblique views. The addition of a 45-degree internally rotated oblique view is recommended by some to detect articular injuries missed by the three standard views. Other imaging techniques such as tomography, stress views, and contralateral digit x-ray can be helpful when a fracture is in question or when joint, epiphyseal, or congenital deformities are suspected.

D. **Diagnosis.** Conclusive diagnosis can be derived only after completion of an adequate history and physical examination, x-ray, and wound exploration. Both physical examination and wound exploration can be impeded unless the digit is anesthetized satisfactorily. The ability to perform digital or wrist nerve blocks is a requirement in order to complete the diagnostic process and before treatment can be implemented. Physicians should therefore be facile in anesthetizing injuries using buffered, long-acting anesthetics without epinephrine (bupivacaine) injected slowly, using a 1- to 1 1/2-inch, 27- to 30-gauge, needle. This may be performed prior to obtaining an x-ray, which will provide anesthesia for exam or treatment. If a block is performed, care should be taken not to overly distend the tissue, which can compromise neurovascular bundles or lead to a compartment syndrome.

Significant crush injury, neurovascular compromise, and multiple digit injuries are indications for wrist nerve blocks.

III. **Treatment**

A. **General guidelines**

1. **Pain management** by the practitioner is always appropriate, since pain motivated the patient to seek treatment. This can be provided by using a local or regional block, as outlined previously, and supplemented by elevation, narcotic analgesics, or nitrous oxide. By providing pain relief, the clinician will maximize diagnosis, therapy, and patient satisfaction.

2. **Wound management** begins with ring removal and gentle skin cleansing to remove grease or soiling, while care is taken not to further disrupt injured tissue. Full-thickness wounds require retraction, so that the wound can be irrigated using copious, pulsatile saline irrigation, in order to remove contaminates from all wound recesses. Lacerations amenable to repair should be closed loosely with as few as possible 5.0 or 6.0 nylon horizontal mattress or simple sutures, using a fine needle. Nail beds are repaired with 6.0 Vicryl or chromic sutures. There is rarely a need for anything other than skin sutures, as more deeply placed sutures may cause neurovascular injury; exceptions include tendon and joint repairs. Wounds may then be covered with antibiotic ointment, a nonadherent dressing, and a loosely applied gauze dressing. Parenteral antibiotic coverage is indicated when there is immune compromise, severe crush injuries, open fractures, tendon lacerations, joint injuries, or delayed wound treatment.

3. **Principles of immobilization**

a. Some fractures are best immobilized with a **long finger splint** that incorporates the digit and metacarpal joint and, at times, the wrist and forearm as well (if deforming forearm tendon forces must be eliminated). If the latter is utilized, the wrist should be kept at approximately 30 degrees of extension for most injuries.

b. A **gauntlet cast** may be useful in immobilizing some fractures when patient reliability is questionable or if the patient is a child, in which case the index through little fingers may be incorporated for protective purposes.

c. Fractures of the ring and little fingers can frequently be treated with an **ulnar gutter splint;** similarly, fractures of the index and

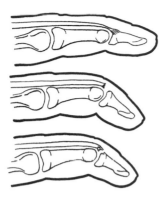

Fig. 1. Mallet-finger deformity resulting from tendon stretch, tendon disruption, and avulsion fracture.

middle fingers can be treated with a **radial gutter splint** with a hole for the thumb.

d. Fractures involving the thumb can be managed with a **radial gutter** or **thumb spica splint** incorporating the entire digit.

e. Splinting the affected digit only with a **foam-backed aluminum splint,** or incorporating the adjacent uninjured digit (buddy splint) for stability and protection, is appropriate for some fractures.

f. **Buddy-taping** to the adjacent uninjured digit may be acceptable in reliable patients with stable, nondisplaced fractures.

B. **Fracture management**

1. **Distal phalanx fractures** occur from a direct blow to the extended tip or dorsal surface. These are divided into comminuted (usually the tuft), transverse, longitudinal, and intraarticular.

a. **Comminuted (tuft) fractures** frequently involve the nail bed. The fracture itself is stable because of fibrous septae and the nail, which acts as a splint. Treatment is 2 to 4 weeks of protection with a cage or molded aluminum splint that encloses the distal phalanx yet allows DIP motion. The presence of a subungual hematoma implies a nail-bed injury that may require surgical repair. Most authors would agree that if the nail plate has been avulsed from its bed or from beneath the eponychial fold, the nail plate should be removed and the nail bed repaired with fine absorbable suture. A subungual hematoma involving 50% or more of the nail bed in some authors' opinions requires nail removal and nail-bed repair.

Other authors recommend simple evacuation by nail trephination, using a nail drill or heated cautery tip. This provides substantial pain relief and, although technically creating an open fracture, is one of the few situations where prophylactic antibiotic coverage is unwarranted. If the nail is removed, a stent should be placed for 10 days beneath the eponychial fold by using the original nail or nonadhering gauze. This prevents nail-bed adhesions, assists in nail regrowth, and may limit new nail deformity.

b. **Transverse fractures** are often nondisplaced, requiring only protective splinting of the distal phalanx for 2 weeks or until the fracture is painless and stable (4 to 6 weeks). Displaced transverse fractures should be reduced, but this may be difficult owing to interposed adipose tissue. If the fracture cannot be reduced by manipulation or remains unstable after reduction, the distal phalanx should be splinted and referred to a surgeon for pinning. If reduction is satisfactory on repeat x-ray, the treatment should proceed as for a nondisplaced fracture. Often, when displaced fractures are treated conservatively, they will heal by a fibrous union that eventually provides a stable, painless phalanx; however, this may take 6 or more months.

c. **Longitudinal fractures** traverse the length of the phalanx and are generally nondisplaced. A splint is placed from the middle to the distal phalanges, leaving the PIP joint free. The splint remains for 3 to 4 weeks followed by passive range-of-motion exercise until the digit is painless. Displaced fractures may be difficult to reduce and are best referred to a surgeon after similar splinting for possible pinning.

d. **Intraarticular fractures** are divided into dorsal injuries (mallet) and volar fractures.

  (1) **Mallet finger** (Fig. 1)

    (a) **Mechanism of injury.** Mallet-finger deformity results from either tendon or bone injuries that prevent full DIP extension and appear to have a DIP flexion deformity. Overstretching or tendon rupture without a fracture may produce a mallet-finger appearance. Exact diagnosis is confirmed by x-ray.

    (b) **Treatment.** Many authors divide these fractures into those involv-

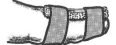

Fig. 2. Proper splinting technique for mallet-finger deformity.

ing less than or greater than 33% of the articular surface. Those fractures involving greater than 33% of the articular surface receive operative fixation with K-wire. This practice is questioned by some authors (Lubahn, Hood, and Schneider), who have had considerable success in treating most mallet-finger injuries conservatively by dorsal splinting, even when the distal phalanx is subluxed volarly. Operative treatment is reserved for those cases that fail conservative treatment. Regardless of the type of injury, mallet-finger deformity should be splinted in slight hyperextension by a middle-to-distal phalangeal splint with the PIP joint free. Several commercial splints are manufactured for such an injury, but a simple aluminum or paper-clip splint may be fashioned and applied as shown (Fig. 2). With conservative treatment, the splint must be left on for 6 to 8 weeks, followed by nocturnal protective splinting for 2 to 4 weeks. The patient must be advised not to "test" the DIP joint prematurely, as such activity will disrupt any bone healing that has occurred and may lead to a failed union; all such fractures require close follow-up. If a failed union does occur, operative treatment is indicated.

(2) **Volar fractures** (Fig. 3) are usually of the avulsion type. As long as there is some DIP joint flexion, these may be treated for 6 to 8 weeks with dorsal or

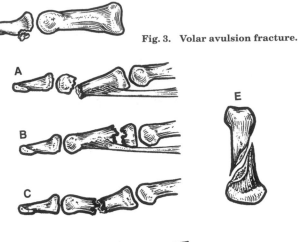

Fig. 3. Volar avulsion fracture.

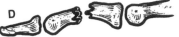

Fig. 4. Displaced angulated, and spiral fractures of the middle phalanx.

volar splinting, with only the DIP joint immobilized and kept in partial flexion (5 to 10 degrees).

(3) **Profundus tendon rupture** from volar injuries or displaced avulsion fractures may be missed unless the function of the profundus tendon is properly tested. Digital x-rays may show minimal bone involvement; on occasion, the avulsed fragment retracts proximally, giving the appearance of an avulsion fracture of the proximal or middle phalanx. These injuries require a splint that incorporates the wrist with the finger maintained in flexion, along with referral (or hospitalization) for prompt surgical repair.

2. **Middle phalangeal fractures** are often caused by a direct blow or by axial loading or hyper-deviation forces. Frequently such fractures involve the neck, proximal waist, or intraarticular structures. These injuries are divided into nondisplaced, stable (usually transverse), and displaced unstable (spiral, oblique, angulated, or intraarticular) fractures. Such unstable or

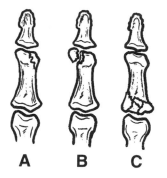

Fig. 5. Intraarticular fractures.
A: Nondisplaced condylar.
B: Displaced condylar.
C: Comminated base.

displaced fractures are often the result of deforming tendon forces across the fracture site.

a. **Nondisplaced stable fractures** are best treated by buddy taping to the adjacent uninjured digit. This provides stability yet allows some joint motion that will limit complications of joint stiffness. These fractures require close follow-up and repeat x-ray in 10 to 14 days to ensure proper alignment. Comminuted fractures may appear stable but are potentially unstable and are best splinted using a gutter splint to incorporate the wrist as well as the injured digit. These fractures should be followed closely, with repeat x-ray performed in 10 to 14 days.

b. **Displaced, spiral, or angulated** (Fig. 4) fractures are generally considered unstable and should be treated as previously discussed by using an ulnar or radial gutter splint and making a referral for surgical stabilization.

c. **Intraarticular (condylar and basilar, Fig. 5; dorsal and volar avulsion, Fig. 6)** involve cartilaginous or ligamentous structures and are at risk for suboptimal outcomes unless treated appropriately. Generally if the fracture is **displaced** (1 mm or more step-off involving the cartilaginous surface), surgical pinning and/or repair of the collateral ligament is indicated. If the fracture is **nondisplaced,** a longer finger splint in the position of function is usually satisfactory, with attempts at early mobilization. Others recommend simple dynamic splinting, an exception being a basilar fracture, which should be placed in a long finger splint and referred, as these

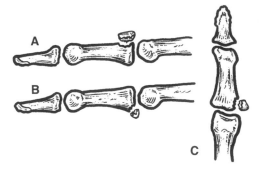

Fig. 6.   Intraarticular fractures. A: volar; B: dorsal; C: marginal.

fractures are prone to healing with complications and may require specialized splinting techniques. Displaced fractures are splinted in radial or ulnar gutter splints and referred.

3. **Proximal phalangeal fractures** result from similar mechanisms as middle phalangeal fractures and are similarly classified. Any fracture, displacement, or instability cannot be tolerated owing to the fact that this bone has the greatest range of motion and is responsible for positioning of the distal phalanx. Proximal phalangeal fractures most often require referral.

a. Any **nondisplaced stable fractures** may be splinted by means of a dorsal long finger splint extending from the metacarpal through the middle phalanx, with the MCP joint at 60 degrees and the PIP joint at 30 degrees of flexion. In the reliable patient, buddy-taping to the adjacent uninjured digit is acceptable.

b. **Displaced** or **unstable fractures** are managed as follows:

(1) **Shaft, oblique, spiral,** or **angulated fractures** may be splinted with radial or ulnar gutter splints, incorporating the wrist to eliminate deforming tendon forces. Reduction by longitudinal traction may be attempted after discussion with the referral physician.

(2) **Intraarticular fractures at the MCP or PIP joints** are splinted similarly; however, some authors prefer buddy-taping if the intraarticular fracture is

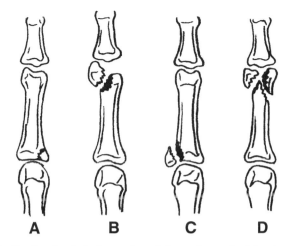

Fig. 7. Proximal phalangeal condylar and marginal fractures.

stable and without a step-off to allow for early range of motion.

    (3) For **displaced fractures (condylar or marginal),** referral is mandatory since they usually require internal fixation (Fig. 7). These may be temporarily splinted by radial or ulnar gutter splints.

  4. **Sesamoid fractures at the thumb** (and less commonly at the index and fifth fingers) MCP joint are uncommon and may be associated with proximal thumb fractures. They are most often encountered in sports when the joint receives a direct blow or is hyperextended. Radiographic detection may be missed unless the injury is sought specifically. Treatment consists of 2 to 3 weeks of immobilization in a dorsal or volar splint from the metacarpal to distal phalanx with the IP joint kept flexed at 10 to 15 degrees.

C. **Referral.** Indications for immediate consultation or referral include:

  1. Oblique, spiral, or rotational deformity fractures.

  2. Intraarticular displaced fractures.

  3. Displaced or angulated fractures that cannot be maintained if reduced.

  4. Multiple fractures where skeleton stabilization is required for one or more fracture sites.

  5. Fractures involving bone loss and requiring mechanical stabilization to maintain length.

6.   Significant skin loss (>1 cm^2) and/or nerve, tendon, or arterial injury.
7.   Open fractures that cannot be adequately
cleaned or covered with soft tissue.
8.   Amputations proximal to the distal phalangeal
waist (see Sec. IX.C).

IV.   **Complications** are similar to those of other fractures;
however, these may be potentially more disabling if the
bones fail to heal normally.

A.   **Infections** are infrequent but do occur, hence the
need for meticulous treatment when the wound is
initially evaluated. Nothing is more important than
thorough wound exploration and irrigation. Prophylactic antibiotic coverage is indicated for open
fractures to prevent osteomyelitis, a rare but feared
complication.

B.   **Nonunion** results from uncorrected displacement
or interposition of soft tissues between fracture
ends and can lead to pseudoarthrosis and chronic
pain. Distal phalangeal fractures commonly show
delayed union; therefore one may be misled on follow-up x-rays looking for callus formation only to
find it lacking. This type of fracture may require additional time (>6 months) to form a bony union.

C.   **Malunion** is most commonly seen in fractures of
the proximal or middle phalanx that were rotated, displaced, shortened, or angulated. For this
reason all fractures so classified require early referral.

D.   **Formation of callus** or **bony exostosis** may interfere with tendon or joint motion due to tendon or
joint impingement.

E.   **Periarticular injuries** can cause chronic joint deformity, stiffness, or arthritis.

F.   **Compartment syndrome** from crush injuries, circumferential bandaging, or casts can occur, so the
patient should be observed for discoloration, pale-
ness, paresthesias, coolness, or worsening of pain
beyond expectation. These symptoms should prompt
removal of coverings to examine the digit.

V.   **Special situations**

A.   **Pediatric injuries** differ from injuries of mature
bone in that the epiphysis is the metabolically active region responsible for longitudinal bone growth.
The periosteum surrounding pediatric bones is
thick, offering protection and plasticity. For this
reason pediatric fractures can be treated conservatively as long as no rotation or displacement exists.
Most fractures, however, should be referred to a
specialist for proper follow-up. At times immobilization of the extremity from the wrist or elbow should
be considered in this potentially active age group.

1.   **Greenstick fractures** may be similarly treated
with buddy-taping to the adjacent digit or gut-

ter splinting with follow-up radiography in 8 to 10 days to exclude displacement or rotation.

2. **Nondisplaced, nonangulated transverse shaft fractures** are often stable and can be treated with buddy-taping or gutter splinting, with follow-up x-ray in 1 week to ensure proper alignment.

3. **Salter-Harris fractures** are classified like other pediatric epiphyseal injuries. Parents should be informed of possible growth disturbance. Lower-numbered fractures (Salter 1 to 3) tend to heal well, but higher ones and those associated with ligamentous disruption may not. Last, one should be aware that "sprained" digits are less common than actual fractures and must be evaluated closely for subtle epiphyseal fractures.

B. **Fractures in the elderly** are often the result of falls and are frequently comminuted owing to the aging process of bone. The digits often show accompanying arthritic changes that lead to complications of joint stiffness even after brief immobilization. It commonly takes a long time to regain motion and reduce stiffness, and the digit may never regain full function. Attempts should be made to avoid unnecessary immobilization of adjacent joints or digits and to actively use the remaining uninjured extremity, including the shoulder.

C. **Amputations** involving the distal portion of the distal phalanx have been found to heal satisfactorily without grafting or primary wound closure even when some bone is exposed. These wounds can be covered with antibiotic ointment and a nonadherent dressing and allowed to heal by secondary intention. This takes several months and—depending on the amount of soft tissue lost—can lead to a cosmetically acceptable appearance. Primary closure can be performed but may require ronguering of the distal bone fragment to provide adequate skin closure. One should discuss such cases with the consultant before proceeding. Protective splinting and prophylactic antibiotics should be provided for these injuries. More proximal digit amputations may be an indication for replantation based on the following criteria if less than 12 hours have elapsed:

1. Single digit amputations distal to the superficialis tendon insertion on the middle phalanx
2. Multiple digits
3. Digits of children
4. Thumb
5. No significant preexisting medical or psychiatric disorder

VI. **Disposition.** All but the most minor fractures will require follow-up evaluation, and most need referral to experienced practitioners. Failure to make appropriate referral may lead to unnecessary morbidity or medical/legal complications. For this reason, a thorough understanding of the fracture type and its subsequent treatment is imperative. Often minimized or overlooked is the need to discuss with the patient the nature of the injury and what the expected outcome and complications may be. Such preemptive discussions may minimize the risk of patient dissatisfaction, medical/legal actions, and colleague criticism of the initially rendered care. The following guidelines should be borne in mind and documented in the record:

A. **Provide adequate analgesics for expected pain.** Most patients will have several hours of pain relief from a nerve block but will require 1 to 2 days of hydrocodone followed by a nonsteroidal anti-inflammatory drug—barring contraindications.

B. **Elevate the extremity for the first 24 hours** to limit swelling and subsequent pain. This must be strongly reinforced.

C. **Tetanus immunization and prophylactic antibiotics for 3 to 5 days** for appropriate injuries should be implemented in the department (preferably parenterally), followed by the first oral dose, which the patient may take later.

D. **Provide standardized wound care, cast, or splint precautions** and emphasize the need to return or seek medical attention promptly should unexpected symptoms or questions arise.

E. **Inform the patient of potential complications** such as infection, stiffness, prolonged rehabilitation, deformity, or the possibility of cosmetically important sequelae. This is especially true of nail or nail-bed injuries, which can cause nail deformity or growth disturbance.

F. **Arrange office appointments with the referral physician** for wound checks, follow-up x-rays, suture removal, and splint checks (within 1 week). Injuries at risk for infection should be checked in 2 to 3 days.

G. **For work-related injuries, avoid extended off duty time beyond 1 to 2 days.** Returning employees back to work as soon as possible should be the rule unless there is a sound medical reason. It is impossible for most physicians to know what form of light duty or modified work is available to an injured employee despite what an employee may say to the contrary. It is best to provide work restrictions such as "one-handed duty" involving the uninjured extremity, even if such work is unavailable. This will limit the employer's need to document lost duty time for Occupational Safety and Health Administration (OSHA)-recordable events even if the company determines that there is no work available with the given restrictions.

H. **Alcohol use or smoking should be discouraged,** as both of these activities impede healing.

VII. **Long-term care and rehabilitation.** Frequently, digit fractures require some rehabilitation, especially after prolonged immobilization. This may necessitate referral to a physical or occupational therapist with expertise in hand injuries. This treatment is best left to the referral physician, who can monitor the patient's progress.

BIBLIOGRAPHY

Carter P, Stein F. *Emerg Med Clin North Am* 1985;3:   .

Chipman C, ed. *Emergency department orthopaedics.* Rockville, MD: Aspen, 1982.

Dong P, Seeger L, Shapiro M, Levere S. Fractures of the sesamoid bones of the thumb. *Am J Sports Med* 1995;23:336–339.

Guly H. Fractures of the terminal phalanx presenting as a paronychia. *Arch Emerg Med* 1993;10:301–305.

Ip W, Ng K, Chow S. A prospective study of 924 digital fractures of the hand. *Injury* 1996;27:279–285.

Lubahn J, Hood J. Fractures of the distal interphalangeal joint. *Clin Orthop Rel Res* 1996;327:12–20.

Mennen U, Wiese A. Fingertip injuries management with semi-occlusive dressing. *Br J Hand Surg* 1993;18B:416.

Morrissy R, Weinstein S, eds. *Lovell and Winter's pediatric orthopaedics,* 4th ed, vol 2. Philadelphia: Lippincott, 1996.

Schenck R. Classification of fractures and dislocations of the proximal interphalangeal joint. *Hand Clin* 1994;10:179–185.

Schneider L. Fractures of the distal phalanx. *Hand Clin* 1988;4:537–547.

Schneider L. Fractures of the distal interphalangeal joint. *Hand Clin* 1994;10:277–285.

Seaberg D. Treatment of subungual hematomas with nail trephination: a prospective study. *Am J Emerg Med* 1991;9:209.

Street J. Radiographs of phalangeal fractures: importance of the internally rotated oblique projection for diagnosis. *Am J Radiol* 1993;160:575.

Acute Joint Injuries of the Hand

Arthur F. Proust

Injuries of the hand lead to many emergency department visits. These injuries can range from the apparent benign sprain to the complex fracture/dislocations and crush injuries. Because no anatomical area is exposed to more potential threats and requires such precision of movement to meet daily demands as the hand, it is important that optimal treatment be initiated at the time of injury.

The severity of injury, however, may not be readily apparent. Subtle injuries, especially to the joint, are often missed as compared with injuries producing gross deformities or radiographic abnormalities. Indeed, since healing of joint structures is often imperfect and unpredictable, early recognition and treatment are key to preventing long-term functional disability.

I. **Evaluation of joint injuries**
  A. **History.** An accurate history will help lead to an accurate diagnosis. Discerning the direction and magnitude of force to the joint is important in determining the type and extent of injury. For example, intraarticular fractures result from an axial load. A lateral force may produce a lateral dislocation or injury of the collateral ligament. Tears of the volar plate or dorsal dislocations are due to a hyperextension mechanism.

    Certain sporting activities or occupations may predispose to specific injuries. For example, injuries of the ulnar collateral ligament of the thumb metacarpophalangeal (MCP) joint often occur when a ski pole causes a radial stress; previously, this injury was known to occur in British gamekeepers. Finally, severity of injury may be predicted by the onset of pain, swelling, and ecchymosis.

  B. **Examination.** Examination of the injured hand may be hindered by the dense sensory fibers producing pain. Deformity, swelling, and ecchymosis on visual inspection may pinpoint the site of injury. Functional impairment is suggested by an abnormal carriage of the hand.

    1. Joint stability is tested by **active range of motion.** Because of the influence of pain, active range of motion is most readily assessed after digital anesthesia. Although significant ligamentous injury may be present, the presence of near normal active range of motion implies that functional recovery will occur with conservative rather than surgical treatment. The point of maximal tenderness should be determined and sensory evaluation completed prior to digital block.

2. The location and degree of ligamentous injury can be assessed by **passive range of motion** and **passive ligament stressing.** The integrity of the volar plate and collateral ligament is tested by anteroposterior and radial-ulnar stress, respectively. This is accomplished in both extension and moderate flexion to eliminate volar plate stabilization. It is also done gently so as to avoid causing a complete tear.

C. **Radiographs.** Indications for radiography include a suspicious mechanism along with swelling and tenderness. Standard views include anteroposterior, oblique, and, most important for individual digits, a true lateral. Many errors are made in the diagnosis of joint injuries because of failure to obtain this radiographic view. Lateral views of the hand are not adequate, as superimposition of the three other digits obscures important details. Whereas oblique views may demonstrate such injuries as condylar fractures, lateral views can delineate the presence or extent of chip fractures at the bases of the phalanges as well as subluxations or fracture-subluxations of the proximal interphalangeal (PIP) joint. Additionally, stress radiographs will help delineate ligamentous disruption.

D. **Management principles.** The majority of joint injuries of the hand are managed by conservative treatment, consisting of a period of buddy-taping or immobilization followed by active range-of-motion exercises. Indications for operative repair include complex or irreducible dislocations, joint instability following reduction, and displaced or large intraarticular fractures. Because of postsurgical periarticular fibrosis, the benefit of the procedure must always outweigh the residual surgical effects of limitation of motion.

Diminished flexion and residual joint stiffness are the usual long-term effects of joint injuries to the hand. With this in mind, immobilization should include 60 to 70 degrees of flexion of the MCP joints, 20 to 30 degrees of flexion of the PIP joints, and 10 to 20 degrees of flexion of the distal interphalangeal (DIP) joints. Uninvolved joints should have minimal if any immobilization. Since prolonged swelling and stiffness accompany even minor joint injuries, therapy guided toward active range of motion is encouraged.

II. **Specific acute joint injuries**
A. **Partial ligamentous injuries.** With incomplete ligamentous tears or sprains, anatomical continuity is maintained. There is sufficient capsular support to resist displacement with stress.
1. **Treatment.** An acutely injured ligament requires 2 to 5 weeks of buddy-taping or immobilization, depending on severity, for optimal healing. The objectives of treatment include time to allow soft tissue healing and proper exercises to restore maximum joint motion.

Interphalangeal joints are best splinted in 30 to 35 degrees of flexion. MCP joints are splinted in 50 degrees of flexion and the thumb MCP joint in 30 degrees of flexion. Volar plaster or aluminum splints can be used.

Active range-of-motion exercises are encouraged following immobilization. A mobile splint with the injured digit taped to an adjacent one for approximately 5 to 7 days may be additionally necessary depending on persistent soft tissue reaction. Alternatively, buddy-taping with active range of motion from the outset has been advocated.

2. **Complications.** The most common complication is persistent swelling and stiffness, which is usually present for 6 to 12 months following severe partial tears. Periarticular fibrosis resulting in some degree of permanent swelling and restriction of joint movement may occur. Also, permanent limitation of range of motion can occur in neglected cases or with patients who fail to exercise properly.

B. **Digital interphalangeal joints.** Structurally, the proximal and distal interphalangeal (IP) joints are identical. The IP joints are **uniaxial hinge joints** which move in a sagittal plane. The **PIP joint** flexes to approximately 105 degrees from full extension compared with the **DIP joint,** which flexes to no more than 90 degrees. This is because the flexor digitorum profundus tendon inserts closer to the articulation of the DIP joint compared to the flexor digitorum superficialis which inserts distal to the volar plate.

The IP joint is stable to lateral and oblique stresses partly because the proximal bicondylar transverse phalangeal diameter doubles its vertical diameter. The central tongue-and-groove mechanism resists shearing and rotary forces.

Strong, quadrangular **collateral ligaments** along with the fibrocartilagenous **volar plate** further enhance IP joint stability and strength (Fig. 1). Arising from the lateral aspect of the proximal condyles, the collateral ligaments are parallel radial and ulnar fibers, which project laterally and distally to insert on the volar base of the more distal phalanx and lateral margins of the volar plate. Extending in a volar fashion are triangular, distinct, thin **accessory collateral ligaments** that insert along the proximal volar plate and complete the lateral wall of the IP joint capsule. The **volar plate** forms the floor of the joint and is 2 to 3 mm thick at its distal phalangeal insertion before tapering to a thin membranous sheet proximally. Thus, the volar plate can fold onto itself during maximal flexion.

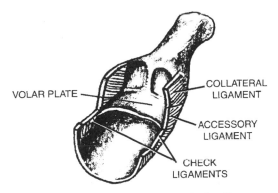

VOLAR PLATE

COLLATERAL
LIGAMENT

ACCESSORY
LIGAMENT

CHECK
LIGAMENTS

Fig. 1. Interphalangeal joint anatomy. Note the boxlike configuration of the collateral ligaments and the accessory ligaments that merge into the volar plate, which is anchored proximally by the check ligaments.

A pair of tough **check ligaments** arise from the radial and ulnar aspects of the proximal volar plate and are firmly attached to the proximal volar periosteum. These ligaments are both supple enough to fold onto themselves during maximal interphalangeal flexion yet strong enough to resist interphalangeal hyperextension.

The interphalangeal joint is stabilized in extension by the taut volar plate and volar fibers of the collateral ligament. In flexion, the joint is stabilized by the capsular fibers stretched over the condylar flare. The volar plate along with the check and accessory ligaments help prevent hyperextension.

1. **DIP joint injuries.** Dislocation of the DIP joint is uncommon. Stability is provided by adjacent flexor and extensor tendon insertions, strong collateral ligaments, and the short lever arm of the distal phalanx. When dislocations do occur, they are almost always dorsal, although they may present laterally in a jackknife fashion. Additionally, these dislocations are frequently open because of skin shear from the underlying, firmly attached osteocutaneous fibers. Radiographs are utilized to determine the presence of commonly associated mallet fracture/dislocations.

   a. **Reduction.** A closed reduction is almost always stable because both flexor and extensor tendons remain attached to the distal phalanx. Reduction, performed after digital nerve block, occurs with hyperextension and application of longitudinal traction, distracting the bayonette opposed distal phalanx.

This is followed by dorsal pressure to the base of the distal phalanx to achieve reduction. Functional stability, tested by active range of motion, reveals that enough ligamentous fibers remain to allow healing with minimal fibrosis and that the volar plate is not interposed within the joint. Two to three weeks of DIP joint immobilization in 5 to 10 degrees of flexion usually suffice.

b. **Open DIP dislocation.** The patient should have treatment directed toward operative debridement of devitalized and contaminated tissue, copious wound irrigation, and gentle reduction. Prophylactic antibiotics are recommended. Immobilization is performed as above. With either open or closed DIP joint dislocations, instability, assessed by active range of motion, indicates complete and multiple ligamentous disruption requiring surgical repair.

   (1) **Irreducible DIP dislocations** require open reduction and have been reported to occur by three mechanisms:

   (a) Dorsal dislocation with the volar plate entrapped in the joint

   (b) Flexor digitorum profundus tendon entrapment seen in DIP dislocations with collateral ligament rupture

   (c) Osteochondral fragment or sesamoid entrapment

   (2) **Chronic (unreduced) DIP dislocations.** Dislocations of 3 weeks or longer duration are considered chronic dislocations. Closed reduction invariably fails, requiring open reduction through a dorsal exposure. This may be technically challenging because of periarticular soft tissue contracture. Prognosis for joint mobility is poor.

2. **PIP joint injuries.** The PIP joint is the most frequently injured joint in the hand; the exact incidence is unknown because reductions frequently occur on the playing field and medical care is never sought. The most common cause is an axial load and hyperextension.

   The PIP joint occupies a position of importance in the hand, with function dependent on mobility. Stability is provided by the junction of the volar plate at the base of the middle phalanx and the collateral ligament system (Fig. 1). This boxlike configuration forms a strong three-dimensional hinge. For joint disruption to take place, at least two sides of the box must be involved.

   Injuries to the PIP joint involve combinations of injuries to the collateral ligament and volar plate, dislocations, and fracture/dislocations. The most important clinical consideration in these injuries is to determine which are stable and which are not. As a general rule, stable injuries have the best outcome.

a. **Lateral PIP joint dislocation**

    (1) **Mechanism of injury.** A lateral dislocation occurs with radial- or ulnar-directed force to the joint. This ruptures one collateral ligament and a major portion of the volar plate insertion, causing the middle phalanx to pivot and assume an oblique orientation. **Ruptures of the radial collateral ligament** occur six times more frequently than those of the **ulnar collateral ligament.**

    (2) **Reduction.** The joint will often reduce spontaneously; otherwise longitudinal traction easily provides reduction. Lateral stability is enhanced by the flexor tendon, its sheath, the lateral bands, and retinacular ligaments of the extensor mechanism. Therefore, following reduction, ligamentous disruption may not be appreciated, as active flexion and extension are usually not limited. Postreduction films are mandatory to confirm completeness of reduction; small avulsion fractures occasionally occur.

        Under digital anesthesia, suspected or confirmed lateral PIP joint dislocations should have each collateral ligament stressed in full extension. The degree of angulation provides an accurate assessment of ligamentous injury that directly relates to the duration of immobilization and prognosis. Complete immobilization for 2 weeks followed by 1 week of partial immobilization (buddy-taping to an adjacent finger on the affected side) at 30 degrees of flexion is indicated if the joint is stable. Joints stable to active range of motion but unstable to stress require 3 weeks of complete immobilization. Joints unstable to active range of motion often require operative repair.

    (3) **Complications.** The patient should be advised that residual stiffness, pain, and swelling may last for a number of months after injury. Use of a protective splint should be encouraged if the patient wishes an early return to the activity that produced the injury.

b. **Dorsal PIP joint dislocation**

    (1) **Mechanism of injury.** Dorsal dislocation is the most common type of disloca-

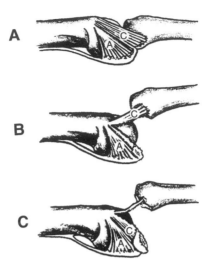

Fig. 2.   Scheme of dorsal interphalangeal joint dislocation. A: Normal anatomy of the joint capsule consisting of the collateral (c) and accessory (a) ligaments. B: Stable dorsal dislocation. The more distal phalanx is displaced dorsally as both the volar plate and one collateral ligament tear. C: Unstable dorsal dislocation. Note the bayonette displacement of the more distal phalanx, with few if any intact ligament fibers. Postreduction stability is unlikely.

tion of the PIP joint. The mechanism of injury is hyperextension of the joint with a concomitant axial load. The physician may not see the dislocation, as it is often reduced by trainers, coaches, or the patient; therefore, it is important for the examining physician to determine the orientation of digit displacement, as dorsal or volar dislocations involve different treatment options.

Rupture of the volar plate with an accompanying collateral ligament tear occurs with PIP joint dislocations (Fig. 2). The middle phalanx assumes a bayonette type of dorsal displacement. The volar plate may be torn at either its membranous and fibrocartilagenous junction proximally or at its distal attachment on the base of the middle phalanx. A small avulsion fracture may occur with the latter, is rarely displaced, and is not an indication for open repair.

(a)   **Fracture/dislocations.** Dorsal fracture/dislocations are potentially the most crippling injuries to the PIP joint. The usual mechanism of injury is an axial load. The fracture occurs at the volar articular surface of the base of the middle phalanx. Fractures involving 33% or greater of the articular surface are unstable because a greater portion of the collateral ligament insertion is detached from the middle phalanx (Fig. 2). Since x-rays fail to show cartilaginous injury, the size of the fracture is not the only criterion determining future joint function. Because of the possibly disabling nature of these injuries, orthopaedic referral is mandatory. Treatment of the acute injury is controversial, and both closed and operative techniques have been described.

   (b) Open dislocations. The severity of open dislocations of the PIP joint is usually underestimated. Debridement, parenteral antibiotics, and operative reduction are recommended.

   (c) Complex dislocations. Irreducible or complex dislocations of the PIP joint are uncommon. The volar plate or the flexor tendons are the structures often blocking reduction.

   (2) Treatment. Closed reduction of the PIP joint is enhanced with digital anesthesia. It is accomplished with mild hyperextension and longitudinal traction applied to the middle phalanx, followed by dorsal pressure to the base of the middle phalanx. Closed reduction is usually easily accomplished and has a good prognosis. Stability assessment, immobilization, and complications are as noted with lateral dislocations.

c. **Volar plate tears.** Disruption of the volar plate can occur without a dislocation of the PIP joint. The mechanism of injury is hyperextension. A horizontal volar skin laceration over the PIP joint should raise one's index of suspicion that this injury has occurred. Even without a laceration, hyperextension at the PIP joint requires assessment of the stability of the volar plate under digital anesthesia.

d. **Volar PIP joint dislocations**

   (1) Mechanism of injury. Volar dislocations of the PIP joint are relatively rare

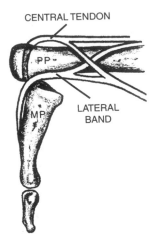

CENTRAL TENDON

PP

MP

LATERAL
BAND

Fig. 3.   Volar dislocation of the PIP
joint. The proximal phalangeal head
ruptures through the retinacular
fibers between the lateral band and
central tendon. The lateral band is
interposed, blocking reduction.

and often missed. They may occur as either pure dislocations or fracture/dislo-
cations. For this injury to occur, the central slip must be disrupted (Fig. 3).
The proximal phalangeal head ruptures
through the retinacular fibers between
the lateral band and central tendon. Additionally, at least one collateral ligament is ruptured, the volar plate may be
torn, or the lateral band may be caught
in the joint resisting reduction. The potential for a boutonniere deformity exists, since the central slip is avulsed at
its insertion.

(2)   **Treatment.** A pitfall of treatment occurs if the patient presents following
field reduction without the presence of a
fracture to indicate that there had been
a volar dislocation. The digit will mistak-
enly be treated as if a dorsal dislocation
had occurred (flexion immobilization),
and a boutonniere deformity may develop. A key finding is to note that the
patient will be unable to extend the PIP
joint against resistance.

Controversy exists in the literature regarding closed versus open reduction.
Some authors advocate open reduction
with repair of the central slip and
transarticular pinning in extension for
all cases of volar PIP dislocation. Others
recommend conservative treatment (as
with closed boutonniere injuries) of the

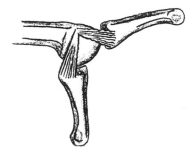

Fig. 4.   Scheme of the collateral ligament of the MCP joint, depicting the dorsal eccentric origin of the collateral ligament attached to the cam-shaped metacarpal head. The collateral ligaments are lax in extension and taut in flexion.

PIP joint in extension for 4 to 6 weeks. This is followed by dynamic PIP extension splinting during the day, static splinting at night, and active range-of-motion exercises. Open reduction is reserved for irreducible dislocations, incongruent joint surfaces following reduction, or active extension lag of more than 30 degrees. All patients must be referred to an orthopaedist.

C.   **Metacarpophalangeal (MCP) joint.** The MCP joint is **condyloid,** with the globular cam-shaped head of the metacarpal articulating with the concave base of the proximal phalanx. In contrast to the interphalangeal joints, full flexion and extension are allowed along with significant abduction, adduction, and limited circumduction. Owing to the configuration of the metacarpal head (broader at its volar surface), the eccentric, dorsally oriented collateral ligaments are taut in flexion and lax in extension (Fig. 4). Therefore, limited lateral movement is allowed only in extension.

The ability to resist hyperextension forces is limited because of the bony contour of the MCP joint, lack of check ligaments, and the thinner proximal volar plate. This is in contrast to the ability of the MCP joint to resist ulnar and radial stress. Strong collateral ligaments are present, along with a thicker distal volar plate that extends between adjacent metacarpals to form the deep **transverse metacarpal ligament.** Also, a buttressing effect occurs between adjacent rays, especially to the third and fourth MCP joints. Finally, flexors and extensors provide dynamic stability; lumbrical and interosseous muscles add to lateral stability.

Primary digital flexion occurs at the MCP joint; therefore, residual stiffness will cause functional impairment. Early diagnosis, appropriate treatment, and rehabilitation are key for optimal recovery.

1. **Collateral ligament injuries.** Because of the protection offered within the web space and adjacent rays, isolated injuries to the collateral ligaments of the MCP joints are uncommon.

   a. **Diagnosis.** Localized swelling and tenderness over the involved metacarpal ligament suggests the diagnosis. The most significant sign is pain to radial or ulnar stress with the MCP joint in extension with or without instability. Usually, no radiographic abnormality is present, although small avulsion fractures of the metacarpal head or intraarticular fractures of the base of the proximal phalanx may be present.

   b. **Treatment.** Conservative treatment with the MCP join splinted in 50 degrees flexion for 3 weeks is recommended if a significant avulsion fracture is not present. Operative treatment is recommended if the fracture is displaced more than 2 to 3 mm or involves more than 20% of the articular surface and is displaced or rotated.

2. **Dorsal metacarpophalangeal MCP dislocations.** There are two types of dorsal MCP dislocations: **simple** and **complex,** both of which are due to **hyperextension forces** resulting in proximal volar plate tears. Simple dislocations can be reduced by closed manipulation, whereas complex dislocations are irreducible and require open reduction.

   a. **Simple dorsal MCP dislocations.** Simple dorsal dislocations of the MCP joint are more accurately termed subluxations, as the articular surfaces are still in partial contact. The proximal phalanx rests in 60 to 90 degrees of hyperextension on the dorsum of the metacarpal head. Clinically, a greater degree of hyperextension exists than in complex MCP dislocations. Radiographically, the joint space is narrow without the presence of an interposed sesamoid.

   Closed reduction is achieved by applying pressure to the dorsum of the proximal phalanx and pushing it over the metacarpal head into flexion. The wrist is flexed during the maneuver to relax the flexor tendons. Traction/countertraction must be avoided, since this may cause the volar plate to be interposed in the joint, converting a reducible to an irreducible dislocation.

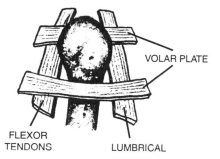

Fig. 5.   Complex dislocation of the MCP joint. The "finger trap" mechanism is depicted, showing the metacarpal head rupturing through the volar plate. Reduction with longitudinal traction tightens the lumbricals and flexors.

Some authors advocate reduction achieved under wrist block, since pain may preclude reduction and lead one to falsely assume that a complex dislocation is present.

Immobilization of the MCP joint for 7 to 10 days in 50 to 70 degrees of flexion is acceptable. Some authors prefer immediate active range-of-motion exercise with hyperextension prevented by buddy-taping. Recurrent simple MCP dislocations are rare.

b.   **Complex dorsal MCP dislocations.** In complex MCP joint dislocations, the metacarpal head ruptures through the volar plate, which then occupies the joint space. The lumbrical on the radial aspect and long flexor tendon on the ulnar aspect further entrap the metacarpal head (Fig. 5). Likened to a "finger trap," the dislocation is irreducible because of the interposition of the volar plate within the MCP joint. Additionally, the ring formed by the lumbrical and long flexor tendon tightens with longitudinal traction.

Complex MCP dislocations can be recognized by noting moderate hyperextension and a dorsal bayonette position. A pathognomonic finding is volar dimpling of the palmar skin.

Another pathognomonic finding is the radiographic presence of a sesamoid within the widened MCP joint space.

Complex MCP dislocations occur most commonly in the index finger, followed by the thumb and little finger. Rarely, MCP dislocations occur in the long and ring fingers.

Reduction of complex MCP dislocations can be accomplished only by open techniques.

Postoperatively, the joint is stable, requiring no immobilization. Early active range-of-motion exercise is encouraged, protecting the affected digit with buddy-taping.

D. Carpometacarpal (CMC) joint dislocations

1. **Anatomy.** The CMC of the index, middle, and ring fingers are **arthrodial diarthroses** or **gliding joints.** The little finger is a **modified saddle joint.** In an interlocking complex configuration, the bases of the metacarpals articulate with each other and the distal carpal row.

   The third metacarpocapitate joint functions as the stable central post of the hand with essentially no movement possible. Limited anteroposterior gliding occurs at the base of the second metacarpotrapezoid joint. The saddle joint articulations between the bases of the fourth and fifth metacarpals are more mobile.

   The joints are bolstered by tough dorsal and volar intermetacarpal and CMC ligaments. Wrist flexors and extensors provide additional support at the bases of the second, third, and fifth metacarpals.

   Two important soft tissue structures are of importance when surgical intervention is necessary. The motor branch of the **ulnar nerve** is found volar to the fifth CMC joint as it winds around the hook of the hamate. The deep palmar arterial arch lies volar to the third CMC joint. **Dislocations** are uncommon and frequently missed.

2. **Mechanism of injury.** These dislocations are usually the result of high-speed trauma as from falls, crushes, or motorcycle accidents. Also, closed-fist trauma may result in CMC dislocations. Every type and combination of CMC dislocations has been described; isolated individual dislocations of the four joints may occur, with the fifth CMC dislocation presenting most frequently. Dorsal dislocations are more common than volar.

3. **Physical examination.** The patient often presents with massive dorsal edema that usually obscures the deformity at the metacarpal base. Maximum tenderness is also elicited at the metacarpal bases. With multiple dislocations, circulatory assessment is extremely important. The integrity of the ulnar nerve should be assessed with fifth metacarpohamate joint dislocations. Additionally, associated injuries to the **median nerve** and avulsions of the **wrist extensor tendons** have been described.

4. **Radiographs.** Initial radiographs should include the posteroanterior, the oblique, and the extremely important lateral views to help demonstrate displacement of the metacarpal base. Other studies including multiple obliques, along

with computed tomography scans have also been helpful in delineating displacement and extent of intraarticular comminution. An important consideration, analogous to the Monteggia and Galleazzi fracture/dislocations of the forearm, is the possibility that the displaced fracture of one metacarpal may coexist with an adjacent CMC joint dislocation. This can occur because the metacarpals are tethered both proximally and distally.

5. **Treatment.** Emergency department treatment consists of ice, elevation, and analgesics. Reduction is difficult to maintain because of joint instability. Various methods of reduction and fixation have been described without a clear consensus. Most authors, however, recommend an attempt at closed reduction followed by percutaneous K-wire fixation.

E. **Joint injuries of the thumb**
   1. **Interphalangeal (IP) joint**
      a. **Anatomy.** The IP joint of the thumb is a **hinge joint** moving in a sagittal plane identical to that of the DIP joints of the fingers. Lateral stability is afforded by the volar plate and configuration of the collateral ligament (Fig. 1). Clelland fibers reinforce lateral stability.
      b. **Dislocation.** IP dislocations of the thumb are uncommon. In **dorsal dislocations,** the volar plate remains attached to the distal phalanx; the tear occurs at the proximal volar plate and the condylar origin of the collateral ligament. Shear stresses on the skin usually produce an open dislocation.
      c. **Reduction.** Closed reduction is usually simple and easily achieved with digital anesthesia. Following reduction, active range-of-motion testing will determine stability and exclude the rare rupture of the flexor pollicis longus tendon. The IP joint should be immobilized in slight flexion for 3 weeks.
   2. **Metacarpophalangeal (MCP) joint**
      a. **Anatomy.** The MCP joint of the thumb is a hybrid of a **ginglymus** and **condyloid joint.** Flexion, extension, abduction, adduction, and limited rotation are allowed. With the most variable range of motion of all the joints in the hand, the maximum extension to maximum flexion varies from 5 to 100 degrees, averaging 75 degrees.

         The broad transverse diameter of the first metacarpal condyle is a major contributor to lateral joint stability. Also, joint stability is provided by the enhanced tensile strength of the volar plate and collateral ligaments. The

intrinsic flexor-adductor muscles adjacent to the sesamoids help to maintain integrity of the proximal volar plate, much like the paired check ligaments at the digital PIP joints. Fibers from the adductor pollicis muscle fuse with the dorsal aponeurosis to form the **adductor aponeurosis.** Overlying the ulnar collateral ligament, the adductor aponeurosis provides active stabilization. Finally, dynamic stability is provided by the **thenar intrinsic muscles,** which are sufficient to stabilize the joint even with volar plate disruption.

b. **Mechanism of injury.** Despite substantial stabilization, the oblique orientation of the thumb makes the MCP joint five times more vulnerable to radially directed stress. The force of strong opposition essential to provide forceful pinch requires strong resistance to hyperextension. Two basic types of ligamentous injury may occur: the **dorsal dislocation** secondary to disruption of the volar plate and **lateral or jackknife dislocation** secondary to a unilateral tear of the collateral ligament.

c. **Dorsal dislocation**

(1) **Mechanism of injury.** Dorsal dislocation of the thumb MCP joint is due either to an **extreme hyperextension** injury or to **shearing stress** causing rupture of the volar supporting structures. Displacement is directly proportional to the degree of disruption. The volar plate ruptures proximal to the sesamoids' insertion. The characteristic bayonette orientation of the phalanx overriding dorsal and parallel to the metacarpal is produced with complete rupture of the volar plate and one of the collateral ligaments.

(2) **Reduction.** Closed reduction can be accomplished following digital block. With the wrist and IP joint flexed to relax the flexor tendons, the thumb is flexed into the palm and dorsal pressure is applied over the proximal phalanx. Reduction is achieved by pushing the base of the proximal phalanx over the metacarpal head. One must avoid traction/countertraction, since this may cause the volar plate to be interposed in the joint, converting a reducible to an irreducible dislocation.

Following reduction, stability is assessed with active range of motion along with stress of the MCP joint to assess ulnar and radial collateral ligament integrity. Immobilization for 4 to 6 weeks in flexion is adequate for stable joints with subsequent orthopaedic referral. Open repair is reserved for an unstable joint, significant lateral instability, or irreducible dislocations.

d. **Lateral dislocations.** Lateral dislocations of the thumb MCP joint are common injuries that present with subtle physical findings. The dislocation that results from rupture of a collateral ligament and volar plate is transient and, in many instances, unrecognized and untreated. The **ulnar collateral ligament ruptures 10 times** more frequently than the radial collateral ligament. Loss of support from the ulnar collateral ligament is quite disabling, since it reduces the thumb's ability to resist stress, which is necessary for a strong pinch.

(1) **Mechanism of injury.** Historically, injury to the ulnar collateral ligament was termed **gamekeeper's thumb,** the result of repeated radial stress from breaking the necks of wild game. The term **ski-pole thumb** currently reflects the most common mechanism of injury and is, in fact, one of the most common ski injuries.

(2) **Examination.** Since the majority of these dislocations reduce spontaneously, the diagnosis is pursued by physical examination and stress radiographs. The patient will present with a painful, swollen MCP joint of the thumb, with the point of maximal tenderness on the ulnar aspect.

(3) **Radiographs** may show an avulsion fracture at the base of the proximal phalanx where the ulnar collateral ligament inserts. More often, stress radiographs are necessary to reveal the injury, as rupture occurs within the ligament itself (Fig. 6). Following radial and median nerve wrist blocks, the ulnar collateral ligament is stressed with the MCP joint in 20 to 30 degrees of flexion to eliminate the stabilizing effect of the volar plate. The uninjured thumb should be tested for comparison because great variability exists in the MCP joint's range of motion.

Greater than 40 degrees of radial deviation indicates complete disruption

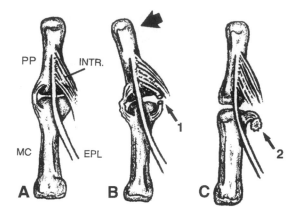

Fig. 6. Ulnar collateral ligament injury to the thumb MCP joint. A: The collateral ligament mechanism. B: Collateral ligament rupture at its insertion. (1) C: Intact ligament but distal attachment avulses a bone fragment. (2)

of the ulnar collateral ligament and is a surgical indication despite stability through active range of motion. Integrity of the ulnar collateral ligament of the thumb is necessary for full function.

The **Stener lesion** is an another indication for surgical repair. Stener noted the adductor aponeurosis becomes interposed between the two ends of the ruptured ligament, preventing adequate healing. The incidence of the Stener lesion ranges from 14% to 83%.

(4) **Treatment.** The thumb is immobilized in a **thumb spica cast** for 3 weeks with the IP joint free for conservative treatment of incomplete ulnar collateral ligament tears and following operative repair of complete tears. A removable splint to allow active range of motion is applied for an additional 5 weeks.

3. **Carpometacarpal (CMC) joint**
   a. **Anatomy.** The carpometacarpal joint (CMC) of the thumb is a biological **universal joint** with the concave metacarpal base seated on the saddle of the trapezium. A wide range of motion is allowed, including circumduction. However, enough stability is present to resist the combined force of the four fingers. The principal ligamentous support is the **anterior oblique CMC ligament.** Its stabilizing

force is equivalent to that of the interphalangeal volar plate. Dorsal support is provided by the posterior oblique CMC ligament, which is reinforced by the insertion of the abductor pollicis longus tendon.

b. Mechanism of injury. Pure CMC thumb dislocations are uncommon. The mechanism is postulated to be secondary to a longitudinal force directed along the metacarpal shaft with the basal joint in slight flexion. The anterior oblique CMC ligament and opponens pollicis muscle are the deterrents to subluxation. Because of the tensile strength of these structures, the longitudinal force more commonly produces fracture/dislocations—i.e., Bennett's fracture.

c. Treatment. Closed reduction of the CMC joint of the thumb is simple but is often unstable, especially to active range of motion. Percutaneous K-wire fixation is utilized to maintain reduction. A **thumb spica cast** is worn for 4 to 6 weeks with the pins then removed; the joint, however, remains protected for an additional 2 to 4 weeks.

III. Summary. Optimal treatment for joint injuries of the hand is essential to prevent long-term functional disability. Complex intraarticular geometry, strong yet flexible supporting ligamentous structures, and dynamic extensors and flexors provide joint stabilization. A thorough history to ascertain the mechanism of injury may be helpful in providing an index of suspicion for specific injuries. Important aspects of the physical exam include assessment for swelling, deformity, and neurovascular status. Active and gentle passive assessment of range of motion under anesthetic block is key to determining joint stability. Standard radiographic views include the anteroposterior, oblique, and—for individual digits—true lateral. Except for rupture of the ulnar collateral ligament of the thumb MCP joint, stable joints are treated by conservative measures that include appropriate immobilization and referral to hand surgeons. Indications for operative repair include complex dislocations, unstable joints, and dislocations associated with large or displaced intraarticular fractures.

BIBLIOGRAPHY

Eaton RG. *Joint injuries of the hand.* Springfield, IL: Thomas, 1972.

Hossfeld GE, Uehara DT. Acute joint injuries of the hand. *Emerg Med Clin North Am* 1993;11:781.

Kahler DM, McCue FC. Metacarpophalangeal and proximal interphalangeal joint injuries of the hand, including the thumb. *Clin Sports Med* 1992;11:57.

Kozin SH, Bishop AT. Gamekeeper's thumb: early diagnosis and treatment. *Orthop Rev* 1994;23:797.

Lamb DW, Kuczynski K, eds. *The practice of hand surgery.* St. Louis: Blackwell Mosby, 1981.

Rockwood CA, Green DP, Bucholz RW, eds. *Rockwood and Green's fractures in adults,* 3rd ed. Philadelphia: Lippincott, 1991.

Viegas SF, Heare TC, Calhoun JH. Complex fracture-dislocation of a fifth metacarpophalangeal joint: case report and literature review. *J Trauma* 1989;29:521.

Wolov RB. Complex dislocations of the metacarpophalangeal joints. *Orthop Rev* 1988;17:770.

Zemel NP. Metacarpophalangeal joint injuries in fingers. *Hand Clin* 1992;8:745.

III

Lower Extremity Orthopaedics

Pelvis

Teresita M. Hogan

The frequency of pelvic fractures is bimodal, with a peak in the second decade of life and in patients over 65 years of age. The epidemiology of pelvic fractures reveals that 60% are caused by motor vehicle accidents (MVAs) and collisions of autos with pedestrians, 30% are due to falls from a height, and 10% are due to falls by the elderly and athletes engaged in both contact and noncontact sports (1,2).

I. **Anatomy.** The pelvis is analogous to an arch and is inherently stable. This arch can be divided into anterior and posterior sections composed of the three innominate bones: the ilium or iliac wings, the ischium, and the pubis. The pelvic bones meet anteriorly at the pubic symphysis. Pelvic stability depends on an intact posterior weight-bearing arch as well as a strong ligamentous connection that provides elasticity and helps absorb impact. Fracture of the pelvis indicates significant external forces transmitted to the body, usually the result of rapid deceleration or crushing injuries. Energy is dispersed to multiple anatomical sites, mandating a search for adjacent and anatomically distant injury in all patients with pelvic fracture (Fig. 1).

II. **Mortality.** In isolated pelvic fracture, mortality is due to hemorrhage from the bone itself as well as the rich vascular plexus feeding the area. Impact forces are not confined to the pelvis, however, and the transmission of forces to vulnerable tissues in areas other than the pelvis contributes to mortality. The most lethal associated injuries are intraabdominal, thoracic aortic, and intracranial. In general, blunt trauma causing pelvic fracture has a mortality of up to 20% (1–3). Fortunately, 80% of patients recover without long-term complications (4). An exception occurs in patients with pelvic fracture who are hypotensive on presentation. This subgroup of patients has a mortality of 40% to 50% (5,6). In patients with open pelvic fractures, mortality approaches 25% (7). Open fractures are associated with a higher incidence of major vessel disruption. Elderly patients suffer greater mortality than age-matched victims with identical injuries. Death occurs in 11% of children with pelvic fractures, usually due to associated head injury (8). Factors influencing mortality at any age include open fracture (mortality rates are 20% to 30%), hemodynamic instability (the mortality rate with hypotension is 42%), and injury severity score (ISS) plus age (ISS plus age >70 years has an 80% mortality rate and ISS plus age <70 years has a 4% mortality rate). Despite these bleak statistics, 75% of pelvic fractures are minor, requiring only conservative orthopaedic management (9).

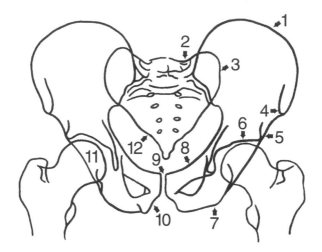

Fig. 1.   The pelvis: *(1)* **iliac crest,** *(2)* **sacrum,** *(3)* **sacroiliac joint,** *(4)* **anterior superior iliac spine,** *(5)* **anterior inferior iliac spine,** *(6)* **acetabulum,** *(7)* **ischial tuberosity,** *(8)* **superior ramus,** *(9)* **symphysis pubis,** *(10)* **inferior ramus,** *(11)* **femoral head,** *(12)* **coccyx.**

III.   Evaluation

    A.   Classification systems. Multiple classification systems developed to guide surgical management have been described for pelvic fractures (10–13). These classification systems do not correlate well with the extent of hemorrhage and are impractical for the initial assessment, stratification, and emergent management of these patients. Emergency physicians must instead focus on rapid diagnosis of associated injuries and the prioritization of multiple management issues.

    B.   Mechanism. The specific mechanism of injury determines the amount of force delivered to the tissues. Pedestrian versus vehicle events cause the most direct tissue trauma. While relatively few pelvic fractures result from this mechanism, it causes 50% of all associated mortality.

    For passengers involved in frontal collisions, an instantaneous deceleration of at least 30 mph is required to produce a major fracture of the pelvis. Side impacts, however, lead to significant pelvic deformation at velocity differentials of only 15 mph (3), resulting in more pelvic injuries (4). Although restraints have a protective effect for brain injury in frontal impact MVAs, they provide no protection to the pelvis or lower extremities in impacts from any direction. Contact intrusion into the occupant compartment as the vehicle is deformed causes most lateral impact pelvic injuries (4).

Lateral compression produces internal rotation of the hemipelvis on the side of impact. Moderate force results in compression of the anterior sacroiliac joint and associated ligaments and puts tension on the posterior ligaments. With greater force, the ilium usually fractures, leaving a fragment attached to the sacrum. Extreme forces produce external rotation of the contralateral hemipelvis and distraction of the sacroiliac joint with or without ilial or sacral fractures.

The transmission of kinetic energy to tissues results in predictable patterns of injury. Therefore, emergency evaluation begins with a history that includes the mechanism of injury. The mechanism will signal the possibility of pelvic fracture and the likelihood of associated injury. Physical examination can confirm these suspicions or raise the question of pathological fracture from a seemingly benign mechanism.

C. **History.** An alert patient can provide complaints that lead to the detection of specific injuries. The presence of back, buttock, pelvic, groin, perineal, hip, or thigh pain as well as any numbness of the lower extremity, paresthesias, or weakness should be noted. Any dysfunction of bowel or bladder or loss of perineal sensation indicates spinal cord involvement. The ability to bear weight or walk excludes all unstable injuries but does not eliminate the possibility of stable fracture.

D. **Physical examination.** Inspection may reveal ecchymosis or abrasions of the pelvis, back, and buttocks. A discoloration of the flanks known as **Grey Turner's sign** is indicative of retroperitoneal hematoma. A hematoma over the inguinal ligament, proximal thigh, and perianal or scrotal areas, known as **Destot's sign**, may result from pelvic fracture. When inspecting the perineum, always note the presence of blood at the anus or urethral meatus. A leg-length discrepancy of 1 cm or greater is significant (14).

Palpating the bony pelvis may demonstrate tenderness or instability. A palpable fracture line or pelvic hematoma (Earle's sign) may be noted. The maneuver of **pelvic springing** is performed by applying alternative compression and distraction forces to the iliac wings in order to detect crepitance or instability. This must be performed gently to prevent further bleeding. Springing of the pelvis and pelvic rock maneuvers are very poor predictors of pelvic fracture. One study showed a specificity of only 71% and sensitivity of only 50% with these maneuvers (15).

The presence of blood on rectal and vaginal examinations is important, as displaced fractures may cause mucosal disruption from within. Complications of exsanguinating hemorrhage as well as subsequent infection in these open injuries mandate early identification of penetration. Rectal penetration mandates colostomy (16). During rectal exam, the physician should check for a high-riding prostate, indicative of urethral tear, and palpate the sacrum for tenderness and asymmetry. The perineum should be examined for the presence of a **perineal butterfly hematoma,** which is highly specific for urethral disruption. Perineal lacerations should not be probed owing to the likelihood of clot disruption, causing extreme bleeding and the introduction of infection to a possible open fracture. Vaginal examination must be gentle to prevent further mucosal injury. During menses, a speculum exam is necessary to ensure that mucosal disruption has not occurred.

Examination of the leg is an important part of the physical exam in pelvic fracture. Awake patients should be evaluated for strength and motor function. Sensation should be checked to detect injury of the sciatic or femoral nerves. As always, pulses and capillary refill in the legs and feet are noted.

A few subtle maneuvers can be employed to detect specific injuries. Adduction/abduction and internal/external hip rotation that demonstrate instability, pain, or crepitus indicate involvement at or near the acetabulum. Specifically useful is the **FABER test** for pubic ramus fracture. Patients experience groin pain when they place the ipsilateral foot on the contralateral knee and the ipsilateral hip is **F**lexed, **AB**ducted, and **E**xternally **R**otated (10). **Axial percussion** through the heel can localize pain to a hip injury or pelvic fracture site and is a useful clinical sign. An unremarkable completed physical examination of an awake, nonimpaired adult patient has a negative predictive value of 99% for pelvic fracture (17).

E. **Radiography.** Radiographs are critical in the diagnosis of pelvic fractures. Ninety percent of all traumatic pelvic injuries can be seen on the anteroposterior (AP) pelvic film alone. The addition of supplemental views increases detection to 94% (18). Plain-film examination is sufficient to identify virtually all clinically significant fractures and dislocations in the acute setting. The AP pelvic film has an accuracy of 88% in detecting ring instability (19). Thaggard (20) defines pelvic instability as a gap or displacement of greater than or equal to 0.5 cm at *any* fracture site on AP view or the presence of an open-book injury. These x-ray findings are associated with the need for blood transfusion. In the sta-

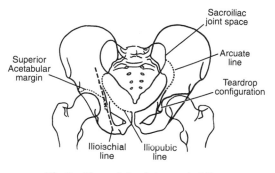

Fig. 2. The pelvis—interrupted lines indicate radiographic projections.

bilized patient, computed tomography (CT) is valuable. It not only defines fracture displacement but, more importantly, delineates associated soft tissue pathology.

In reading the AP pelvic film, a systematic approach is necessary. The x-ray should be examined carefully for symmetry and cortical and trabecular integrity. Displacement of soft tissue lines and intrapelvic fat pads are indirect signs of hematoma formation. Note that single breaks in the adult pelvic ring are exceptional and that a second break is usually present. Children, however, have a disproportionately high rate of single bone injuries with intact pelvic rings.

Normal radiographic projections are depicted in Fig. 2. The arcuate, iliopubic, ilioischial, and acetabular teardrop lines, the sacral foramina, and the sacroiliac joints should be reviewed systematically. Deviations from the normal projections signal underlying fracture.

1. **AP pelvic films should be screened for the following:**
    a. Bilateral symmetry of the hemipelvis.
    b. Sacroiliac width >4 mm.
    c. Symphyseal widening >5 to 8 mm in adults and >10 mm in children.
    d. Symphyseal offset >2 mm.
    e. Symphyseal overlapping, which is always abnormal.
    f. Fractures of the iliac wing and pubic rami.
    g. Avulsion of the iliac spine and ischial tuberosities.
    h. Sacrum: check the arcuate lines of the neural foramina to detect transverse fracture, which is difficult to visualize. These are best seen on lateral views.

      i. Fracture of the fifth lumbar transverse process is often seen with sacroiliac (SI) joint disruption.

      j. Superior displacement of one iliac wing or the pubis suggests a diastasis of the SI joint or symphysis.

      k. Acetabular fractures are difficult to detect. Following the iliopectineal and ilioischeal lines will help discern cortical discontinuities. Forty-five-degree oblique views and Judet views may further assist in diagnosis (22).

    2. Augmented plain views are done to enhance visualization of fractures.

      a. The **pelvic inlet** view, angled 35 to 40 degrees caudally, helps define the pelvic rim or acetabulum as well as central displacement of fractures of the posterior and anterior arches.

      b. The **pelvic outlet** or tangential views, angled 35 to 40 degrees cephalad, give additional definition to the sacrum and SI joints.

      c. The **Judet** view, a three-quarters internal and external oblique view, highlights the acetabulum.

IV. **Management.** As with all trauma, a rapid primary survey is done and life-threatening conditions are addressed as they are discovered. Excluding associated trauma, the only immediate life-threatening aspect of pelvic fracture is exsanguinating hemorrhage. Hemorrhage is the cause of death in 65% of all patients who die of pelvic fracture (23,24). Exsanguinating pelvic fractures can be treated by five basic modalities:

- Fluid resuscitation/transfusion
- Pneumatic antishock garments (e.g., military antishock trousers (MAST)
- External fixation
- Angiographic embolization
- Internal fixation

    A. **Fluid resuscitation/transfusion.** Concealed hemorrhage due to pelvic fracture can be extensive; the retroperitoneal space can hold up to 4 L of blood. The standard use of large volumes of crystalloid for fluid resuscitation has recently been questioned with regard to dilution of blood components, dislodgement of tamponading clots, and worsened survival rates (24,25). Early blood transfusion in hemodynamically unstable patients, however, is *not* controversial in light of the potential for exsanguinating hemorrhage in pelvic fracture. Fortunately, the need for early initial transfusion is not predictive of exsanguinating hemorrhage. One study has shown that two-thirds of patients with initial hemodynamic compromise, were completely stabilized with infusion of only 1 to 2 units of packed red blood cells (27).

In children, exsanguination from pelvic fracture is less common than in adults, despite their having similar fracture patterns. A child's nonatherosclerotic vessels constrict more completely and fracture displacement is more limited due to more developed and adherent periosteum, contributing to greater hemostasis. ISS, age, sex, and mechanism all fail to predict the child at risk for hemorrhage. Only pelvic fracture symmetry is predictive of hemorrhage in children. Displaced or unstable fragments correlate most highly with life-threatening hemorrhage (28).

Response to volume replacement is an important determinant of further management of ongoing hemorrhage. In adults with hypotension or other signs of decreased organ perfusion, the failure to gain hemodynamic stability after 2 to 3 L of crystalloid and 4 to 6 units of blood requires that additional steps be taken to control bleeding. In children with hypotension, failure to establish stability after 40 mL/kg of volume replacement is an ominous sign, demanding other strategies to promote hemostasis.

B. **Pneumatic antishock garment (PASG) or military antishock trousers (MAST).** Once utilized for all types of shock, the primary indication for PASG is now the stabilization/immobilization of pelvic fractures in the prehospital and emergency department settings, especially in the presence of hypotension. The PASG stabilizes pelvic bony fragments, decreases hemorrhage and pain, and helps prevent clot dislodgment and further vessel disruption. PASGs have been used for up to 48 hours to effectively control hemorrhaging after pelvic fracture (9,29,30). In these cases, the bony prominences of the iliac crests, knees, and ankles should be well padded and inflation pressure maintained at <40 mm Hg. Other options for definitive fracture management can then be utilized. Respiratory problems, often requiring mechanical ventilation, and leg compartment syndromes often complicate extended use of PASG support.

C. **External fixation.** Anterior external fixation through pins placed in the iliac crests and fixed to an external frame is useful in hemodynamically unstable patients with displaced pelvic fractures, reducing mortality from 22% to 8% (31,32). External fixation can be applied rapidly in the emergency department. The only absolute contraindication is bony comminution that mechanically prevents splinting. The **Ganz antishock pelvic clamp** is another technically simple external fixator that can provide adequate hemodynamic control in the acute phase of care. In vertical fractures, external fixation is only temporary and used to help control hemorrhage. Internal fixation is required for definitive management.

D. **Angiographic embolization.** Early angiography is indicated when hypovolemia persists in spite of vigorous fluid and blood resuscitation and non-pelvic sources of hemorrhage have been excluded or controlled. To avoid the complications of mass transfusion, angiography should be performed within 6 hours of injury (33). Only 5% to 15% of pelvic fracture hemorrhage occurs from identifiable arterial vessels, but in these patients, early use of angiography can be lifesaving. Selective angiographic embolization offers advantages over open surgical ligation of the internal iliac or hypogastric artery (10,34,35). If angiography reveals disruption of major vessels such as the aorta, common iliac, femoral, or external iliac arteries, surgical repair is required (34–36). Medium-sized and small arteries can be tamponaded angiographically with coils or foam. In many cases, identification of significant arterial hemorrhage cannot be made until either angiography or surgery is performed. Therefore, some centers utilize a combined approach with rapid application of an external fixator under fluoroscopic guidance in the angiography suite (37).

The greatest impediment to angiographic embolization is that up to 85% of retroperitoneal hemorrhage in pelvic fracture results from venous sources. Owing to the extensive anastomoses and valveless collateral vessels of the pelvic venous plexus, the most effective method for controlling such hemorrhage remains pelvic stabilization (37).

Prioritizing the role of external fixation, laparotomy, and angiography is difficult in the hemodynamically unstable pelvic fracture patient. Diagnostic peritoneal lavage (DPL) is useful in establishing these priorities (see Sec. VI.B.1):

1. **Negative DPL.** External fixation and angiography are suggested. Although DPL can result in false-positive results, there have been no false-negative DPLs in numerous studies (29, 38–46).

2. **Grossly positive DPL.** Immediate laparotomy is mandatory (38). External fixators may be applied in the operative suite.

3. **DPL positive by microscopic evaluation.** External fixation should precede angiography. Laparotomy is used only if angiographic control fails (30,38,40).

V. **Specific pelvic fractures.** The most serious of pelvic fractures are those involving a double break in the pelvic ring.

A. **Double breaks in the ring—i.e., the "bucket-handle" fracture (see Fig. 6).** Double breaks in the pelvic ring occur in about 33% of all pelvic fractures (8). They develop as the result of severe trauma, particularly in ejection from MVAs. These fractures

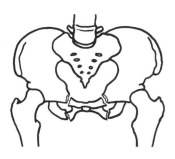

Fig. 3.   Straddle fracture.

are the result of disruption of both ischiopubic rami on one side with either disruption of the ipsilateral SI joint or fracture of the posterior sacroiliac region. Double breaks in the pelvic ring are unstable by definition, as two fractures cause collapse of the ring. Patients with these fractures will be unable to bear weight. These fractures are associated with frequent intraperitoneal injury as well as retroperitoneal hematomas and urinary injuries. Patients with these fractures usually have massive blood loss and require blood transfusion. Some examples of double breaks in the pelvic ring fractures follow.

1. **Straddle fractures (Fig. 3)**
   a. Straddle fractures comprise 30% of all unstable fractures (8).
   b. They are the result of fractures of all four ischiopubic rami simultaneously.
   c. Straddle fractures are disruptions of the *anterior* arch only.
   d. They occur when patients land with the perineum straddling a solid object.
   e. They may also occur from extreme lateral compression, such as a side-impact MVA.
   f. Patients with straddle fractures may demonstrate an inability to void.
   g. Thirty-three percent of cases are associated with urinary tract injury, such as disruption of the bladder or the proximal urethra.
   h. Associated abdominal injuries occur in another 33% of patients.
   i. Weight bearing and leg length, which both emanate from the posterior arch, are unaffected.
   j. Straddle fractures associated with rupture of the posterior sacroiliac ligaments will produce an unstable injury.
   k. Disruption of the ischial rami can damage pudendal vessels and nerves. Careful neurovascular evaluation of the legs is required with this injury.

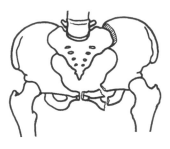

Fig. 4.   Malgaigne fracture.

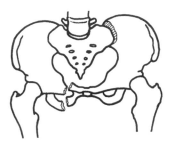

Fig. 5.   Bucket-handle fracture.

2. **Malgaigne fracture (Fig. 4)**
   a. These fractures result from vertical shear forces applied to the pelvis.
   b. They result when unilateral vertical fractures of the pubic rami are accompanied by vertical ipsilateral sacral fractures, ilial fractures, or SI separations.
   c. Malgaigne fractures are associated with a 20% mortality.
   d. Local nerve or vessel injury is common.
   e. Hemorrhage with hypotension is frequent.
   f. Patients with Malgaigne fractures may have bony instability on examination.
   g. Damage to the posterior arch results in inability to bear weight.
   h. When vertical fractures are contralateral to the rami fractures, it is termed a **bucket-handle fracture** (Fig. 5).
3. **Open-book or sprung pelvis (Fig. 6)**
   a. These injuries result from AP compression, driving the iliac wings apart.
   b. They result in disruption of the symphysis and the sacroiliac complex.
   c. Radiographic separation of the pubic symphysis of greater than 5 to 8 mm is diagnostic of an open-book or sprung pelvis.

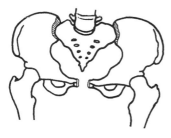

Fig. 6. Sprung pelvis.

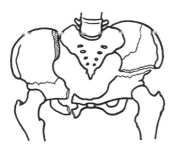

Fig. 7. Multiple fractures.

    d. Widening of the pubic symphysis to greater than 2.5 cm is associated with SI disruption.

    e. The stability of these fractures depends on intact posterior sacroiliac ligaments.

    f. Open-book fractures are often associated with bladder rupture, mandating cystourethrography. Physical exam may reveal extravasated urine in the scrotum or subcutaneous tissues of the penis and abdominal wall.

    g. Fractures of the posterior arch are associated with retroperitoneal hematomas.

4. Severe multiple fractures (see Fig. 7)

    a. These fractures are the result of high-speed MVAs, falls from great heights, or crush injuries by great weights.

    b. They are associated with the highest mortality of all pelvic fractures, ranging from 50% to 70% (7,47).

    c. Bony instability is common and often detectable on physical examination.

    d. Open fractures may result in hematuria and hematochezia.

    e. Patients with severe multiple fractures usually have a complicated recovery with permanent gait disturbances and chronic low back pain.

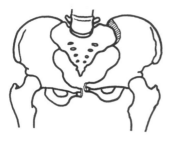

Fig. 8.   **Dislocation of the pubic symphysis and sacroiliac joint.**

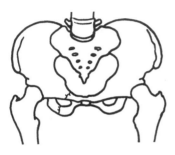

Fig. 9.   **Nondisplaced fracture of the pubic rami.**

5.   **Sacroiliac dislocations (Fig. 8)**
     a.   The radiographic appearance of these injuries will show cephalad migration of the hemipelvis, which indicates complete SI disruption.
     b.   If these injuries reveal greater than 2.5 cm of pubic diastasis, the anterior ring is also disrupted.
     c.   Untreated patients have an extremely poor outcome, with inability to ambulate. Most are treated with internal fixation under direct visualization.
B.   **Single breaks in the ring.** Fractures of only one segment of the pelvic ring are unusual owing to the rigid structure of the pelvis. However, they can rarely be seen because of the slight laxity of the SI joints and pubic symphysis. A double break must be sought out before accepting that an isolated disruption of the ring has occurred.
     1.   **Ipsilateral superior and inferior pubic rami (Fig. 9)**
          a.   These are stable and respond to conservative management.
          b.   Patients can be managed at home with pain control, rest, and ice in the initial period.

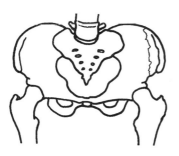

Fig. 10. Duverney fracture.

    c. Displacement at the fracture site is suggestive of an associated posterior component fracture, requiring CT scan of the pelvis to assess this possibility.

    d. Whenever these fractures are seen, careful examination for occult injury of the SI joint or symphysis pubis must be made.

    e. On physical examination, pudendal nerve injury must be evaluated.

C. **Fractures of individual pelvic bones with an intact pelvic ring.** Fractures of the individual pelvic bones comprise one-third of all pelvic fractures. These are inherently stable and have low morbidity and mortality. Isolated individual fractures occur from falls from a standing height, bed, or wheelchair. In young patients, they may occur as avulsions from violent muscle contractions or extreme strain. In children, these fractures should not be confused with normal unfused apophyses and ossicles, or the triradiate cartilage or ischiopubic synchondrosis. The iliac spines, ischial tuberosities, superior pubic rami, and coccyx are often involved as individual fractures, especially in osteoporotic patients. The potential for associated injuries is small owing to the relative lack of force involved. The exception to this is the **iliac wing** fracture.

    1. **Iliac wing fracture (Duverney fracture) (Fig. 10)**

        a. Direct trauma to the iliac crest may result in an unstable bony fragment. However, because the stability of the pelvis and the ability to bear weight remain uncompromised, this is considered a stable fracture.

        b. Iliac wing fractures are notable for local hemorrhage, possibility of adjacent visceral injury, and subsequent severe ileus, necessitating intravenous hydration and nothing-by-mouth (NPO) status.

        c. Some iliac wing fractures may extend into the acetabulum, complicating management.

      d. Patients with iliac wing fractures require complete evaluation for associated intraabdominal injuries and should be admitted to the hospital with orthopaedic consultation. Most are treated conservatively, with no operative management of the fracture required.

2. Isolated ramus fracture

      a. Isolated ramus fractures are the most common pelvic fracture (48).

      b. These fractures are inherently stable.

      c. They may be associated with hip or sacroiliac pain.

      d. Management is conservative and consists of pain medication and limited ambulation.

3. Coccygeal fracture

      a. These fractures are inherently stable.

      b. Treatment consists of rest, stool softeners, analgesics, and donut cushions for sitting. Outpatient management is typical.

      c. Coccygeal fractures are rarely complicated by rectal penetration; however, rectal examination for occult blood must be done to rule out this possibility.

4. Sacral fracture

      a. Sacral fractures are extremely rare, with an incidence of less than 8% of all pelvic fractures (49). They are associated with other pelvic fractures in 80% to 90% of cases (8), especially if the sacral fracture is vertical.

      b. There are three types of sacral fractures: upper, lower, and vertical.

      c. Upper fractures are associated with buttock or perianal pain. They are typically difficult to visualize on plain film, and may require CT or MRI for appropriate imaging. Twenty-five percent will have associated neurological deficits (8). These fractures may damage the sacral nerve, causing loss of bowel and bladder function, sexual dysfunction, sciatica and, rarely, leakage of cerebrospinal fluid (50,51).

      d. Lower sacral fractures are equally painful but rarely complicated by any neurological injury.

      e. Management of sacral fractures requires orthopaedic evaluation and admission for pain control. Unstable fractures require internal fixation. Patients with neurological complications will have poor neurological recovery in spite of maximal treatment.

5. Avulsion fractures (Fig. 11)

      a. The sites of avulsion fractures in order of frequency are the anterosuperior iliac spine, anteroinferior iliac spine, and the ischial tuberosity.

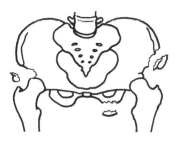

Fig. 11.   Avulsion fractures.

    b. These fractures result from extreme muscle strain or violent contraction, as in hurdlers and long-jumpers. They are also seen in children prior to physeal closure.

    c. Patients present with local pain and swelling, limiting range of motion about the hip.

    d. Treatment consists of analgesia, ice, and rest. Most patients will recover without sequelae.

6. **Diastasis of the pubic symphysis**

    a. Diastasis of the symphysis is usually an isolated stable injury.

    b. It may be complicated by injury to the posterior urethra or the pudendal neurovasculature. Therefore appropriate neurological and genitourinary exams are required.

    c. A separation of greater than 2.5 cm on the AP pelvic film indicates associated posterior injury and an unstable pelvis.

7. **Acetabular fracture**

    a. Acetabular fractures usually result from AP compressive forces. They are often seen in pedestrians struck by motor vehicles or in drivers whose knees strike the dashboard.

    b. Acetabular fractures comprise approximately 20% of all pelvic fractures. Thirty-three percent of these fractures are *not* visible on routine AP pelvic films (52), and visible findings may be extremely subtle, limited to a jagged shadowing of the normally smooth posterior acetabular margin line.

    c. Most often acetabular fractures occur in the posterior lip. These can be associated with posterior dislocation of the femoral head and may hinder or prevent closed reduction.

    d. With acetabular fractures, the physician must always check for associated injury to the femoral head.

    e. Sciatic nerve damage is also seen, requiring careful neurological evaluation.

VI. Associated injuries. Pelvic fractures in elderly fallers or from sports involve low energy and are usually not complicated by additional injuries. Pelvic fracture from high-energy forces (e.g., MVAs, pedestrian-MVA collisions) are frequently complicated by additional pathology.

   A. **Musculoskeletal.** The most common injuries associated with pelvic fracture involve trauma to the extremities. In decreasing frequency, fractures occur in the femoral shaft, tibia/fibula, hip, foot, ankle, and patella (39), followed by dislocation of the hip, knee, and ankle. Fractures of the vertebral column are associated with neurological sequelae and are a further source of retroperitoneal blood loss.

   B. **Intraabdominal.** The next most common associated injuries are intraabdominal, with the most consistent predictor of abdominal injury being the presence of multiple pelvic fractures. Eighty percent of children and 50% of adults with multiple pelvic fracture will have intraabdominal injury (2, 6, 53), including disruption of major vessels and damage of solid viscera. Massive blood loss in children with pelvic fracture, in contrast to that in adults, is usually the result of solid viscus injury rather than peripelvic hemorrhage. Segments of bowel that lie in the false pelvis are subject to bony penetration during pelvic fracture.

      1. **Diagnostic peritoneal lavage.** DPL to rule out concomitant intraabdominal injury is suggested in pelvic fracture patients who are hemodynamically unstable (2). It should be performed early to minimize false-positive results from the diapedesis of red blood cells from a retroperitoneal hematoma. False-positives can also result from tears in the posterior peritoneum that contain retroperitoneal hematomas or from passing the catheter through an anteriorly extending retroperitoneal hematoma. Patients subjected to negative abdominal exploration after pelvic fracture have a high incidence of mortality (8,39). Use of the supraumbilical open technique for DPL reduces the numbers of false-positives to between 9% and 12.5% (27, 29, 39, 40).

      2. **Computed tomography.** CT is useful in diagnosing intraabdominal injuries. It can demonstrate retroperitoneal hematomas and define fractures, especially acetabular disruptions and sacral fractures. CT is further useful in defining disruption of the superior and posterior arch and intraarticular loose bodies. Its use, however, is limited in the presence of hemodynamic instability. CT is not required in the application of external fixators but is essential before internal fixation for posterior pelvic reconstruction.

C. **Urological injuries.** Any pelvic fracture may result in urological injury, and 17% of patients with pelvic fracture will have such injuries, including rupture of the urethra, penetration of the bladder, and renal injury. Straddle fractures are frequently associated with severe urological injury, as are fractures of the symphysis pubis and Malgaigne fractures. Extravasated urine may be detected in the scrotum, subcutaneous tissues of the penis, the subcutaneous plane of the abdominal wall, or in DPL or chest tube drainage. Gross hematuria or blood at the urethral meatus necessitates retrograde urethrography and cystography. Microscopic hematuria alone in the absence of clinical signs of urological injury is a poor predictor of urological injury and does not require emergent study (54,55). Urethral injuries in males with pelvic fractures occur in up to 25% but are rare in women (56). Bladder injuries occur equally in both sexes. Genitourinary injuries are uncommon in children. A high-riding prostate is an often looked for but seldom found indicator of a urethral tear.

The sequence of retrograde urethrogram (RGU), cystogram, or intravenous pyelogram (IVP) must be individualized to each case. The RGU is performed gently to avoid completing a partial urethral tear. A Foley catheter is inserted 1 to 2 cm beyond the meatus and the balloon inflated with 1 to 2 cm of sterile saline to create a seal. AP and oblique radiographs are taken as contrast fills the urethra. Any extravasation indicates urethral injury. If normal anatomy is demonstrated, the Foley can then be passed into the bladder for cystography.

D. **Thoracic aorta.** The extreme force required for pelvic fracture mandates a search for clinical as well as radiographic evidence of injury to the thoracic aorta, particularly when a deceleration mechanism is involved. These injuries are life-threatening and obvious management priorities.

VII. **Complications of pelvic fractures.** Most complications of pelvic fracture patients result from associated injuries rather than the fracture itself. Several studies have shown the incidence of complication ranging from 43% to 73%, with pulmonary pathology occurring in about 50% (47,57,58). The most common complications described with pelvic fracture include acute respiratory distress syndrome, atelectasis, fat embolism, pneumonia, urinary tract infection, wound infection, sepsis, coagulopathy, and pulmonary embolism.

In general, patients with complications have higher ISS, lower trauma scores, increased transfusion requirements, and longer hospital stays than patients without complications. No association of complications exists regarding age, sex, mechanism, site of injury, amount of fracture displacement, or vector of injury. Unstable fractures are more likely to be associated with complications than stable fractures. Early death usually results from hemorrhage. Later mortality results from intracranial trauma, sepsis, or multiple organ failure.

VIII. **Nontraumatic skeletal causes of pelvic pain**

A. **Osteitis pubis** is an inflammation of unknown cause of the symphysis pubis. The condition is self-limited. It can be extremely painful and is associated with repetitive stress to the area, as occurs in laborers and athletes. It is often seen after childbirth and can occur following urinary tract infections. Pain is of gradual onset, exacerbated with tensing of the abdominal muscles for the Valsalva maneuver or cough. Ambulation becomes very painful. On physical exam, the symphysis is tender. Even passive abduction of the hips induces pain. Radiographs are initially normal; after several days, spotty demineralization and widening of the symphysis may be seen. These changes resolve after 6 to 8 months. Treatment consists of rest and pain relief, preferably with nonsteroidal antiinflammatory drugs (NSAIDs). Oral prednisone and local infiltration with a steroid can be beneficial. Symptoms typically abate in 1 to 2 weeks but may last longer.

B. **Coccygodynia** is characterized by coccygeal pain resulting from fibrosis after trauma or fracture. It is often seen as a result of multiple childbirth. Pain with sitting, exacerbated by slumping forward, is typical. Palpation reveals local pain, tenderness, and inflammation, both externally and on rectal exam. Radiographs may show degenerative changes or a new fracture. Treatment consists of analgesia, sitzbaths, and a foam- or air-filled doughnut pillow for sitting. Stool softeners may be helpful. Extreme cases may benefit from local steroid injection. Conservative treatment is utilized for at least 6 months before surgical coccygectomy is considered.

IX. **Summary.** The management priority in pelvic fracture must begin with identifying and controlling sources of hemorrhage, before hemodynamic instability, failure of organ perfusion, and coagulopathy develop. Associated injuries must be evaluated. Pelvic motion must be kept to a minimum. Early transfusion is important.

Clinically, all unresponsive patients must be treated as if they were specifically complaining of pelvic pain. All alert patients must be asked about the presence of pain to the pelvis, back, buttock, groin, hip, thigh, and perineal area as well as the association of numbness or weakness in legs and loss of bowel or bladder sensation or control. The ability to ambulate after injury excludes the existence of unstable fractures, but stable fractures may still be present.

Mortality is directly altered by the timing to intervention. Mortality due to pelvic fractures has been reduced through the use of an aggressive multidisciplinary approach. Emergency physicians need to orchestrate a team of general, vascular and orthopaedic surgeons, radiologists, and urologists to maximize early lifesaving interventions.

Nontraumatic disorders should be identified so early treatment can begin.

REFERENCES

1. Kinzl L, Burri C, Coldeway J. Fractures of the pelvis and associated intrapelvic injuries. *Injury* 1982;14:63–69.
2. Jerrard DA. Pelvic fractures. *Emerg Med Clin North Am* 1993; 11: 147–163.
3. McCoy GF, Johnstone RA, Kenwright J. Biomechanical aspects of pelvic and hip injuries in road traffic accidents. *J Orthop Trauma* 1080;0:110 120.
4. Siegel JH, Mason-Gonzalez S, Dischinger P, et al. Safety belt restraints and compartment intrusions in frontal and lateral vehicle crashes: mechanisms of injuries, complications and acute care costs (see comments). *J Trauma* 1993;34:736–758.
5. Mucha PJ, Farnell MB. Analysis of pelvic fracture management. *J Trauma* 1984;24:379–386.
6. Rothenberger DA, Fischer RP, Strate RG, Velasco R, Perry JFJ. The mortality associated with pelvic fractures. *Sugery* 1978;84:356–361.
7. McMurtry R, Walton D, Dickinson D, Kellam J, Tile M. Pelvic disruption in the polytraumatized patient: a management protocol. *Clin Orthop* 1980;22–30.
8. Kricun ME. Fractures of the pelvis. *Orthop Clin North Am* 1990;21:573–590.
9. Klein SR, Saroyan RM, Baumgartner F, Bongard FS. Management strategy of vascular injuries associated with pelvic fractures. *J Cardiovasc Surg (Torino)* 1992;33:349–357.
10. Kane WJ. Fractures of the pelvis. In: Rockwood CA, Green DP, eds. *Fractures in adults,* 2nd ed. Philadelphia: JB Lippincott, 1984:1093.
11. Conwell HE, Reynolds FC, eds. *Key and Conwell's management of fractures, dislocations and sprains,* 7th ed. St Louis, CV Mosby, 1961.
12. Tile M. Pelvic ring fractures: should they be fixed? *J Bone Joint Surg* 1988;70B(1):1–2.
13. Connolly JF, ed. *DePalma's the management of fractures and dislocations,* 3rd ed. Philadelphia: WB Saunders, 1981.
14. Kellam J, Browner B. Fractures of the pelvic ring. In: Browner B, Jupiter J, Levine A, et al, eds. *Skeletal trauma.* Philadelphia: WB Saunders, 1992:872.
15. Grant PT. The diagnosis of pelvic fractures by "springing." *Arch Emerg Med* 1990;7:178–182.
16. Maull KI, Sachatello CR, Ernst CB. The deep perineal laceration—an injury frequently associated with open pelvic fractures: a need for aggressive surgical management. A report of 12 cases and review of the literature. *J Trauma* 1977;17:685–696.
17. Yugueros P, Sarmiento JM, Garcia AF, Ferrada R. Unnecessary use of pelvic x-ray in blunt trauma. *J Trauma* 1995;39:722–725.

18. Young JW, Burgess AR. *Radiographic management of pelvic fractures: a need for aggressive surgical management.* Baltimore: Urban and Schwarzenberg, 1987.
19. Edeiken-Monroe BS, Browner BD, Jackson H. The role of standard roentgenograms in the evaluation of instability of pelvic ring disruption. *Clin Orthop Rel Res* 1989;240:63–76.
20. Thaggard A, Harle TS, Carlson V. Fractures and dislocations of the bony pelvis and hip. *Semin Roentgenol* 1978;13:117–134.
21. Baumgartner F, White GH, White RA, et al. Delayed exsanguinating pelvic hemorrhage after blunt trauma without bone fracture: case report (see comments). *J Trauma* 1990;30:1603–1065.
22. Judet R, Judet J, Letournel E. Fractures of the acetabulum: classicfication and surgical approaches for open reduction. Preliminary report. *J Bone Joint Surg Am* 1964;46:1615–1646.
23. Brown JJ, Greene FL, McMillin RD. Vascular injuries asociated with pelvic fractures. *Am Surg* 1984;50:150–154.
24. Cryer HM, Miller FB, Evers BM. Pelvic fracture classification: correlation with hemorrhage. *J Trauma* 1988;28:973–980.
25. Shoemaker WC, Peitzman AB, Bellamy R, et al. Resuscitation from severe homorrhage. *Crit Care Med* 1996;24 (supply):S12–S23.
26. Bickell WH, Wall MJ, Pepe PE, et al. Immediate vs. delayed fluid resuscitation for hypotensive patients with penetrating torso injuries. *N Engl J Med* 1994;331:1105–1109.
27. Flint L, Babikian G, Anders M, Rodriguez J, Steinberg S. Defintive control of mortality from severe pelvic fractures. *Ann Surg* 1990;211:703–716.
28. McIntyne RC Jr., Bensard DD, Moore EE, et al. Pelvic fracture geometry predicts risk of life-threatening hemorrhage in children. *J Trauma* 1993;35:423–429.
29. Flint LMJ, Brown A, Richardson JD, Polk HC. Definitive control of bleeding from severe pelvic fractures. *Ann Surg* 1979;189:709–716.
30. Mucha P, Welch TJ. Hemorrhage in major pelvic fractures. *Surg Clin North Am* 1988;68:757.
31. Iannacone WM, Brathwite CEM. Use of the external fixation frame for acute stabilization of unstable pelvic fractures. *Tech Orthop* 1993. In press.
32. Mears DC, Rubash HE. *Pelvic and acetabular fractures.* Thorofare NJ: Slack, 1986.
33. Holting T, Buhr H, Richter G, et al. Diagnosis and treatment of retroperitoneal hematoma in multiple trauma patients. *Arch Orthop Trauma Surg* 1992;111:323–326.
34. Reynolds BM, Balsano NA. Venography in pelvic fractures: a clinical evaluation. *Ann Surg* 1971;173:104–106.
35. Matalon TS, Athanasoulis CA, Margolies MN. Hemorrhage with pelvic fractures: efficacy of transcatheter embolization. *AJR* 1979;133:859–864.
36. Rafii M, Firooznia H, Golimbu C, Waugh JG, Naidich D. The impact of CT in clinical management of pelvic and acetabular fractures. *Clin Orthop* 1983;178:228.
37. Patterson BM. Pelvic ring injury and associated trauma: an orthopaedic perspective. *Semin Urol.* 1995;13(1):25–33.

38. Moreno C, Moore EE, Roenberger A, Cleveland HC. Hemorrhage associated with major pelvic fracture: a multispecialty challenge. *J Trauma* 1986;26:987–994.
39. Gilliland MD, Ward RE, Barton RM, Miller PW, Duke JH. Factors affecting mortality in pelvic fractures. *J Trauma* 1982;22:691–693.
40. Evers BM, Cryer HM, Miller FB. Pelvic fracture hemorrhage: priorities in management. *Arch Surg* 1989;124:422–424.
41. Hubbard SG, Bivins BA, Sachatello CR, Griffen WO Jr. Diagnostic errors with peritoneal lavage in patients with pelvic fractures. *Arch Surg* 1979;114:844–846.
42. Gilliland MG, Ward RE, Flynn TC, Miller PW, Ben-Menachem Y, Duke JH Jr. Peritoneal lavage and angiography in the management of patients with pelvic fractures. *Am J Surg* 1982;114:744–747.
43. Moore JD, Moore EE, Markovchick VJ, Rosen P. Diagnostic peritoneal lavage for abdominal trauma: superiority of the open technique at the infraumbilical ring. *J Trauma* 1981;21:570–572.
44. Markovchick VJ, Elerding SC, Moore EE, Rosen P. Diagnostic peritoneal lavage. *JACEP* 1979;8:326–328.
45. Lazarus HM, Nelson JA. Technique for peritoneal lavage when a pelvic fracture and suspected hematoma are present. *Surg Gynecol Obstet* 1981;153:403.
46. Soderstom CA. Severe pelvic fractures: problems and possible solutions. *Am Surg* 1982;48:441–446.
47. Trunkey DD, Chapman MW, Lim RCJ, Dunphy JE. Management of pelvic fractures in blunt trauma injury. *J Trauma* 1974;14:912–923.
48. Rogers LF. *Radiology of skeletal trauma*. New York: Churchill Livingstone, 1992.
49. Tile M. *Fractures of the pelvis and acetabulum*, 2nd ed. Baltimore: Williams & Wilkins, 1995.
50. Byrnes DP, Russo GL, Ducker TB, Cowley RA. Sacrum fractures and neurologic damage. *J Neurosurg* 1977;47:459.
51. Weaver EN, England GD, Richardson DE. Sacral fracture: case presentation and review. *Neurology* 1981;9:725–728.
52. Pearson JR, Hargadon EJ. Fractures of the pelvis involving the floor of the acetabulum. *J Bone Joint Surg AM* 1962;44B:550–561.
53. Bond SJ, Gotschall CS, Eichelberger MR. Predictors of abdominal injury in children with pelvic fracture. *J Trauma* 1993;31:1169–1173.
54. Fallon B, Wendt JC, Hawtrey CE. Urological injury and assessment in patients with fractured pelvis. *J Urol* 1984;131:712–714.
55. Antoci JP, Schiff M Jr. Bladder and urethral injuries in patients with pelvic fractures. *J Urol* 1982;128:25–26.
56. Carter CT, Schafer N. Incidence of utethral disruption in females with traumatic pelvic fractures. *Am J Emerg Med* 1993;11:218–220.
57. Looser KG, Crombie HD Jr. Pelvic fractures: an anatomic guide to severity of injury: review of 100 cases. *Am J Surg* 1976;132:638–642.
58. Poole GV, Frazier EF, Griswold J, et al. Complications of pelvic fractures from blunt trauma. *Am Surg* 1992;58:225–231.

Hip and Femur

Teresita M. Hogan

I. **Femur**
   A. **Fractures.** The femur is the largest and strongest of all skeletal bones (Fig. 1). Despite this, the femoral head is relatively vulnerable. Its anatomical orientation, mobility, and load-bearing role subject it to extreme shearing forces. The head's vascular supply is easily disrupted, causing ischemic complications after fracture. In contrast, the femoral shaft has an anatomic bend for structural reinforcement and an abundant vascular supply, which promotes healing. Over 250,000 femoral fractures occur in the United States annually. The overwhelming majority are seen in elderly osteoporotic patients as a result of relatively minor trauma. As the population ages, over 500,000 femoral fractures are expected annually by 2050 (1). The mean age of occurrence is 76 years, with the fracture rate doubling in each decade after the age of 50. The risk of a second hip fracture in elderly patients is twice that of the first because of their increased likelihood of falling. Fractures of the femur fall into two broad categories: fractures of the proximal femur, including subcapital, neck, intertrochanteric, and subtrochanteric, and those of the shaft (Fig. 2).
      1. **Proximal femoral fractures** include those of the femoral head and neck as well as intertrochanteric and subtrochanteric fractures. Table 1 compares and contrasts the major characteristics of these injuries. Suspected injury of the proximal femur can be evaluated using anteroposterior (AP) and lateral views of the hip. The AP pelvic view is extremely informative. Evaluation of Shenton's line can reveal subtle changes in anatomical relationships (Fig. 3). Femoral shaft injuries require AP and lateral views that include the knee and hip joint. Elderly patients sustaining hip fracture require a three-pronged emergency evaluation focusing on fracture diagnosis, assessment for associated injury, and an investigation into possible medical problems contributing to a fall.
         a. **Femoral head**
            (1) **Mechanism.** Since fractures of the femoral head often result from high-velocity mechanisms, an evaluation for associated trauma is required. High velocity is defined by the force transmitted to the patient. Typically, high velocity forces occur in MVAs, vehicle versus pedestrian and falls from height. Full Advanced Trauma Life Support (ATLS) principles must be

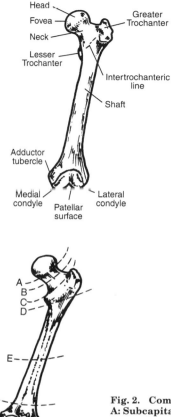

Fig. 1. The femur.

**Fig. 2. Common fractures of the femur:
A: Subcapital. B: Neck. C: In-
tertrochanteric. D: Subtrochanteric.
E: Shaft. F: Supracondylar. G: Condylar.**

applied. Femoral head fractures typically
occur in conjunction with dislocation of the
hip, a true orthopaedic emergency, as discussed in Sec. II of this chapter.

Isolated fractures of the femoral head
present with localized hip pain, which
may or may not prevent ambulation.
There is no shortening or rotation of
the affected leg (Fig. 4). Blood loss from
this injury is limited by containment
within the hip capsule, so discoloration
and swelling of surrounding tissues are
slight. There can be associated spasm of
the hip flexors. Young patients with
femoral head fractures are usually the
victims of high-velocity trauma. Isolated

Table 1.   Proximal femur fractures

	Femoral head	Femoral neck	Intertrochanteric	Subtrochanteric
Mechanism	Extreme shearing force from high energy trauma	Falls, causing direct trauma to greater trochanter or forced lateral rotation	>90% from falls, with direct trauma to greater trochanter	Fall with extreme force
Epidemiology	Mainly young patients Isolated fractures are rare; most occur with dislocation 75% from MVAs	Bone demineralization Women >>men Whites >>>blacks Mean age 74–78 years fairly common	Very common—98/100,000 population due to bone demineralization Mean age 75–81 years Women >>men Whites >>>blacks	Represent 11% of all proximal femur fractures, 89% high-velocity injury. Stress fractures in runners or pathologic fracture from CA (usually breast)
Clinical presentation	Complete immobility of hip With anterior dislocation—abducted and externally rotated With posterior dislocation—thigh is adducted, internally rotated and shortened	Nondisplaced—minimal symptoms, occasionally ambulatory with antalgic gait Displaced—moderate to severe pain, nonambulatory, external rotation, abduction of leg, shortening	Severe pain, all nonambulatory, extreme external rotation and abduction of leg, earlier swelling and ecchymosis of hip	Severe pain on flexion, abduction, and external rotation Thigh tenderness and swelling

Associated injury	Hip dislocation Anterior (22–77% have fracture) Posterior (10–16% have fracture) 70% of patients have remote injuries	Rare	Rare	Other extremity fractures in 30% Intraabdominal, neurologic or GU injury in 15%
Classification	Two types: Single fracture fragment Comminuted fracture	*Garden* I. Impacted/incomplete displacement II. Complete without displacement III. Complete/partial displacement IV. Complete/total displacement	*Evans Modified†* I. Nondisplaced two fragments II. Displaced/two fragments III. Three fragments/ detached greater trochanter IV. Four fragments/ detached lesser trochanter V. Four fragments/both trochanters detached	*Seinheimer‡* I. Nondisplaced II. Two-part fractures III. Three-part fractures IV. Comminuted V. Extension into the greater trochanter
Complications	Avascular necrosis, arthritis, myositis ossificans, recurrent dislocation	Avascular necrosis	Rare due to excellent blood supply	Rare due to excellent blood supply

*Mattox KL, et al. Prospective mast study in 911 patients. *J Trauma* 1989;29:1104.
†Flaherty JJ, et al. Relationship of pelvic bone fracture patterns to injuries of urethra and bladder. *J Urol* 1968;99:297.
‡Seinheimer F. Subtrochanteric fractures of the femur. *J Bone Joint Surg* 1978;60A:300–306.

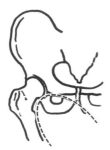

Fig. 3.   Shenton's line.

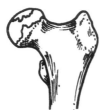

Fig. 4.   Femoral head fractures.

fracture of the femoral head may be difficult to diagnose, as a significant proportion of these are missed on plain film alone (3). In young patients, fracture lines can be quite fine or impacted. In the elderly, osteophytes and general osteoporosis can obscure fractures. If clinical suspicion is high, magnetic resonance imaging (MRI) or a bone scan is necessary to confirm and delineate the extent of injury. Associated acetabular fractures must also be sought.

Occult fractures occur in both the femoral head and neck and should be suspected in patients with persistent posttraumatic hip pain and normal plain radiography. Approximately 50% of these patients will have an occult fracture of the pelvis or proximal femur detected on MRI (4). The sensitivity and specificity of MRI are better than those of bone scan (5), especially within the first 24 hours, and in the elderly.

(2)   **Management.** When there is no associated dislocation, emergency department management of femoral head fracture consists of radiologic diagnosis, bed rest, and pain control. Acute medical con-

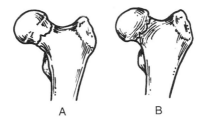

Fig. 5. Femoral neck fractures: A: Nondisplaced neck fracture. B: Impacted subcapital fracture.

ditions that may have contributed to the fall must be considered. Early orthopaedic evaluation is important, as most patients will require open reduction to minimize complications of avascular necrosis or osteoarthritis. Elderly patients cannot tolerate prolonged bed rest and their survival is improved by open reduction, internal fixation, and early ambulation.

b. **Femoral neck (Fig. 5)**

(1) **Mechanism.** Femoral neck fractures are primarily the result of minor trauma in elderly osteoporotic patients.

(2) **History and physical examination.** Symptoms vary depending on the degree of displacement. Nondisplaced fractures may present with minimal discomfort. These patients may even be able to ambulate. However, most will have an antalgic gait. Displaced fractures are more dramatic in presentation. Patients are nonambulatory and experience severe pain with any motion of the hip. On exam, they usually exhibit external rotation, abduction, and slight shortening of the affected leg. There is tenderness to percussion over the greater trochanter.

Although associated injury must be considered, most patients suffer isolated fracture of the femoral neck. As with any hip fracture in the elderly patient, any medical condition that may have led to the fall must be adequately investigated. Only if the history is consistent with a simple mechanical fall should a more extensive medical workup be avoided. When acute medical deterioration or syncope is suspected, the appropriate evaluation and hospitalization should ensue.

(3) **Radiography.** Plain radiographs are usually diagnostic. If clinical suspicion is high and standard AP and lateral films are negative, a view with 15° to 20° of internal rotation provides improved visualization of the bony anatomy. When suspicion is high, computed tomography (CT) or MRI of the hip may reveal a fracture.

(4) **Treatment.** If no medical condition exists and no associated trauma is found, emergency treatment consists of pain control, bed rest, and admission with immediate orthopaedic consultation for definitive open repair. Open reduction and internal fixation (ORIF) can often be accomplished with bone screws or pins. In patients whose general health is poor, who are relatively inactive, or who are approximately 70 years or more, endoprosthetic replacement may be the preferred method of repair.

c. **Stress fractures of the femoral neck**

(1) **Mechanism.** Stress fractures often develop insidiously. Any patient subjected to chronic and repetitive mechanical stress about the joint (athletes, military recruits, joggers) who is complaining of persistent pain should be evaluated for a stress fracture of the femoral neck.

(2) **History and physical examination.** Initial symptoms of stress fracture of the femoral neck may be limited to vague groin pain or referred knee pain. Early-morning stiffness progressing over days to weeks and causing an antalgic gait is common. Pain is often attributed to a "muscle pull," delaying medical consultation. Physicians can be easily lulled into the same mistaken diagnosis because the physical findings early in the course can be subtle. Minor discomfort is produced with range of motion, and some spasm is usually seen at extremes of range. Spasm and typical tenderness to percussion over the greater trochanter may be the only early clues suggesting proximal stress fracture. Later, the anterior hip may become tender to palpation and develop induration or edema.

(3) **Radiography.** X-rays may be negative in the first 2 weeks. Oblique views or to-

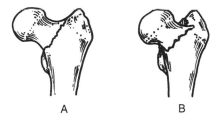

Fig. 6.   Intertrochanteric fractures: A: Nondisplaced. B: Displaced.

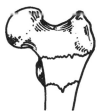

Fig. 7.   Subtrochanteric fractures.

mography can enhance detection. Recently, MRI has been found superior to bone scan for diagnosis of Femoral neck and all occult hip fractures (6,7).

(4) **Treatment** is usually conservative; up to 6 weeks without weight bearing may be required. Rehabilitation is usually needed before full function is recovered. Patients with suspected stress fracture should be given analgesia, ice, and orthopaedic follow-up; they should also avoid weight bearing.

d. **Intertrochanteric and subtrochanteric (Figs. 6 and 7)**

(1) **Mechanism.** Subtrochanteric fractures make up 10% of all fractures of the proximal femur. They represent a transition between fractures of the proximal femur and femoral shaft fractures (Fig. 7). Because of the intertrochanteric bone mass and density, they occur in the face of much greater forces than neck fractures in 90% of cases. The remaining 10% are stress fractures or pathological fractures from metastatic cancer, usually of the breast. Thirty percent of patients with subtrochanteric fractures have another

long- bone fracture, while 5% have intraabdominal injury and 6% have neurological injury.

(2) **History and physical examination.** Although blood loss is greater because of the extracapsular location of these fractures, a search for intraabdominal or intrathoracic hemorrhage must always be done in the presence of vascular instability. Hypotension due to the fracture alone is unlikely.

(3) **Treatment.** Urgent surgical repair of all hip fractures should be performed soon after injury. Delays beyond 48 hours increase the risk of postoperative complications as well as the 1-year mortality (8). This treatment interval is generally adequate to address coexistent medical conditions and stabilize patients preoperatively. Patients with recent or concurrent myocardial infarction, however, are an exception, and in this subset of patients, surgery must be delayed owing to a nearly 40% risk of postoperative reinfarction within 3 months. To minimize delays, the emergency physician should make immediate orthopaedic contact and initiate any necessary preoperative medical interventions, such as the reversal of anticoagulation (9). As in the case of fractures of the femoral neck, the treatment goal in treating intertrochanteric fractures is restoring functional status as quickly as possible; this is usually best achieved with urgent reduction and internal fixation using a nail plate or intermedullary devices.

e. **Greater trochanteric injury**

(1) **Mechanism.** Avulsions of the greater trochanteric apophysis occur in young athletes after forceful muscle contraction. Fracture may also result from a direct blow to the area.

(2) **History and physical examination.** Both injuries will show local tenderness; however, discoloration over the trochanter is unusual (10). Pain increases with abduction against resistance. Spasm may cause forced hip flexion, making localization of the injury quite simple.

(3) **Radiography.** AP and lateral views are adequate for visualization. When direct trauma is involved, comminution of the fracture fragment may be seen.

(4) **Treatment.** The prognosis is good in these injuries. Ice, analgesics, and initial bed rest are followed by partial weight bearing for 3 to 4 weeks. A large, intact, displaced fracture may be amenable to ORIF.

f. **Lesser trochanter injury**

(1) **Mechanism.** As with greater trochanteric injury, the majority of these injuries occur in aggressive young athletes who tend to strain the hip flexors maximally. Eighty-five percent occur in patients under 20 years of age (11). A lesser trochanteric avulsion or fracture in a relatively inactive adult should signal possible pathological fracture.

(2) **History and physical examination.** Patients with isolated trochanteric injuries exhibit **Ludloff's sign** of iliopsoas insufficiency—an inability to raise the affected leg while seated because of hip pain.

(3) **Radiography.** AP and lateral views of the femur typically reveal an avulsed fragment from the lesser trochanter.

(4) **Treatment.** Lesser trochanteric injury is often treated with initial bed rest and pain medication. Partial weight bearing with or without casting may then be employed. Failure of conservative treatment, unreliable patients, or patients with large degrees of separation on x-ray may require operative intervention. Recovery in these cases is usually complete.

2. **Distal femoral fractures**

a. **Femoral shaft**

(1) **Mechanism.** The femoral shaft begins 5 cm distal to the lesser trochanter and ends 6 cm proximal to the adductor tubercle. It is intrinsically more stable than the proximal femur, necessitating even greater energy to fracture.

(2) **History and physical examination.** Femoral fractures are clinically obvious; patients are in extreme pain, nonambulatory, and unable to move the ipsilateral hip or knee. Any thigh deformity reflects the location of the fracture, the mechanical pull of surrounding musculature, and the extent of hemorrhage.

Although patients with femoral fractures can lose 1 L or more of blood into the thigh, other causes of shock must always be suspected and ruled out before attributing hemodynamic instability to the fracture alone. All patients must be carefully evaluated for associated injuries. The same leg may sustain additional fractures to the femoral neck, supracondylar area, or patella. As many as one-third of patients with femoral fractures will also have ligamentous injury of the ipsilateral knee.

(3) **Treatment.** These patients require immobilization of the leg for pain control and to limit further blood loss or soft tissue injury. Immobilization can be achieved with sandbags or by using Hare or Buck traction devices. Ice should be applied to the thigh intermittently to limit swelling and hemorrhage. A presurgical workup should be initiated while arranging orthopaedic admission for reduction and stabilization. Early care includes skeletal traction via pins installed in the distal femur or tibia or in an applied cast. Although traction applied for weeks once constituted definitive care, the last several decades have witnessed ever-increasing use of internal fixation with plates or intermedullary nails.

B. **Avascular necrosis of the femoral head.** Avascular necrosis (AVN) of the femoral head complicates many conditions from infancy to old age. Males between ages 40 and 50 are primarily affected, and the condition is bilateral in 40% to 80% of patients (12).

1. **Mechanism.** Trauma is the most common cause of AVN of the hip. Fractures of the vulnerable femoral neck or head or dislocations can disrupt branches of the medial and lateral circumflex arteries. Systemic disorders such as sickle cell disease, hemophilia, gout, and collagen vascular disorders such as systemic lupus erythematosus can also result in avascular necrosis of the femoral head.

2. **History, physical examination, and radiography.** Clinically, AVN evolves in four stages. In stage 1, the patient has minimal symptoms of pain only with exertion and a normal radiograph. In stage 2, there are more moderate symptoms, with increased pain and limitation of joint motion. Films demonstrate decreased bone density of the femoral head. In stage 3, patients have an antalgic limp and pain, limiting the activities of daily living. X-rays demonstrate collapse of the femoral head. In stage 4, patients are likely incapacitated and radiographs show loss of joint space and degenerative involvement of the acetabulum.

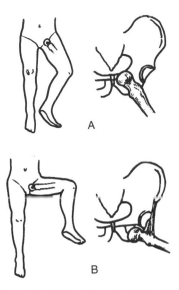

Fig. 8. Anterior hip dislocations: A: Pubic. B: Obturator.

   3. **Treatment.** Emergency department treatment consists of pain medication, bed rest, and orthopaedic consultation. Workup focuses on early identification of the causative process or inciting metabolic condition. Surgical correction depends on the stage of the disease, but eventual total hip replacement is typically necessary.

II. **Hip**
   A. **Dislocations.** Hip dislocations are true orthopaedic emergencies. These major injuries are always the result of extreme force and are highly associated with other serious injury. Up to 50% of patients have associated fractures (6). Reduction of the hip is a priority once life threatening injuries are identified and addressed. The dislocation may result in ischemia of the leg; the development of avascular necrosis of the femoral head is directly related to the duration of the dislocation.

   1. **Mechanism.** Hip dislocations are described as anterior or posterior. In **anterior dislocations** (Fig. 8), the femoral head lies anterior to the coronal plane of the acetabulum, while **posterior dislocations** (Fig. 9) lie posterior to the coronal plane. If the femoral head remains centered in the coronal plane of the acetabulum but displaces superiorly, the dislocation is described as central. **Central superior dislocations** are all associated with medial or superior acetabular fractures.

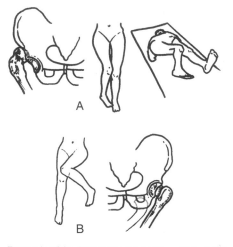

Fig. 9. Posterior hip dislocations: A: Iliac. B: Ischial.

The hip capsule is a strong fibrous structure, attached anteriorly at the intertrochanteric line. The posterolateral half of the femoral neck lies outside the capsule, creating a predisposition for posterior dislocation. Only 10% to 15% of hip dislocations are anterior (13). Posterior and anterior dislocations often result from MVAs in which a front-seated passenger's knee strikes the dashboard (posterior dislocation results when the thigh is adducted or neutral, while anterior dislocation results when the thigh is in abduction). The degree of hip flexion at impact determines if the dislocation will move superiorly or inferiorly. Fractures of the femoral head may result from these forces as the head impacts the acetabular rim. The greater the degree of hip flexion, the less likely is an associated femoral head fracture (14). These are usually evident on x-ray (13). Visualizing fractures of the acetabulum, however, may require special views. Posterior dislocations are associated with ipsilateral fracture of the femur and patella (15). Since dislocation often occurs as dashboard injuries, ligamentous injuries of the knee are common.

a. **Anterior dislocations fall into one of three categories.**

   (1) Anterior **obturator** hip dislocation. The femoral head displaces medially and lies in the obturator foramen (Fig. 8B).

   (2) Anterior **iliac** hip dislocation. The femoral head moves superiorly and lies over the iliac wing.

(3) Anterior **pubic** hip dislocation. The femoral head moves inferiorly over the inferior pubic ramus (Fig. 8A).

b. **Posterior dislocations fall into one of two categories**

(1) Posterior **ischial** hip dislocation. The femoral head is displaced inferiorly and lies over the ischium (Fig. 8B).

(2) Posterior **iliac** hip dislocation. The femoral head is displaced superiorly and lies over the iliac wing (Fig. 9A). See Table 2 for clinical presentations of each type of hip dislocation.

2. **History and physical examination.** Hip dislocations result in characteristic limb findings. After anterior dislocation, the leg is externally rotated and shortened, with slight knee flexion. The femoral head may be visible and palpable over the anterior iliac crest or the inguinal area. Posterior dislocations result in internal rotation of the entire leg with marked knee flexion and adduction of the thigh. The femoral head is rarely visible but often palpable in the buttock.

In all hip dislocations, a full neurovascular exam of the leg is necessary. The femoral artery, vein, and nerve may all be injured with anterior hip dislocation. Conversely, the sciatic nerve is injured in 10% to 14% of posterior dislocations (16). Because of the severity of the force required for a hip dislocation, a complete trauma evaluation is done to identify and treat associated injury.

3. **Radiography.** Once the patient has been adequately stabilized, radiographic evaluations must include the entire femur as well as the knee joint.

4. **Reduction.** Early diagnosis and immediate **closed reduction** of the dislocated hip is the treatment of choice. **Open reduction** is reserved for cases in which closed reduction has failed, the reduction is unstable, or fracture fragments cause separation of the acetabulum and femoral head. Most authorities on orthopaedics recommend closed reduction only with the use of general or spinal anesthesia to prevent articular damage, which may occur from forceful reduction in patients with contracted thigh and hip muscles (14). Conscious sedation techniques may be employed in attempting reduction in the emergency department, but repeated attempts or undue force should be avoided.

a. **Methods of reducing hip dislocations**

(1) **Gravity method of Stimson.** This method produces the best results in posterior dislocation but can be used in anterior dislocation as well. The patient lies prone with both thighs hanging over the edge of a cart or table. An assistant stabilizes the

Table 2.   Characteristics of hip dislocations

Type	Femoral Head	Clinical Posture	Reduction Technique
Anterior obturator	Medial displacement into obturator foramen; head not palpable	Hip and knee flexed at 90°, mild external rotation of leg	Allis maneuver
Anterior iliac	Superior displacement over iliac wing; head palpable and visible over iliac crest	Midposition between that of anterior iliac and anterior pubic dislocation	Allis maneuver or modified Allis maneuver
Anterior pubic	Inferior displacement over inferior pubic ramus; head palpable in inguinal area	Slight knee flexion, extreme external rotation, slight shortening of leg	Allis maneuver
Posterior ischial	Inferior displacement over the ischium; head easily palpable in low buttock	Extreme adduction, internal rotation, and knee flexion with knee crossing over contralateral thigh and foot near contralateral knee	Stimson method
Posterior iliac	Superior displacement over iliac wing; head may be palpable over the midbuttock	Moderate adduction, slight internal rotation, and knee flexion with knee just touching the contralateral thigh. 1–2 cm of shortening of affected leg	Stimson method, Allis maneuver, or modified Allis maneuver

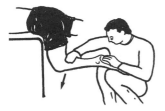

Fig. 10.   Posterior hip dislocation: reduction using Stimson's method.

pelvis by pressing the sacrum down to the table. The physician then flexes the knee to 90°and applies gentle downward traction. A subtle rotary motion may help to move the femoral head over the acetabular rim (Fig. 10). Stimson's maneuver may be precluded by associated injuries that prevent placing the patient prone.

(2) **Allis maneuver.** This technique is best for superior riding dislocations. The patient is placed supine with the knee flexed at 90°. An assistant stabilizes the pelvis by pressing down on the anterior iliac spines. Lateral traction must also be applied to the affected inner thigh, and this may require a second assistant. The physician then applies longitudinal traction to the thigh, followed by adduction and internal rotation as the hip is flexed to 90 degrees (Fig. 11).

In the **modified Allis maneuver,** the patient's hip is flexed to 90 degrees but then placed in *maximum adduction.* Longitudinal traction is then applied while an assistant presses down on the pelvis with one hand and pushes the head of the femur into the acetabulum with the other.

5. **Postreduction care.** After successful reduction of any dislocation, repeat assessment of neurovascular function is required, as is a postreduction radiograph. Postreduction CT will identify acetabular or osschondral fractures. Failure of closed reduction necessitates open reduction. All patients require admission and traction ranging from days to weeks. Complications include transient and permanent sciatic nerve injury, aseptic necrosis of the femoral head, posttraumatic arthritis, recurrent dislocation, and myositis ossificans (16,17). Complications may occur despite the most expedient treatment, and prosthetic hip replacement may eventually become necessary.

B. **Bursitis.** Three bursae of the hip are often affected with bursitis (Fig. 12).

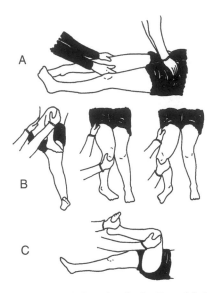

Fig. 11. Allis maneuver: A: Traction in the line of deformity. B: The hip is flexed, gently alternating internal and external rotation as well as abduction and adduction. C: The limb is rotated and extended while force on the trochanter reduces the femoral head.

1. The **deep trochanteric bursa** located between the greater trochanter and the gluteus maximus tendon is commonly involved. Symptoms of trochanteric bursitis consist of pain over the greater trochanter that often radiates along the lateral thigh to the knee. Internal rotation, abduction, and flexion of the hip will typically exacerbate pain. The trochanteric bursa also has a superficial component that lies between the greater trochanter and the skin. **Superficial trochanteric bursitis** is exacerbated with hip adduction. Treatment includes rest, heat, and nonsteroidal antiinflammatory drugs (NSAIDs). Patients may benefit from intrabursal steroid injections or ultrasound therapy.

2. **Ischial gluteal bursitis (weaver's bottom)** is seen in patients subjected to prolonged sitting. Pain radiates down the back of the thigh and is reproduced with pressure over the ischial tuberosity. A cushion or sitting pillow treats pain and may help prevent recurrence. This adjunct should be used in all patients with gluteal bursitis in conjunction with rest and NSAIDs.

3. **Ileopectineal bursitis** causes pain in the area of the femoral triangle, lateral to the femoral ves-

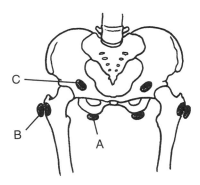

Fig. 19. Bursae of the hip: A: Ischiogluteal
B: Trochanteric. C: Iliopectineal.

sels and just inferior to the middle of the inguinal ligament. Pain is eased by flexion, abduction, and external rotation and exacerbated by adduction, extension, and internal rotation of the hip.

4. **Infectious bursitis about the hip** is difficult to diagnose owing to its insidious nature. Emergent incision and drainage are necessary. Parenteral antibiotics should be administered concurrently. Clues to infectious cases are fever, redness, and warmth of the overlying skin, and an elevated white blood cell count.

III. **Summary.** The hip and femur present multiple challenges to emergency physicians. Fracture detection and management include review of possible medical cause of the fall and likely associated injury.

Dislocations are true medical emergencies that require full ATLS evaluation prior to rapid reduction.

REFERENCES

1. Koval KJ, Zuckerman JD. Functional recovery after hip fracture. *J Bone Joint Surg Am* 1994;77:751–758.
2. Alba E, Youngberg R. Occult fractures of the femoral neck. *Am J Emerg Med* 1992;10:64–68.
3. Bogost GA, Lizerbaum EK, Crues JV. MR imaging in evaluation of suspected hip fracture: frequency of unsuspected bone and soft-tissue injury. *Radiology* 1995;197:263–267.
4. Matin P. The appearance of bone scans following fractures, including immediate and long-term studies. *J Nucl Med* 1979;20:1227–1231.
5. Gaunche CA, Kozin SH, Levy AS, Brody LA. The use of MRI in the diagnosis of occult hip fractures in the elderly: a preliminary review (see comments). *Orthopedics* 1994;17:327–330.
6. Evans PD, Wilson C, Lyons K. Comparison of MRI with bone scanning for suspected hip fracture in elderly patients. *J Bone Joint Surg BR* 1994;76:158–159.

7. Zuckerman JD, Skovron ML, Koval KJ, et al. Postoperative complications and mortality associated with operative delay in older patients who have a fracture of the hip (see comments). *J Bone Joint Surg AM* 1995;177:1551–1556.

8. Zuckerman JD. Hip fracture (see comments). *N Engl J Med* 1996;334:1519– 1525.

9. Milch H. Avulsion fracture of the great trochanter. *Arch Surg* 1939;38:334–350.

10. Eikenbary CF. Avulsion or fracture of the lesser trochanter. *J Orthop Surg* 1921;3:464–468.

11. Ware HE, Brooks AP, Toye R, Berney SI. Sickle cell disease and silent avascular necrosis of the hip. *J Bone Joint Surg* 1991;73B(6):947–949.

12. Delee JC, Evans JA, Thomas J. Anterior dislocation of the hip and associated femoral-head fractures. *J Bone Joint Surg* 1980;62(A):960–964.

13. Epstein HC. *Traumatic dislocation of the hip*. Baltimore: Williams & Wilkins, 1980.

14. Dehne E, Immerman EW. Dislocation of the hip combined with fracture of the shaft of the femur on the same side. *J Bone Joint Surg* 1951;33(A):731–745.

15. Epstein HC. Traumatic dislocations of the hip. *Clin Orthop* 1973;92:116–142.

16. Brav EA. Traumatic dislocation of the hip. *J Bone Joint Surg* 1962;44(A):1115–1134.

The Knee and Lower Leg

Patricia Lee

The knee is a remarkable and complex weight-bearing joint. It allows considerable flexion, limited rotation, and variable load bearing simultaneously and with surprising stability, considering the architecture of its bony parts.

I. **Anatomy.** The distal femur, the proximal tibia, and the posterior aspect of the patella make up the bony portion of the knee. Although the proximal fibula does not articulate with the knee joint, it does provide for attachment of the collateral ligament. The meniscal cartilages serve as cushions, while the muscles of the quadriceps femoris muscle group (superficial rectus femoris, vastus medialis, vastus lateralis, and vastus intermedius), quadriceps tendon, patella, and patellar tendon make up the extensor mechanism (Fig. 1).

II. **Mechanism of injury.** The knee is frequently injured in daily activities, falls, motor vehicle crashes, and sports. Injury to any of the bones (femur, tibia, patella), ligaments (anterior cruciate, posterior cruciate, medial collateral, lateral collateral), and cartilages that make up the knee may result in pain or long-term disability. Some mechanisms of injury lead to specific pathology, such as a football tackle from the side associated with a medial collateral ligament (MCL) injury, while "catching" a ski tip may cause injury to the anterior cruciate ligament (ACL); a head-on collision with the knee striking the dashboard may cause a posterior cruciate ligament (PCL) injury.

III. **Physical examination.** The knee is examined with the patient supine and compared with the uninjured knee.

    A. **Inspection.** Note any swelling ecchymoses, effusion, or deformity.

    B. **Palpation.** Tenderness over collateral ligaments, the joint line (meniscus, tibial plateau), the patella, or the patellar tendon should be checked. A ballottable patella may indicate a joint effusion.

    C. **Range of motion.** Normally from 0 to 140 degrees of flexion; any limitation should be recorded.

    D. **Varus and valgus stress test.** With injury, applying varus or valgus stress with the knee at 30 degrees of flexion and in full extension will cause localizing pain of the lateral or medial collateral structures, respectively (Fig. 2).

    E. **Extensor mechanism.** Pain or inability to raise the straight leg against resistance may indicate patellar fracture or injury to the quadriceps or patellar tendons.

    F. **McMurray test.** With the knee in flexion, it is slowly extended while applying an internal or external rotational stress to isolate the lateral or medial meniscus

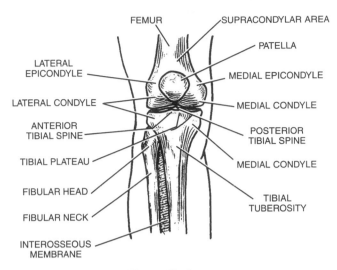

Fig. 1.   The knee.

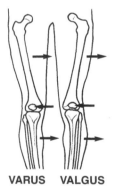

VARUS   VALGUS

Fig. 2.   Varus and valgus stress testing. Arrows indicate applied forces.

respectively. A positive test suggesting meniscal injury is signaled by a pop, crunch, or crepitance (Fig. 3).

G. **Drawer test.** Flexing the hip to 45 degrees and the knee to 90 degrees, the thumbs are placed over the anterior joint line of the proximal tibia. A gentle pull anteriorly and push posteriorly gauges stability of the anterior or posterior cruciate ligament as firm, loose, or "mushy." Comparison with the uninjured knee is useful (Fig. 4).

H. **Lachman test.** The knee is flexed to 15 to 20 degrees. While holding the femur firmly with one hand,

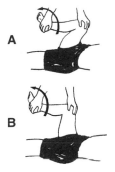

A

B

Fig. 3. The McMurray test.

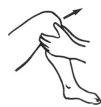

Fig. 4. The Drawer test.

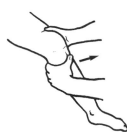

Fig. 5. The Lachman test.

the examiner places the other hand at the level of the tibial tuberosity and tries to move the tibia anteriorly. Laxity indicates an ACL disruption (Fig. 5).

I. **Patellar apprehension test.** As the examiner attempts to displace the patella laterally with the knee in full extension, the patient's "apprehension" or resistance to the examiner's hand suggests a recent patellar dislocation.

IV. **Radiography.** Plain film radiographs should include three views of the knee as well as the "sunrise" view of the patella. Computed tomography (CT) and magnetic reso-

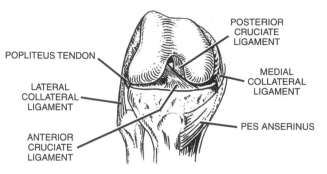

POSTERIOR CRUCIATE LIGAMENT

POPLITEUS TENDON

MEDIAL COLLATERAL LIGAMENT

LATERAL COLLATERAL LIGAMENT

PES ANSERINUS

ANTERIOR CRUCIATE LIGAMENT

Fig. 6.   Ligaments of the knee.

nance imaging (MRI) rarely change emergency department management and are not usually done acutely.

V. **Knee**

A. **Ligamentous injuries.** The ACL and PCL provide anterior and posterior stability, while side-to-side stability is provided by the MCL and lateral collateral ligaments (LCL). Frequently a combination of ligaments may be injured. Injuries may be classified **grade I,** fibers stretched but not torn; **grade II,** partial tear; and **grade III,** complete rupture. Grade III injuries may be painless. Grade I and II injuries are managed conservatively. Grade III injuries usually require surgical repair (Fig. 6).

1. **Anterior cruciate ligament (ACL)** injury is the most common severe knee injury. The ACL attaches to the posterior lateral femoral condyle and anterior lateral tibial spine.

a. **Mechanism.** ACL injury often results from deceleration, flexion, and rotation with or without external force, as upon running at full speed followed by a sudden stop. The patient may hear a "pop" at the time of injury, with immediate swelling of the knee due to hemarthrosis.

b. **Physical examination.** Severe swelling within hours due to hemarthrosis is common. The Lachman and anterior drawer tests will be positive.

c. **Radiography.** Plain films are generally unremarkable, although an avulsion fracture of the lateral tibial plateau, called the **lateral capsular sign,** may be seen. MRI may be useful.

d. **Treatment options.** If a tense effusion is present, joint aspiration will relieve pain. If the patient is an athlete or the knee is unstable, operative repair may be necessary.

However, management is generally conservative.

e. **Complications** include subsequent knee dislocation and degenerative joint disease.

f. **Disposition.** A compressive bandage, knee immobilizer, crutches, pain management, ice, elevation, and urgent orthopaedic referral are appropriate.

2. **Posterior cruciate ligament** injury is rarely an isolated injury, as the PCL is stronger than the ACL or collateral ligaments. The PCL attaches to the anterior femoral condyle and posterior tibial spine.

a. **Mechanism.** More force is required than for other ligamentous injuries, such as that generated in a "dashboard injury" (flexed knee with violent anterior force to the tibia). The PCL may tear due to hyperextension only after the ACL is torn.

b. **Physical examination.** Abrasions, lacerations, or ecchymosis may be noted about the tibial tubercle. The patient may walk with a slightly flexed knee. When the posterior drawer maneuver is positive, the possibility of popliteal artery injury is high, mandating careful evaluation and observation of the distal circulation.

c. **Radiography.** Plain films are unremarkable. MRI is confirmatory.

d. **Treatment options.** Clinical judgment regarding the degree of long-term disability dictates whether operative management is required. If a PCL tear is associated with other ligamentous injuries, a spontaneous reduced dislocation should be suspected and an arteriogram of the popliteal artery strongly considered.

e. **Complications** include knee dislocation, degenerative joint disease, and popliteal artery injury.

f. **Disposition.** In the absence of knee instability, a compressive bandage, knee immobilizer, crutches, ice, elevation, pain management, and urgent referral to an orthopaedist is appropriate. Admission with vascular consultation is reserved for injuries associated with joint instability or suspected spontaneously reduced knee dislocation.

3. **The medial collateral ligament** is the most commonly injured knee ligament. MCL injuries often accompany ACL injury and can cause joint instability.

a. **Mechanism.** Trauma to the lateral aspect of knee or valgus force with or without rotation may cause MCL injury. The patient may describe a tearing sensation with immediate pain.

b. **Physical examination** reveals tenderness over the medial femoral condyle extending into the joint line. A hemarthrosis may occur if the ACL or capsular portion of the MCL is torn.

c. **Radiography.** Plain films are usually normal.

d. **Treatment options.** Grade I (stretch) and II (partial tear) sprains are treated conservatively. Grade III injury (complete tear) may require surgery.

e. **Complications** include joint instability and chronic pain.

f. **Disposition** should include a knee immobilizer and compressive bandage, ice, elevation, and pain control. The patient uses crutches and avoids weight bearing until urgent orthopaedic follow-up can occur.

4. **Lateral collateral ligament** injury is uncommon. The LCL is wider than the MCL and usually is only partially torn, causing no knee instability. Associated common peroneal nerve injury may occur.

a. **Mechanism.** Trauma to the medial side of the knee or varus stress with or without rotation can cause LCL injury.

b. **Physical examination.** Tenderness is found at the lateral femoral condyle extending into the joint line.

c. **Radiography.** Plain films may be normal.

d. **Treatment options.** Grade I and II sprains are treated conservatively. Grade III injury may require surgery.

e. **Complications** include joint instability and chronic pain.

f. **Disposition** is similar to that for MCL injuries, discussed above.

B. **Dislocations** of the knee imply extreme forces and extensive injury to the ligamentous stabilizers of the knee. They are fortunately rare. They are true orthopaedic emergencies, as they are associated with major neurovascular injury in the popliteal fossa.

1. **Anterior knee** dislocation is most common, although posterior, lateral, and medial dislocations can also occur. Because they frequently reduce spontaneously in the field, it is important that this diagnosis be considered in all severe knee trauma.

a. **Mechanism.** Hyperextension results in a posterior capsular tear, rupture of the ACL, and partial tear of the PCL, leading to anterior dislocation. Posterior dislocations may result from direct force to the anterior tibia with the knee in flexion, resulting in rupture of the posterior capsule and cruciates.

b. **Physical examination.** Careful inspection, palpation, and distal neurovascular assessment are critical. If the knee is unstable after a traumatic injury, one must assume that a dislocation with spontaneous reduction has occurred. Anterior subluxation of the tibia with or without applied stress indicates an anterior dislocation, while posterior subluxation is found in posterior knee dislocation. Swelling in the popliteal fossa may indicate a popliteal artery injury that must be repaired immediately. The absence of distal pulses indicates a true vascular emergency, as spasm of the popliteal artery is unlikely.

c. **Radiography.** Anteroposterior (AP) and lateral knee films may show subluxation or an associated fracture. Arteriography is indicated.

d. **Complications.** Of all knee dislocations, 30% to 40% are associated with injury to the popliteal artery. Injuries to the peroneal and tibial nerves may occur. Persistent joint instability and eventual degenerative arthritis are likely.

e. **Treatment options.** Immediate reduction is indicated. Avoidance of direct pressure on the popliteal fossa and traction accompanied by the appropriate anterior or posterior forces returns the leg to its normal position, reestablishing the normal joint relationship. A long leg posterior splint is applied with the knee in 15 degrees of flexion, avoiding compression of the leg and popliteal fossa and thereby eliminating any iatrogenic risk of compartment syndrome.

f. **Complications.** Deep vein thrombosis and compartment syndrome may occur. Injury of the popliteal artery is most likely with anterior knee dislocation.

g. **Disposition.** Admission with immediate orthopaedic evaluation is necessary, with care to address any associated injuries.

2. **Patellar** dislocation is seen in patients with abnormal patellofemoral anatomy (flattening of the lateral femoral condyle, patella alta, genu valgum). Dislocations and subluxation tend to be recurrent because of ligamentous laxity. Patellar dislocation is typically lateral, although horizontal, superior, or intercondylar dislocation may occur. The patient will usually say that the

knee "went out," followed by deformity and swelling. These injuries may reduce spontaneously prior to evaluation.

a. **Mechanism.** In the presence of abnormal patellofemoral architecture, dislocation may occur with simultaneous external rotation and flexion at the knee. Direct trauma is a less common cause.

b. **Physical examination.** A lateral patellar dislocation is obvious unless spontaneous reduction has occurred. In this event, tenderness and swelling are noted along the medial aspect of the patella. If the examiner attempts to push the patella laterally, the patient may try to prevent the motion (a positive patellar apprehension test).

c. **Radiography.** Knee views will show the grossly dislocated patella or, in the event of spontaneous reduction, the patella may appear normal. A fracture of the inferomedial aspect of the patella, best seen on the "sunrise view," is pathognomonic for a reduced lateral patellar dislocation. Presence of a fat/fluid level is indicative of an associated osteochondral fracture.

d. **Treatment options.** With a straight leg upon the gurney, the seated patient leans forward. This maximizes hip flexion and knee extension, relaxing the extensor mechanism and allowing easy reduction with medially directed force to the patella. Intraarticular, horizontal, and superior dislocations may require surgical reduction.

e. **Complications.** Degenerative arthritis, osteochondral fractures (5%), and recurrent dislocation or subluxation may occur.

f. **Disposition.** Patients with lateral dislocations reduced in the emergency department can be discharged to orthopaedic follow-up with compressive dressings, knee immobilizers, and crutches to prevent weight bearing.

C. **Cartilaginous injuries**

1. **Meniscal injuries.** The menisci are fibrous cartilages that act as joint spacers, providing knee stability, lubrication, shock absorption, and load distribution. The central portions are avascular, with the entire blood supply arising from peripheral attachments. The most common types of injuries are the "bucket-handle" or the "flap tear," where only one portion has torn free. The **medial meniscus** is most frequently injured, since it attaches to the MCL capsule and may be damaged in MCL tears. The popliteal tendon passes posteriorly and laterally through the at-

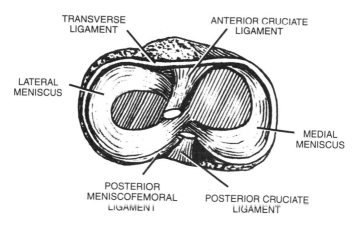

Fig. 7. The menisci.

tachments of the lateral collateral ligament, and thus the lateral meniscus is less frequently injured (Fig. 7).

a. **Mechanism.** The patient may describe seemingly trivial twisting of a flexed knee.

b. **Physical examination.** An effusion may be clear or bloody and is usually delayed. A positive McMurray test may accompany the patient's complaint of "locking" of the knee. Tenderness along the medial joint line may occur.

c. **Radiography.** Plain films are normal.

d. **Treatment options** are nonoperative or operative, depending on the specific injury.

e. **Complications** include degenerative arthritis and long-term disability. Meniscectomy may improve disability if the repair is done within 2 months of injury.

f. **Disposition.** Knee immobilizer, compressive bandage, crutches, rest, ice, elevation, pain management, and urgent orthopaedic referral are indicated.

2. **Osteochondritis dissecans** is a separation of bone and its overlying cartilage, usually from the medial femoral condyle and less frequently from the lateral femoral condyle. It is more common in males during late childhood or adolescence and may occur bilaterally (10%). Patients may complain of chronic pain or joint locking (Fig. 8).

a. **Mechanism.** Although repeated trauma or ischemia has been implicated, the cause is not known.

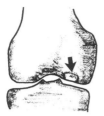

Fig. 8. Osteochondritis dissecans.

   b. **Physical examination.** With the knee flexed, localized tenderness of the medial condyle may be the only finding. Joint locking may occur with rang-of-motion exercise.

   c. **Radiography.** Plain films show a thin, radiolucent line that represents the separation of a rounded, subchondral bone island from the condyle.

   d. **Treatment options.** Children under the age of 12 may require only a period of cast immobilization without weight bearing. In older children and adults, arthroscopy with debridement or, if possible, pin fixation is necessary.

   e. **Complications** include degenerative joint disease and chronic pain.

   f. **Disposition.** Asymptomatic patients discovered fortuitously during radiographic evaluation need only orthopaedic referral. Those with severe pain and/or joint locking are discharged with a knee immobilizer and kept non-weight-bearing until their orthopaedic evaluation.

3. **Osteochondral** and **chondral fractures.** Chondral fractures occur in cartilage while osteochondral fractures involve the cartilage and subchondral bone. These may occur in the femoral condyles or the patella.

   a. **Mechanism.** Most of these fractures are the result of direct trauma, compression and rotation, and patellar dislocation.

   b. **Physical examination.** Persistent significant pain and tenderness after injury, joint locking, and hemarthrosis are often confused with a meniscal tear.

   c. **Radiography** may reveal small bone fragments or may appear normal.

   d. **Treatment options.** Displaced osteochondral fractures may be amenable to surgical fixation or require arthroscopic debridement.

   e. **Complications.** Chondromalacia or osteochondritis dissecans with pain, locking, and effusions may result.

f. **Disposition.** Prompt orthopaedic referral is necessary for possible arthroscopic fixation of an osteochondral fracture. Patients may be discharged with a knee immobilizer, crutches, and pain medication with instruction to rest, elevate the limb, and apply ice.

4. **Chondromalacia patellae,** also known as **patellar malalignment syndrome,** is often seen in young adults, especially women. Progressive peripatellar pain with exertion such as stair climbing as well as deep aching in the knees occurs without history of recent trauma and is recurrent.

   a. **Mechanism.** Premature degeneration of the patellar cartilage due to patellar malalignment, direct trauma, congenital abnormality, recurrent patellar subluxation, or excessive knee strain leads to pain.

   b. **Physical examination.** The patella may seem to face medially, which is known as "squinting of the kneecaps." The patella may be hypermobile through flexion and extension, with tenderness of the patella or medial aspect of the knee upon compression of the patella into the medial femoral groove. Knee extension against resistance may be painful through the terminal 30 degrees.

   c. **Radiographs** are unremarkable.

   d. **Treatment options.** Conservative measures—rest, analgesia, and isometric quadriceps-strengthening exercises—provide symptomatic relief.

   e. **Complications.** Chronic pain may progress.

   f. **Disposition.** Squatting, running, kneeling, or climbing steps should be avoided. Severe cases may benefit from immobilization, avoidance of weight bearing, and nonsteroidal antiinflammatory drugs (NSAIDs) pending orthopaedic follow-up.

5. **Bursitis.** The synovium-lined periarticular sacs about the knee allow smooth skin movement over bony and tendinous prominences (Fig. 9).

   a. **Mechanism.** Inflammation of the bursa due to acute trauma, chronic repetitive use, or infection or secondary to systemic arthritides may occur. Bursitis may arise in a delayed fashion 1 to 2 weeks following direct trauma.

   b. **Physical examination** demonstrates pain, redness, swelling, warmth of the overlying skin, and sometimes crepitus with palpation. Range of motion of the knee is maintained until the skin is stretched and pain occurs.

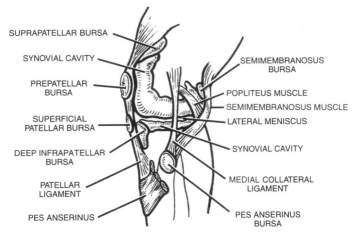

SUPRAPATELLAR BURSA

SYNOVIAL CAVITY

PREPATELLAR BURSA

SUPERFICIAL PATELLAR BURSA

DEEP INFRAPATELLAR BURSA

PATELLAR LIGAMENT

PES ANSERINUS

SEMIMEMBRANOSUS BURSA

POPLITEUS MUSCLE

SEMIMEMBRANOSUS MUSCLE

LATERAL MENISCUS

SYNOVIAL CAVITY

MEDIAL COLLATERAL LIGAMENT

PES ANSERINUS BURSA

Fig. 9. The bursae of the knee.

(1) **Acute prepatellar bursitis ("housemaid's knee").** Tenderness of the prepatellar bursa is found superficial to the patella.

(2) **Superficial infrapatellar bursitis.** Tenderness of the bursa over the tibial tubercle may be misdiagnosed as Osgood-Schlatter disease.

(3) **Deep infrapatellar bursitis.** Tenderness of the bursa beneath the patellar tendon (which separates it from the underlying fat pad and tibia) is noted. Pain occurs with active movements, but passive flexion and extension will be painless.

(4) **Anserine bursitis.** Tenderness of the bursa located between the fibers of the medial collateral ligament and the pes anserinus tendon is rare and is due to direct trauma or repetitive friction. This may be confused with an injury of the medial collateral ligament. Pain is increased during flexion or extension.

(5) **Baker's cyst (popliteal cyst).** Located in the popliteal area at the posteromedial aspect of the knee, between the medial head of the gastrocnemius and the semimembranosus tendon, this bursa often communicates with the joint space. Inflammation of the bursa

may result from a torn meniscus, loose body, degenerative changes, chondromalacia, or rheumatoid arthritis. Because there is no posterior limiting structure, the cyst may become quite large. Popliteal cysts in children are benign and require no treatment. Symptoms consist of intermittent swelling and pain, which can limit range of motion and occasionally cause venous obstruction. Rupture of a Baker's cyst may mimic deep venous thrombosis of the calf.

(6) **Popliteal bursitis.** Tenderness occurs along the lateral joint line located proximal to the fibular collateral ligament and the popliteal tendon.

c. **Treatment options.** NSAIDs as well as treatment of any underlying condition are the mainstays of conservative treatment. Aspiration is indicated if pronounced swelling is extremely painful or if an infectious bursitis (typically prepatellar) is suspected.

6. **Traumatic prepatellar neuralgia** presents as persistent pain over the patella with point tenderness limited to the middle and outer patellar edges. The pain may be exacerbated with the very slight pressure of overlying clothing. Because the condition is the result of repeated direct trauma to the prepatellar neurovascular bundle, treatment with local injections of lidocaine-hydrocortisone may be beneficial.

7. **Fat-pad syndrome.** Pain due to swelling of the infrapatellar fat pad located below the patellar tendon may result from premenstrual fluid retention.

8. **Jumper's knee.** Focal tendinitis with localized tenderness along the superior or inferior patellar pole increases with active resistance against extension. Treatment with rest, NSAIDs, and isometric quadriceps exercises is indicated.

9. **Extensor mechanism injuries.** The quadriceps complex may sustain injury through rupture of the quadriceps tendon, fracture of the patella, patellar tendon rupture, or avulsion of the tibial tuberosity. The patient may report a sudden buckling of the knee with extreme pain.

a. **Mechanism.** Indirect injury is secondary to forced flexion against a contracted quadriceps. Occasionally direct trauma is the cause.

b. **Physical examination.** Absent or markedly reduced active extension indicates a complete or partial rupture. An inferiorly displaced patella with proximal ecchymosis, localized swelling, and a palpable supra-patellar defect indicates a quadriceps tendon rupture. Proximal displacement of the patella along with inferior pole tenderness and swelling indicates a rupture of the patellar tendon.

c. **Radiographs.** An inferiorly displaced patella, sometimes associated with a superior pole bony avulsion fragment, suggests a quadriceps tendon rupture. Superior patella displacement with an inferior bony avulsion fragment indicates a patellar tendon rupture.

d. **Treatment options.** A partial quadriceps tendon rupture requires a long leg cast with the knee in extension for 6 weeks. Patellar tendon rupture, patellar avulsion fracture, or complete quadriceps tendon tears require early surgical repair.

e. **Disposition.** Knee immobilization, crutches, and pain management with prompt orthopaedic referral are indicated.

10. **Biceps femoris and medial flexor injuries.** The medial knee flexors are the gracilis, sartorius, and semitendinosus muscles. The biceps tendon inserts on the fibular head and the lateral collateral ligament.

a. **Mechanism.** Sudden contraction against resistance, as occurs in running or jumping, can lead to partial or complete muscle tears.

b. **Physical examination.** Pain and swelling are noted over involved muscle areas.

c. **Treatment options** include 3 to 4 weeks of rest, analgesics, and heat in partial ruptures. Surgical repair is indicated for complete ruptures.

d. **Disposition.** Immobilization and avoidance of weight bearing prevent further injury until urgent orthopaedic follow-up occurs.

11. **Overuse syndromes** consist of a combination of symptoms that are commonly associated with running and may represent more than one injury.

a. **Iliotibial band friction syndrome or iliotibial tract tendinitis** is seen in long distance runners as a gradual, progressive pain with tenderness over the lateral epicondyle of the femur. During extension, the iliotibial band lies anterior to the lateral femoral epicondyle, but in flexion, it moves posteriorly over the epicondyle. This condition generally presents between 21 to 25 years of age as a painful limp that is worsened with running, walking, and stair climbing and is improved with straight-leg walking.

(1) **Mechanism.** Repetitive flexion and extension causes chronic tendon trauma and eventual inflammation.

(2) **Physical examination.** Discrete tenderness is noted over the lateral femoral epicondyle approximately 3 cm proximal to the joint line. Pain is increased with weight bearing on the flexed knee.

(3) **Treatment options.** Antiinflammatory medication and rest are usually adequate, although lidocaine-hydrocortisone injection may be necessary.

(4) **Disposition.** Cessation of inciting activities is accompanied by NSAID treatment and orthopaedic follow-up.

b. **Semimembranosus tendinitis** is similar to iliotibial tract tendinitis except pain is noted medially at the joint line.

12. **Fabella syndrome.** The fabella is a sesamoid bone found in 10% of patients; it lies embedded in the tendon of the lateral head of the gastrocnemius. It articulates with the posterior lateral femoral condyle and is bilateral in 50% of cases.

a. **Mechanism.** Degenerative or inflammatory changes lead to pain.

b. **Physical examination.** Intermittent posterolateral knee pain is worse in extension. Tenderness is increased with compression of the fabella against the condyle.

c. **Treatment options.** Conservative treatment with NSAIDs and rest is helpful in most cases.

d. **Disposition.** Orthopaedic referral for surgical repair may be necessary in severe and unremitting cases.

13. **Compartment syndromes.** The **anterior** compartment contains the tibialis anterior, extensor hallucis longus, and extensor digitorum longus muscles, the anterior tibial artery, and the deep peroneal nerve. It is the most common leg compartment affected. The **lateral** compartment includes the peroneus longus and peroneus brevis muscles as well as the superficial peroneal nerve. The **superficial posterior** compartment includes the soleus, gastrocnemius, and sural nerve. The deep posterior compartment contains the tibialis posterior, flexor hallucis longus, and flexor digitorum longus muscles as well as the posterior tibial nerve and artery. Compartment syndromes are true orthopaedic emergencies (Fig. 10).

a. **Mechanism.** Circulatory embarrassment occurs because of direct vascular compromise (arterial injury or extrinsic compression) or secondary to posttraumatic tissue swelling within the restricted space of the

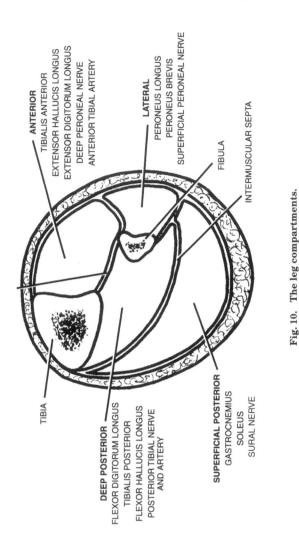

ANTERIOR
TIBIALIS ANTERIOR
EXTENSOR HALLUCIS LONGUS
EXTENSOR DIGITORUM LONGUS
DEEP PERONEAL NERVE
ANTERIOR TIBIAL ARTERY

LATERAL
PERONEUS LONGUS
PERONEUS BREVIS
SUPERFICIAL PERONEAL NERVE

FIBULA

INTERMUSCULAR SEPTA

TIBIA

DEEP POSTERIOR
FLEXOR DIGITORUM LONGUS
TIBIALIS POSTERIOR
FLEXOR HALLUCIS LONGUS
POSTERIOR TIBIAL NERVE
AND ARTERY

SUPERFICIAL POSTERIOR
GASTROCNEMIUS
SOLEUS
SURAL NERVE

Fig. 10.   The leg compartments.

compartment. As edema increases, the compartment pressure increases, further decreasing tissue perfusion. This progresses to ischemia and eventual necrosis of intercompartmental tissue. It is most commonly seen after fracture of the tibia, rarely the fibula, and may be seen in soft tissue trauma alone.

b. **Physical examination.** Of the six classic signs of compartment syndrome—pain, pallor, paralysis, pulselessness, paresthesias, and pain on passive movement—it is the latter two signs that allow early diagnosis. Severe calf pain with passive range of motion of the ankle and toes or impaired function of the peroneal nerve—as indicated by decreased sensation on the dorsum of the foot at the web space of the great and second toes—are the best early indicators of impending compartment syndrome. Measurement of compartment pressure using a variety of available monitors is indicated. In most cases the calf will be notably firm to palpation.

c. **Treatment and disposition.** Any patient with signs and symptoms of impending compartment syndrome requires admission and emergency orthopaedic consultation. Compartmental pressure greater than 30 mm Hg requires emergent fasciotomy. Any fracture or injury prone to developing compartment syndrome must be immobilized with care, preventing unnecessary circumferential constriction of the calf or popliteal fossa, which could prove contributory.

14. **Fractures**

a. **Patellar** fractures may be transverse (most common), stellate (comminuted), longitudinal, or vertical. Because the blood supply to the patella derives centrally and from the distal poles, fractures may result in ischemia and the development of avascular necrosis.

(1) **Mechanism.** Direct trauma to the patella is often associated with distraction forces from quadriceps contraction.

(2) **Radiographs.** Routine knee views typically reveal obvious patellar fractures. A bipartite patella is a normal variant that may be mistaken for a fracture, usually occurring superolaterally. Some 50% are bilateral and comparison views may be useful. An osteochondral fracture may appear as a small defect on the underside of the patella or as a fat/fluid level.

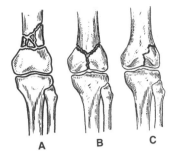

Fig. 11. Distal femoral fractures.
A: Comminuted supracondylar.
B: Intercondylar. C: Condylar.

    (3) **Treatment options.** A nonsurgical approach with long leg casting is reserved for nondisplaced fracture (less than 2 mm of articular displacement and 3 mm of fragment separation) with intact extensor function. All others require open reduction and internal fixation (ORIF).

    (4) **Complications** include traumatic chondromalacia, degenerative arthritis, and rarely nonunion or avascular necrosis.

    (5) **Disposition.** Immediate orthopaedic consultation is necessary, as many orthopaedists may elect admission for immediate repair. If repair is to occur in the next few days, patients are discharged with a posterior leg splint or knee immobilizer and kept non-weight-bearing.

  b. **Distal femur (Fig. 11)**

    (1) **Mechanism.** Axial loading with varus or valgus rotation may cause supracondylar, intercondylar, or condylar fractures. These are uncommon injuries.

    (2) **Physical examination.** Tenderness, swelling, and deformity of the distal femur.

    (3) **Radiograph.** Routine knee views reveal the fracture. Condylar fractures may need MRI or CT scan to establish the extent of articular surface involvement.

    (4) **Treatment options.** All but incomplete or nondisplaced fractures require operative repair.

    (5) **Complications.** The popliteal artery may be injured, especially when an associated knee dislocation has occurred.

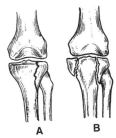

A   **B**   Fig. 12. Tibial condylar fractures.

(6) Disposition A long leg posterior splint is placed prior to admission, with care not to compress the popliteal fossa.

c. **Proximal tibia. Tibial plateau** and **tibial condylar** fractures are common and highly variable fractures involving the proximal tibia and extending to the articular surface. Most involve the lateral tibial plateau (Fig. 12).

  (1) **Mechanism.** Strong valgus or varus forces accompanied by an axial load are involved. Fracture fragments are often depressed as they are impacted by the femoral condyles. These injuries may result from pedestrian "bumper" injuries, falls, or sports injuries.

  (2) **Physical examination** reveals a swollen, painful knee with inability to bear weight. Tenderness is found along the joint line. Care must be taken to assess the distal neurovascular status and examine the leg for compartment syndrome.

  (3) **Radiographs.** Routine views are generally adequate to define all but subtle injuries. CT or MRI may be necessary to evaluate very subtle or very complex fractures.

  (4) **Treatment** options vary greatly depending on fracture type, associated injuries, patient, and orthopaedist. Approaches range from conservative closed treatment to ORIF. Depression of the articular surface >4 mm will typically require ORIF.

  (5) **Complications.** Fractures of the tibial plateau and condyle are often due to high-energy mechanisms and are frequently associated with soft tissue in-

juries. Any fracture of the proximal third of the tibia may be associated with injury to the popliteal or anterior tibial artery, leading to ischemia or compartment syndrome. Long-term disability and degenerative arthritis may occur.

(6) **Disposition.** Patients are hospitalized with a long leg posterior mold for observation of their neurovascular status.

d. **Tibial spine** fractures are rarely isolated injuries and are frequently associated with ACL disruption, MCL tears, or tibial condylar fracture. They represent an avulsion and indicate loss of ACL function.

(1) **Mechanism.** Sudden knee extension with internal rotation may result in fracture of the tibial spine.

(2) **Physical examination** is similar to that for ACL tears, demonstrating effusion with positive posterior or anterior drawer signs.

(3) **Radiograph.** Findings on routine views may be subtle, revealing only an irregular articular surface or intraarticular calcific density, best seen in oblique or tunnel views. A fabella should not be mistaken for an intraarticular fracture fragment (see Sec. v. C.12).

(4) **Treatment options.** A long leg cast with full knee extension for 4 to 6 weeks may be used in nondisplaced fractures. Displaced fractures will require ORIF prior to immobilization.

(5) **Complications.** Collateral and cruciate ligament injuries are common. Chronic pain and knee instability are frequently encountered.

(6) **Disposition.** A long leg posterior plaster splint, pain medication, and crutches to avoid weight bearing are used, with urgent orthopaedic consultation.

VI. **Lower leg.** Because the tibia and fibula are parallel bones connected by ligaments, a displaced fracture of one bone will usually result in the fracture or displacement of the other. The tibia is the primary weight-bearing bone, while the fibula is important for ankle stability. Tibial fractures are the most common long bone fracture of the lower leg. The outcome of tibial fractures is determined by the degree of initial displacement, comminution, and integrity of the overlying soft tissue and skin. Isolated fibular fractures are uncommon and will generally heal without treatment (Fig. 13).

A. **Tibial tuberosity fracture.** The tibial tuberosity, which is the insertion point of the patellar tendon, is

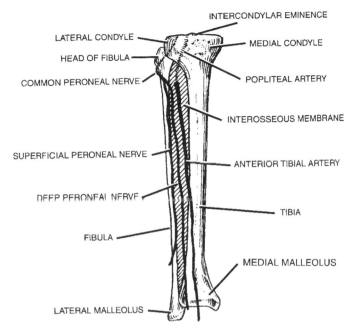

Fig. 13. The leg.

not commonly fractured. This injury is typically seen in young patients.

    1. **Mechanism.** Sudden flexion at the knee coupled with contraction of the quadriceps muscle may cause avulsion.

    2. **Physical examination.** Knee extension may be partially or completely impaired. There is tenderness and swelling over the tibial tuberosity.

    3. **Radiographs.** Routine views reveal avulsion of the tibial tuberosity. In children and adolescents, the variable appearance of the unfused ossification center of the tibial tubercle may be mistaken for an avulsion fracture.

    4. **Treatment options.** Displaced fractures may require ORIF.

    5. **Complications.** This injury may be associated with tears of the MCL, ACL, or patellar tendon.

    6. **Disposition.** Immobilization with avoidance of weight bearing and urgent orthopaedic referral are indicated.

B. Subcondylar fractures include transverse or oblique fracture of the proximal tibial metaphysis (Fig. 14).

    1. **Mechanism of injury.** Rotation or angular stress with concurrent vertical load as well as

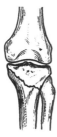

Fig. 14.   Subcondylar fracture of the tibia.

direct trauma, as incurred in motor vehicle accidents, may lead to subcondylar fracture.

2. **Physical examination** may range from local
   tenderness and swelling to gross deformity with
   extensive soft tissue injury.
3. **Radiographs.** Routine views, which should include the entire tibia, typically reveal an obvious
   fracture.
4. **Treatment options.** Displaced fractures may
   require ORIF.
5. **Complications** include neurovascular injury
   and compartment syndrome of the calf.
6. **Disposition.** Patients should have a long leg
   posterior splint carefully placed to avoid excessive compression of the calf or popliteal fossa
   and be admitted for neurovascular observation
   and definitive orthopaedic care.

C. **Tibial shaft fractures.** Fractures produced by indirect trauma heal better than those produced by direct
trauma; comminution increases the risk of delayed
union or nonunion.

1. **Mechanism of injury.** Direct trauma, as in motor vehicle accidents, or "boot-top" fracture from
   skiing is most commonly responsible. Indirect
   trauma due to rotational and compressive forces
   may create a spiral or oblique fracture.
2. **Physical examination.** Tenderness, swelling,
   and deformity are obvious.
3. **Radiographs.** Routine views include AP and
   lateral views of the entire tibia and fibula.
4. **Treatment options** vary and are controversial.
   Fractures of the tibial shaft in good position may
   be treated conservatively, while more displaced
   or unstable fractures will require internal or external fixation.
5. **Complications** are common in fractures of the
   tibial shaft and include injury of the anterior
   tibial artery, compartment syndrome, and injury
   of the peroneal nerve. Patients presenting with
   increased pain 1 to 2 days after casting should

be evaluated for compartment syndrome after the cast is bivalved. Nonunion or delayed union is common with severe displacement, comminution, open fracture, osteomyelitis, or neurovascular compromise. Deep venous thrombosis is another complication.

6. **Disposition.** Emergent orthopaedic consultation is necessary. Because of the high incidence of compartment syndrome, any patient with a displaced fracture of the tibial shaft will be immobilized in a long leg splint and hospitalized for observation.

D. **Proximal fibular fracture.** An isolated proximal fibular fracture is frequently associated with other serious knee injuries.

1. **Mechanism.** Direct trauma to the fibular head or a varus stress resulting in an avulsion fracture may occur. A valgus stress to the knee may result in a tibial condylar fracture with an associated proximal fibular fracture.

2. **Physical examination.** There is pain and tenderness of the fibular head. A complete knee and ankle exam is mandatory to rule out a serious associated injury.

3. **Radiographs.** AP and lateral views demonstrate the fracture.

4. **Treatment options.** As the proximal fibula has little role in weight bearing, casting is largely for comfort.

5. **Complications.** Common peroneal nerve injury, collateral ligament tear, ACL injury, or anterior tibial artery thrombosis may accompany proximal fibular fracture.

6. **Disposition.** In the absence of associated injuries, the patient is kept non-weight bearing until urgent orthopaedic follow-up can occur.

E. **Fibular shaft fracture.** Because of the fibula's close relation to the tibia, an isolated fibular fracture is common.

1. **Mechanism.** Fracture may occur with direct trauma or indirectly. While a varus force may avulse a proximal fragment of the fibula, a valgus force may produce fracture of the fibular shaft in association with lateral fracture of the tibial plateau or injury of the medial collateral ligament. A fracture of the fibular shaft may result from the transmission of forces via the interosseous membrane from primary ankle stress, as in the Maisonneuve fracture (see Chapter 21).

2. **Physical examination.** Fractures of the fibular shaft will cause painful walking even in the absence of a deformity. There is tenderness and swelling at the fracture site. Any fracture of the

fibular shaft requires complete examination of
the ankle, with attention to the medial structures.
3. **Radiography.** AP and lateral tibial/fibular
views are indicated. Any symptoms or findings
localized to the ankle require complete ankle
views.
4. **Treatment options.** Isolated fractures of the
fibular shaft greater than 3 cm proximal to the
lateral malleolus are treated symptomatically,
with casting largely for comfort.
5. **Disposition.** In most cases, the patient may be
discharged with an elastic bandage. Crutches
and splinting are reserved for those with severe
pain.

BIBLIOGRAPHY

Mercer LR. *Practical orthopaedics,* 4th ed. St Louis: Mosby, 1995.

Rosen P, Barkin RM, Braen GR, et al. *Emergency medicine concepts
and clinical practice,* 3rd ed. St Louis: Mosby, 1996. (In Mosby's
Emergency Medicine Electronic Library.)

Rosen P, Doris PE, Barkin RM, et al. *Diagnostic radiology in emergency medicine.* St Louis: Mosby, 1996. (In Mosby's Emergency
Medicine Electronic Library.)

Sonzongni JJ. Examining the injured knee. *Emerg Med* 1996;
28: 76–86.

Stewart C. Knee injuries: diagnosis and repair. *EM Reports. American Health Consultants,* 1997; 18: 1–12.

21

The Ankle

Felix Ankel

Ankle injuries are among the most common injuries seen in the emergency department. The evaluation of ankle injuries in systemic fashion requires a working knowledge of ankle anatomy, mechanisms of injury, physical examination techniques, indications for radiographs, and acute treatment modalities.

I. **Anatomy**
   A. **Bones.** The ankle is a modified hinge joint formed by three bones: the **tibia, fibula,** and **talus.** The tibia forms the **medial malleolus** and the **plafond** (ceiling). The fibula forms the **lateral malleolus.** The posterior aspect of the tibia is often called the **posterior malleolus.** The superior portion of the talus, the talar dome, articulates with the distal tibia and fibula to form the ankle mortise joint (Fig. 1).
   B. **Ligaments.** Between the distal tibia and fibula is a fibrous **syndesmosis** consisting of the anterior tibiofibular, posterior tibiofibular, transverse tibiofibular, and interosseus ligaments as well as the interosseus membrane (Fig. 2). The medial and lateral ligamentous structures stabilize the talus within the mortise, maintaining the ankle joint. Medially, the **deltoid ligament** group consists of the tibionavicular, tibiocalcaneal, and anterior and posterior tibiotalar ligaments. The lateral ligament group consists of the **anterior talofibular** (ATFL), **calcaneofibular** (CFL), and **posterior talofibular** (PTFL) ligaments (Fig. 3).
   C. **Muscles.** Muscles around the ankle are derived from the anterior, posterior, and lateral compartments of the leg. The anterior muscles (tibialis anterior, extensor digitorum longus, peroneus tertius, and extensor hallucis longus) are involved in dorsiflexion and are innervated by the deep peroneal nerve. The posterior muscles are separated into the superficial (gastrocnemius, plantaris, and soleus) and deep groups (flexor digitorum longus, flexor hallucis longus, and tibialis posterior). They are involved in plantarflexion and inversion and are innervated by the tibial nerve. Finally, the lateral muscles (peroneus longus and brevis) are involved in plantarflexion and eversion and are supplied by the superficial peroneal nerve. The tendons of the peroneus muscles pass below the lateral malleolus and underneath the peroneal retinaculum. The peroneus brevis attaches to the base of the fifth metatarsal, a common site of avulsion injury.
   D. **Nerves.** The saphenous, sural, and deep peroneal nerves provide cutaneous sensation around the an-

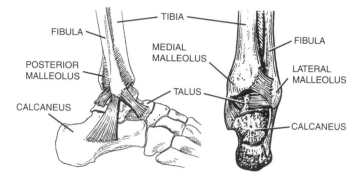

Fig. 1.   The ankle.

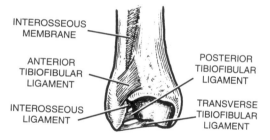

Fig. 2.   The ankle ligaments: anterior view.

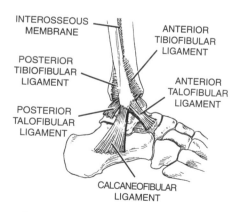

Fig. 3.   The ankle ligaments: lateral view.

kle, while the tibial, superficial, and deep peroneal nerves supply motor branches to nearby muscles.

E. **Arteries.** The posterior tibial artery courses behind the medial malleolus and separates into its medial and lateral plantar branches. The dorsalis pedis artery is a continuation of the anterior tibial artery, which extends anteriorly to the foot, where it is palpated lateral to the extensor hallucis tendon.

II. **History and mechanism of injury**

A. **History.** The history should delineate the activity leading to the injury, the onset of pain or swelling, and the ability to ambulate. Patients often describe a "pop" or "crack" upon injury, which may indicate damage to a ligament, tendon, or bone. The presence or absence of a previous ankle injury should be noted.

B. **Mechanism of injury.** The ankle joint is used primarily in dorsiflexion and plantarflexion. Abduction, adduction, and internal and external rotation occur in a limited fashion. The terms *inversion* and *eversion* describe motion at the tarsal joints rather than the ankle. Supination is the combination of adduction and inversion, while pronation is the combination of abduction and eversion. In dorsiflexion, the ankle is "locked" as the wider anterior portion of the talus occupies the mortise joint. The collateral ligaments are more taut in this position. In plantarflexion, the mortise joint has less intrinsic stability and relies on the collateral ligaments for support. It is important to determine the position of the ankle and the direction of stressors during injury.

III. **Physical examination.** A systematic physical examination should include assessment of ligamentous and joint stability, soft tissue injury, and neurovascular function. The entire leg from the knee to the toe should be exposed and examined to avoid missing associated pathology.

A. **Inspection.** Check for swelling, ecchymosis, deformity, skin color, and integrity.

B. **Palpation.** Sites remote from the injury, such as the proximal fibula or the base of the fifth metatarsal, are palpated first, proceeding to the areas that are most tender. This should include both malleoli as well as the lateral, deltoid, and syndesmotic ligaments.

C. **Neurovascular.** Palpate the dorsalis pedis and posterior tibial pulses, and document distal capillary refill. Any deficits in motor and/or sensory function are noted.

D. **Range of motion.** Normal range of motion of the ankle extends from 45 degrees of plantarflexion and 20 degrees of dorsiflexion.

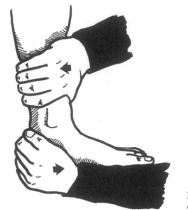

Fig. 4.   The anterior drawer test.

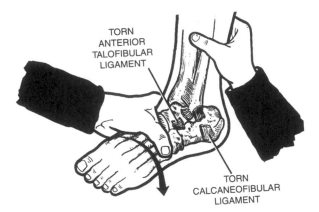

TORN
ANTERIOR
TALOFIBULAR
LIGAMENT

TORN
CALCANEOFIBULAR
LIGAMENT

Fig. 5.   The talar tilt test.

E. **Specific maneuvers**
   1. **The anterior drawer test** (Fig. 4) is performed to assess the integrity of the ATFL. The foot is placed in neutral position, cupping the heel with one hand while applying a posterior force to the distal tibia with the other. The extremity is compared with that on the opposite side and the test is considered positive if greater subluxation is noted at the injury.
   2. **The talar tilt test** (Fig. 5) is performed to assess the integrity of the ATFL and CFL. The patient's foot is placed in neutral position and the heel and distal tibia plantarflexed and inverted

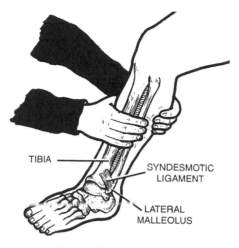

Fig. 6. The squeeze test.

by the examiner, noting any differences between the affected and unaffected side. A talar tilt test that is positive when the foot is everted suggests disruption of the deltoid ligament.

3. **The squeeze test** (Fig. 6) is performed to assess the tibiofibular syndesmosis. The patient's calf is held with one hand and the distal tibia and fibula are squeezed together with the other. A positive test causes pain at the distal syndesmosis.

4. **Thompson's test** is performed to determine if there is an Achilles tendon rupture. The patient is placed in a prone position with the knee flexed. Failure to dorsiflex the foot by squeezing the gastrocnemius and soleus muscles in the calf indicates rupture.

5. **Weight bearing.** The taking of two unassisted steps with each foot determines ability to bear weight.

IV. **Radiography.** The decision to order a radiograph should be based on physical findings. The **Ottawa rules** (Table 1) propose clinical indications for obtaining ankle films. Standard views include anteroposterior (AP), lateral, and mortise views. The mortise view is obtained with the leg rotated inward 15 degrees and provides the best view of the ankle joint spaces. It visualizes both malleoli, the talar dome, the tibial plafond, and the entire mortise joint. On the mortise view, the width of the medial clear space (between the medial malleolus and the medial aspect of the talus) should be equal to that of the superior clear space (between the talar dome and

Table 1.   Ottawa criteria for ankle radiographs

An ankle radiographic series is required in patients aged 18–55 only if there is any malleolar pain and any of the following findings:

Bone tenderness at the posterior edge or tip of the medial malleolus

Bone tenderness at the posterior edge or tip of the lateral malleolus

Inability to bear weight for four steps both immediately and in the emergency department

tibial plafond). Widening of the medial clear space indicates likely instability of the mortise joint due to ligamentous disruption. Patients with tenderness over the navicular or base of the fifth metatarsal may also need foot x-rays. Stress radiographs are rarely obtained in the acute setting but can be used in assessing and documenting movement with anterior drawer and talar tilt testing. Other diagnostic modalities such as computed tomography (CT), magnetic resonance imaging (MRI), arthrography, and bone scanning may also be of use but are infrequently necessary on initial evaluation.

V.   **Treatment**

   A.   **Ankle sprains** are encountered daily in the emergency department. Before making a final diagnosis of ankle sprain, more serious injuries are ruled out by physical exam and, as necessary, radiographs.

   1.   **Lateral sprains.** The majority of ankle sprains involve the lateral ligaments (ATFL, CFL, and PTFL) and are inversion injuries. They are classified as grade I, II, or III, depending on clinical findings (Table 2).

   a.   **Grade I.** Patients with grade I ankle sprains have mild pain and swelling. Commonly the ATFL is minimally torn. Anterior drawer and talar tilt testing are normal. Treatment includes rest, ice, compressive dressing, and elevation (RICE). Patients are discharged with crutches and analgesics and told to follow up in 1 to 2 weeks with their physicians.

   b.   **Grade II.** Patients with grade II ankle sprains have moderate pain and swelling. On physical exam, there may be a positive anterior drawer and/or talar tilt test. Patients are discharged with RICE, rigid splinting, and analgesics and told to follow up with an orthopaedist or sports medicine specialist in 1 week.

   c.   **Grade III.** Patients with grade III ankle sprains have marked pain, swelling, and ecchymosis. They are unable to bear weight

Table 2. Classification of ankle sprains

Severity	Symptoms	Signs	Examination	Treatment
Grade I	Mild pain and swelling, able to bear weight	Slight edema	Negative anterior drawer and talar tilt	RICE* and referral to primary care physician in 1 week
Grade II	Moderate pain and swelling, difficulty bearing weight	Moderate edema and ecchymosis	Positive anterior drawer (4–14 mm) and talar tilt test (5–15 degrees)	Rigid splint and referral to orthopaedist in a week
Grade III	Severe pain and swelling, inability to bear weight	Severe edema and ecchymosis	Positive anterior (>15 mm) and tilt test (>15 degrees)	Rigid splint and referral to orthopaedist within a week

*Rest, ice, compressive dressing, and elevation.

and have more marked ankle laxity, with positive anterior drawer and talar tilt tests. Treatment and disposition are those of grade II sprains.

2. **Medial sprains.** Medial ankle sprains are eversion injuries. They are less common than lateral sprains because the ankle intrinsically limits eversion and because the **deltoid ligament** is very strong. The significant force needed to injure the deltoid ligament makes associated injuries common, including proximal fibular fractures, syndesmotic tears, and lateral malleolar fractures. Physical exam reveals swelling and tenderness over the deltoid ligament. Radiographs may demonstrate an inconstant superior or medial clear space. Treatment for mild and moderate deltoid ligament sprains is RICE and analgesics, with follow-up with a primary care physician. Sprains with more extensive ligamentous disruption should be splinted and referred to an orthopaedist within a week.

3. **Syndesmotic sprains.** Syndesmotic injuries often occur in competitive sports and are associated with malleolar fractures. Common mechanisms include axial loading and external rotation upon an ankle in neutral position. Patients complain of pain over the anterior and posterior superior tibiofibular ligaments. The **squeeze test** (Sec. III.E.3) is used to diagnose syndesmotic injuries. An **external rotation test** (Fig. 7) can also aid in the diagnosis. This test is positive if pain is elicited in the tibiofibular ligament and interosseous membrane upon external rotation of the ankle with the foot in neutral position and the knee flexed at 90 degrees. Radiographic examination may reveal abnormal spacing of the mortise joint or between the distal tibia and fibula. Initial therapy includes RICE, a rigid ankle splint, and analgesics with referral to an orthopaedist for definitive treatment.

B. **Ankle fractures.** The ankle joint may be envisioned as a ring consisting of three bones (tibia, fibula, and talus) and three ligament groups (medial, lateral, and syndesmotic) (Fig. 8). The majority of ankle fractures are caused by abnormal motion of the talus within the mortise. A single break in the ring does not cause a talar shift; two breaks in the ring (bones and/or ligaments) lead to talar instability and a possible shift. The stability of the talus within the mortise has important implications for management. The primary mechanisms of injury in ankle fractures are external rotation, abduction, adduction, and vertical compression. Generally,

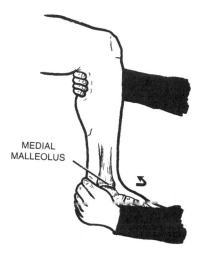

MEDIAL
MALLEOLUS

Fig. 7.   The external rotation test.

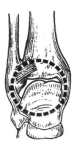

Fig. 8.   The ankle mortise conceptualized as a ring.

fractures caused by ligamentous avulsion are transverse, while fractures caused by talar impaction are oblique.

The two classification systems for ankle fractures most commonly used are those of **Lauge-Hansen** and **Danis-Weber.** The Lauge-Hansen classification (Table 3) distinguishes stages of injury within four groups of fracture. The groups are named by the position of the foot during injury (first word) and the direction of the stressors during injury (second word). They include supination-adduction, supination–external rotation, pronation-abduction, and pronation–external rotation. The Danis-Weber classification is simpler and is based on the location of the fibular fracture (Fig. 9). A Weber type A fracture is a fibular avulsion fracture below the tibiotalar joint

Table 3.   Lauge-Hansen classification of ankle injuries

Severity	Supination-Adduction	Supination–External Rotation	Pronation-Abduction	Pronation–External Rotation
Stage I	Transverse fracture of the lateral malleolus or collateral ligament tear	Anterior syndesmotic injury	Transverse fracture of medial malleolus or deltoid ligament tear	Transverse fracture of medial malleolus or deltoid ligament tear
Stage II	Oblique fracture of the medial malleolus	Spiral fracture of distal fibula	Syndesmotic injury with or without avulsion of posterior malleolus	Anterior syndesmotic injury
Stage III		Posterior syndesmotic injury with or without avulsion of posterior malleolus	Oblique fracture of distal fibula	High fracture of fibula
Stage IV		Oblique fracture of the medial malleolus		Posterior syndesmotic injury with or without avulsion of posterior malleolus

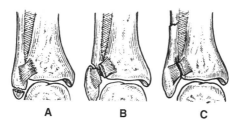

Fig. 9. The Weber classification.

line, a Weber type B fracture is an oblique fracture
arising from the joint line, and a Weber type C frac
ture is a more proximal fracture of the fibula associated with syndesmotic injury. The goals of ankle
fracture treatment are reestablishing the exact positioning of the talus within the mortise and a
smooth articular surface.

1. **Lateral malleolar fracture.** The most common fracture of the ankle is a lateral malleolar
   fracture. Although this is usually an inversion
   injury, the lateral malleolus can also be fractured through internal rotation, direct trauma,
   or after impact by the talus during a severe
   eversion injury. Patients often present with
   signs and symptoms similar to those of ankle
   sprain. Inability to bear weight increases the
   probability of fracture and warrants radiographic evaluation. Patients with small chip
   fractures require a short leg splint and RICE,
   remaining non-weight bearing until seen by an
   orthopaedist within a week. More severe lateral
   malleolar fractures with disruption of the mortise and widening of the tibiofibular joint indicate potential joint instability. These require
   immediate orthopaedic consultation and immobilization in a long leg posterior splint.

2. **Medial malleolar fracture.** The prognosis for
   a medial malleolar fracture is more guarded
   than for an isolated lateral malleolar fracture.
   Medial malleolar fractures are often associated
   with lateral or posterior malleolar fractures.
   Isolated medial fractures can occur with inversion, eversion, or direct-blow mechanisms. Patients present with medial ankle pain, swelling,
   ecchymosis, and a decreased range of motion.
   They may be unable to bear weight. Isolated
   fractures involving the medial articulation war-
   rant consultation with an orthopaedist. The patient with an isolated medial malleolar fracture
   and no evidence of joint instability should have
   a bulky short leg splint applied and treated

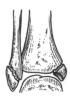

Fig. 10. **Bimalleolar fracture.**

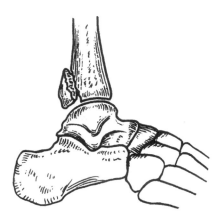

Fig. 11. **Posterior marginal fracture.**

with RICE and analgesics while avoiding weight bearing until seen by an orthopaedist.

3. **Bi- and trimalleolar fractures.** Medial malleolar fractures often represent one component of a bi- or trimalleolar fracture (Fig. 10). In trimalleolar fractures, all three malleoli (lateral, medial, and posterior) are fractured. Patients will have severe pain, swelling, and ecchymosis. In cases of bi- or trimalleolar fracture/dislocation, the obviously deformed joint should be reduced immediately in the emergency department prior to hospitalization for operative fixation. Adequate analgesia and conscious sedation technique should be employed. Closed injuries are typically unaccompanied by vascular compromise, and traction with the appropriate manipulation to correct the deformity is usually successful. Open fractures are common and more likely to have associated vascular compromise. Reduction in the emergency department after surgical cleansing and copious irrigation is necessary unless immediate or-

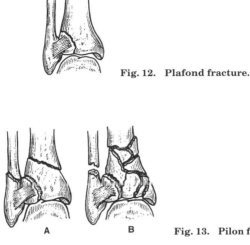

Fig. 12.   Plafond fracture.

A   B   **Fig. 13.   Pilon fracture.**

thopaedic operative care is available. In both closed and open fracture/dislocations, a long leg posterior splint is placed followed by postreduction radiographs and vascular checks.

4. **Posterior marginal fractures.** Isolated posterior marginal tibial fractures are rare. They occur by ligamentous avulsion or by axial loading. Nondisplaced fractures involving less than 25% of the articular surface can be treated with a non-weight-bearing short leg cast for a month. Displaced fractures or fractures involving a large part of the articular surface are often managed with open reduction and internal fixation (Fig. 11).

5. **Plafond fractures (Fig. 12).** Plafond fractures are also known as anterior marginal tibial fractures. They usually occur when the talus hits the distal tibia due to a high-energy dorsiflexion force. These fractures require orthopaedic consultation, and operative intervention is often necessary.

6. **Pilon fracture (Fig. 13).** Pilon fractures are ankle fractures resulting from axial compression that directs force vertically into the tibial plafond. Pilon fractures are sometimes confused with trimalleolar fractures. However, the mechanisms of action are different and the fractures of the malleoli in trimalleolar fractures are usually displaced from their anatomical position. In pilon fractures, there is severe comminution

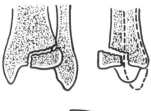

Fig. 14.   Tillaux fracture.

of the distal tibia and fibula with the malleoli generally maintained in their usual anatomical position. Sometimes CT is necessary to differentiate a pilon fracture from a trimalleolar fracture. Pilon fractures require orthopaedic consultation from the emergency department and hospitalization for operative fixation. A long leg posterior splint provides adequate stabilization.

7. **Tillaux fracture (Fig. 14).** A Tillaux fracture is an avulsion fracture of the anterolateral aspect of the distal tibia. The fracture line starts at the joint line and extends vertically, exiting at or distal to the fused physis. The juvenile Tillaux fracture is similar but is a Salter III injury involving the distal physis prior to bony fusion (see Chapter 27). The usual mechanism of this injury is external rotation and abduction, leading to avulsion of the bone element by the ATFL. If closed reduction is unsuccessful, open reduction and internal fixation is used. RICE, analgesics, and prompt orthopaedic referral are indicated.

8. **Talar dome fractures.** Fractures of the talar dome include **osteochondritis dissecans** of the talus, osteochondral fractures, and transchondral fractures. These lesions are typically small and may be overlooked on initial radiographs. The most common sites involved are the superolateral and superomedial margins of the dome. Lateral lesions are usually anterior while medial lesions are usually posterior. Lateral osteochondral fractures occur with extreme dorsiflexion. Medial osteochondral fractures occur with supination leading to impaction. Patients may present describing a persisting ankle sprain that will not heal. Prolonged pain, swelling, and crepitus should raise the suspicion of this injury. Palpating the dome of the

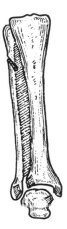

Fig. 15. Maisonneuve fracture.

talus with the foot plantarflexed may localize the tenderness. Most nondisplaced fractures of the talar dome can be treated conservatively without surgery. Displaced fractures should receive operative management for debridement and removal of any loose body.

9. **Maisonneuve fracture.** The Maisonneuve fracture is an oblique fracture of the proximal fibula with either disruption of the deltoid ligament or fracture of the medial malleolus (Fig. 15). The mechanism of injury is external rotation upon an inverted or adducted foot. Patients present with complaints of pain around the ankle radiating proximally, with an inability to bear weight. Palpation reveals tenderness about the medial malleolus and the proximal fibula. AP and lateral views of the tibia and fibula are necessary to complement ankle views. These injuries are easily missed, supporting routine palpation of the proximal fibula in all patients with ankle sprains. Treatment is based on the integrity of the ankle joint and presence of a medial malleolar fracture. If the mortise joint is disrupted or there is a fracture of the medial malleolus, operative fixation is necessary. If the superior and medial clear spaces are within normal limits and there is no malleolar fracture, the patient can be treated in a long leg cast for 6 to 12 weeks.

C. **Ankle dislocations.** Isolated ankle dislocation is rare, and most ankle dislocations are associated with fractures involving the malleoli. Posterior dislocations are most common. Care is similar to that of bimalleolar fracture/dislocations.

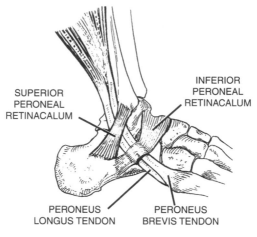

SUPERIOR
PERONEAL
RETINACALUM

INFERIOR
PERONEAL
RETINACALUM

PERONEUS
LONGUS TENDON

PERONEUS
BREVIS TENDON

Fig. 16.   Peroneal joint and retinacula.

D.   **Peroneal tendon subluxation (Fig. 16).** Peroneal tendon subluxation is caused by dorsiflexion
and eversion of the ankle with forceful contraction
of the peroneal muscle. The peroneal retinaculum is
disrupted, with resultant subluxation of the peroneal tendon from its shallow groove at the posterior lateral fibula to a position overlying the lateral
malleolus. Patients present with posterior lateral
ankle swelling, tenderness, and ecchymosis. Treatment consists of a stirrup splint with adequate
malleolar padding and referral to an orthopaedist.
Subsequent treatment by the orthopaedist may include casting and avoidance of weight bearing for 4
weeks or operative management.

VI.   **Conclusion.** Ankle injuries are commonplace in the
emergency department. An understanding of ankle
anatomy is integral to the accurate assessment and care
of these injuries. A systematic approach in the history
and physical examination and the selective use of radiographs will prevent the clinician from overlooking commonly missed injuries. Appropriate splinting and timely
consultation and referral will help reduce the morbidity
associated with many ankle injuries.

BIBLIOGRAPHY
Hoppenfeld S. *Physical examination of the spine and extremities.*
Norwalk, CT: Appleton-Century-Crofts, 1976.
Reisdorff E, Cowling K. The injured ankle: new twists to a familiar
problem. *EM Reports* 1995;16:39–48.
Rockwood C, Green D. *Fractures in adults,* 3rd ed. Philadelphia:
Lippincott, 1991.

Rosen P, Barkin RM, et al. *Emergency medicine concepts and clinical practice,* 3rd ed. St Louis: Mosby, 1992.

Ruiz E, Cicero J. *Emergency management of skeletal injuries.* St Louis: Mosby, 1995.

Simon R, Koenigsknecht S. *Orthopaedics in emergency medicine: the extremities,* 3rd ed. Norwalk, CT: Appleton-Century-Crofts, 1995.

Stiell IG, Greenberg GH, McKnight RD, et al. Decision rules for the use of radiography in acute ankle injuries. Refinement and prospective validation. *JAMA* 1993;269:1127–1132.

Tintinalli J, Krome R, Ruiz E. *Emergency medicine: a comprehensive study guide,* 4th ed. New York: McGraw-Hill, 1996.

The Foot

Felix Ankel

Functions of the foot include weight bearing, balance, and leverage for walking and running.

I. **Anatomy.** The foot contains 28 bones and 57 joints (Fig. 1). It is divided into the **hindfoot, midfoot,** and **forefoot. Chopart's joint** is the joint between the hindfoot and the midfoot. **Lisfranc's joint** is between the midfoot and forefoot.

   A. **Bones.** The hindfoot consists of the calcaneus and the talus. The calcaneus is the largest bone in the foot and forms the heel. The medial part of the calcaneus has a shelf-like portion called the **sustentaculum tali,** which helps support the talus. The talus has a head, neck, and body. The distal head articulates with the navicular. The lower surface of the neck has a deep groove that forms the **sinus tarsi** with the calcaneus and contains a strong interosseus talocalcaneal ligament. The talar body is cuboidal in shape and articulates with the distal tibia. The midfoot consists of the navicular, cuboid, and cuneiforms. The navicular is located medially, with the three cuneiform bones lying distal to the navicular. The cuboid bone lies laterally. The forefoot consists of 5 metatarsal and 14 phalangeal bones, 2 for the large toe and 3 for the rest. Two sesamoid bones are located within the flexor hallucis brevis tendon beneath the first metatarsophalangeal joint.

   B. **Arteries.** Blood supply is derived from the posterior tibial and the dorsalis pedis arteries. The **posterior tibial** courses behind the medial malleolus and separates into the medial and lateral plantar arteries. The **dorsalis pedis** is a continuation of the anterior tibial artery and extends down the foot, where it joins the lateral plantar artery to form the **plantar arch.**

   C. **Nerves.** The sensory fibers to the heel arise from the **tibial nerve.** The medial and lateral plantar nerves, which arise from the tibial nerve, innervate the more distal part of the sole. The dorsum of the foot is innervated by the saphenous, sural, superficial, and deep peroneal nerves. The **saphenous** nerve supplies skin sensation along the proximal and medial sides of the foot. The **sural** nerve supplies the skin along the lateral margins of the forefoot. The superficial and deep **peroneal nerves** supply the rest of the foot's dorsum.

   D. **Muscles.** The muscles involved in plantar flexion, abduction, and adduction of the toes are located on the plantar surface of the foot. Extensor tendons are located on the dorsal aspect of the foot and are held in place by an extensor retinaculum.

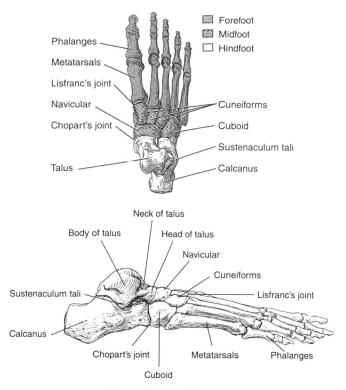

Fig. 1. **Bones of the foot.**

E. **Arches and soft tissue.** Arches maintain the shape of the foot. The **longitudinal arch** starts at the posterior calcaneus and extends anteriorly via the medial and lateral columns. The horizontal relationships of the five metatarsals describe the transverse arch. There is a thick **plantar fascia** that extends from the calcaneus to the heads of the metatarsals. Weight is equally distributed between the heel and forefoot by the longitudinal arches. The integrity of the **longitudinal arch** depends on the position and alignment of the bones rather than the soft tissue. The medial column of the longitudinal arch goes to the medial three toes and carries the most weight. The lateral column goes to the two lateral toes and maintains balance. The **transverse arch** allows for flexibility and stability and is aided by the wedge shapes of the midfoot bones.

II. **Mechanism of injury.** Foot injuries are generally the result of direct trauma, indirect trauma, or overuse injury.

It is important for the examiner to ask about activity during injury and ability to ambulate afterward. An adequate history will often help the physician determine the location of the injury and predict which injury may be present. The following are examples of mechanisms of injury that can alert the clinician to specific pathology.

A. **Fall from height on heel.** Heel pain from a fall warrants inspection of both extremities and the lower spine.

B. **Axial compression on plantarflexed foot.** This may happen in an auto accident and should raise the possibility of a tarsometatarsal joint injury.

C. **Sudden increase in training.** A sudden increase in training vigor in a competitive runner may suggest a stress fracture as the possible etiology for foot pain.

Keeping in mind the general load-bearing relationships of the foot is also helpful in understanding mechanisms of injury. At the forefoot, weight is not distributed equally. The first metatarsal head bears twice as much weight as the other metatarsal heads combined, making injuries of the first metatarsal head particularly significant. Push-off forces are concentrated on the second metatarsal during locomotion, making stress fractures of this bone common.

III. **Physical examination.** Physical examination is done in a thorough and systematic fashion. It includes assessment for ligamentous and joint stability, neurovascular compromise, and soft tissue injury. Comparison to the unaffected side can aid examination. Areas seemingly remote from the apparent injury may have associated pathology (e.g., fracture of the lumbar spine in a patient with bilateral calcaneal fractures). Examination and documentation should include the following.

A. **Inspection.** Inspect for swelling, ecchymosis, deformity, color, and skin integrity.

B. **Palpation.** Palpate for tenderness and crepitus at sites remote from the injury, then proceed to the presumed injury. Medially, palpate the medial malleolus, sustentaculum tali, head of the talus, navicular tuberosity, and head of the first metatarsal. Laterally, palpate the lateral malleolus, peroneus longus and brevis tendons, and the base of the fifth metatarsal. Dorsally, the tibialis anterior, extensor digitorum longus, and extensor hallucis longus tendons are examined. Axial compression of the metatarsals will exacerbate pain with metatarsal fractures.

C. **Range of motion.** Range of motion is assessed, anticipating approximately 45 degrees of plantarflexion, 20 degrees of dorsiflexion, 30 degrees of inversion, 20 degrees of eversion, 20 degrees of internal rotation, and 10 degrees of external rotation.

D. **Neurovascular examination.** Palpation of the dorsalis pedis and posterior tibial pulses as well as assessment of distal capillary refill is followed by a

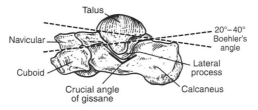

Fig. 2. Boehler's angle.

motor and sensory exam, including two-point discrimination when applicable.

IV. **Radiography.** Radiographic interpretation of the foot is difficult because of overlapping shadows, secondary ossification centers, and sesamoid bones. A thorough physical exam and knowledge of the radiographic anatomy will facilitate correct interpretation.

A. **Foot.** X-rays usually include **anteroposterior (AP), lateral,** and **oblique** views. Two views are inadequate to diagnose foot fractures and dislocations in a consistent fashion. An oblique view is often necessary to sort out the shadows of the overlapping small bones.

B. **Calcaneus.** Calcaneal views are ordered when evaluating calcaneal injuries. These include AP, lateral, and axial calcaneal views. Calculating **Boehler's angle** (Fig. 2) on the lateral view aids in the diagnosis of occult calcaneal fracture. A normal Boehler's angle is between 20 and 40 degrees and can readily be compared with that of the uninvolved side.

C. **Toes.** Toe x-rays suffice in injuries limited to the toes.

D. **Bone scan.** Bone scans can aid in the diagnosis of occult or stress fractures that are not radiographically apparent. They are not typically used in the acute setting.

V. **Treatment and disposition**

A. **Hindfoot**

1. **Fractures**

a. **Talus.** The talus is the second most commonly fractured tarsal bone. It supports and distributes the weight of the body and articulates with the tibia, calcaneus, and midfoot. It is held in place by ligaments and has no muscular attachments. The neck of the talus connects the more proximal body to the distal head. The trochlea articulates with the tibia superiorly. The medial and lateral facets articulate with the medial and lateral malleoli. The head of the talus articulates with the tarsal navicular bone distally. More than half of the talus is covered by articular cartilage.

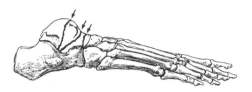

Fig. 3.   Talar fractures.

The vascular supply to the talus is easily compromised. Injuries to the talus, especially dislocated fractures of the talar neck, can cause avascular necrosis.

(1) **Osteochondral.** Osteochondral fractures are common injuries that present after an inversion or eversion injury of the ankle (see Chapter 21).

(2) **Body.** Fractures of the talar body are typically the result of high-impact injuries causing compression of the talus between the tibia and the calcaneus. There is usually considerable displacement of fracture fragments with dislocation of both the ankle and subtalar joint. These injuries should be evaluated by an orthopaedist and often require operative reduction and internal fixation. Nondisplaced body fractures can be treated by a short leg nonwalking cast for 6 to 8 weeks (Fig. 3).

(3) **Neck.** The talar neck is the most commonly fractured part of the talus. It may be associated with subtalar dislocation. The talar neck is fractured when the foot is in extreme dorsiflexion, as in a motor vehicle accident or a fall from a height. With this injury the posterior ligaments are torn and the anterior distal tibia wedges itself into the talar neck. The **Hawkins classification** of talar neck fractures is based on fracture displacement. Fractures without displacement (Hawkins I) require immobilization with a short leg cast for 8 to 12 weeks, with an initial non-weight-bearing period. Talar neck fractures with displacement (Hawkins II and III) frequently cause skin tension and subsequent necrosis, converting a closed fracture into an open one. Such displaced talar fractures mandate immediate evaluation of the circulatory status of the foot and early re-

duction. Open dislocated fractures are orthopaedic emergencies, requiring irrigation, broad-spectrum antibiotics, and operative debridement. Because they are often associated with talar neck fractures, medial malleolar fractures require careful scrutiny of the talar neck. Closed type II and III fractures need prompt open reduction and internal fixation (ORIF) to minimize complications. Even with ideal care, fractures of the talar neck are fraught with complications that seem proportional to initial displacement, including skin necrosis, infection, delayed union, malunion, and osteoarthritis. Avascular necrosis of the talus occurs in up to 50% of type II fractures and over 80% of type III fractures.

(4) **Posterior process.** Fractures of the medial or lateral tubercle of the posterior process are caused by abrupt plantarflexion of the foot. Fracture may be confused with a normal variant of the **os trigonum** tarsi. The os trigonum is one of the 21 inconstant accessory bones in the foot and is located at the posterior aspect of the talus. This os is frequently encountered and often bilateral. Fractures of the posterior tubercle that do not affect range of motion can be treated by initial splinting and subsequent immobilization in a short leg cast for 4 to 6 weeks.

(5) **Head.** Fractures of the talar head are rare. They are caused by forces transmitted longitudinally through the metatarsal and navicular bones compressing the head. Most nondisplaced fractures can be treated with ice, elevation, immobilization with a bulky compression dressing, and orthopaedic follow-up. Subsequent treatment may consist of a short leg cast with or without weight bearing. Displaced fractures may necessitate open reduction.

b. **Calcaneus.** The calcaneus is the largest bone in the foot and absorbs most of the body's weight with walking. It is the most commonly fractured tarsal bone. It articulates with the cuboid anteriorly and the talus superiorly. The medial and lateral processes on its plantar aspect serve as insertion points for muscles and the plantar fascia. The calcaneus has a thin cortex and contains trabeculae that sometimes make radiographic interpretation of subtle fractures difficult. Calcaneal fractures frequently occur with falls from a height and are associated with compression fractures of the lumbar spine. The management of calcaneal fractures is challenging because often treatment results are not optimal (see Fig. 2).

(1) **Intraarticular.** Intraarticular calcaneal fractures involving the **subtalar joint** are usually caused by extreme axial loading, with the talus splitting the calcaneous into two major fragments at the **crucial angle of Gissane.** These fractures are best seen on lateral radiographs and are associated with a decrease in **Boehler's angle.** Treatment and prognosis vary depending on the extent of the fracture. Early orthopaedic consultation is mandatory, as a significant percentage of patients have a poor outcome with this injury.

(2) **Extraarticular.** Extraarticular calcaneal fractures not involving the subtalar joint have less long-term morbidity. Fractures of the calcaneal tuberosity are rare. Localized pain, swelling, and ecchymosis are found on exam. Fractures of the **medial** or **lateral tuberosity** are caused by abduction or adduction when the heel strikes the ground. Treatment for nondisplaced fractures includes immobilization with a bulky compression dressing, rest, elevation, and ice for 1 to 2 weeks, with orthopaedic follow-up. Subsequent treatment with a walking cast and partial weight bearing for at least 8 weeks, until the fragments are united, is suggested. Displaced fractures require either closed or open reduction and fixation. Fractures of the **posterior tuberosity** can occur with an avulsion of the Achilles tendon. Nondisplaced fractures are treated with immobilization in a slight equinus position for 6 to 8 weeks, while displaced fragments may require surgical fixation. Stress from the **bifurcate ligament,** which attaches the calcaneus to the cuboid and navicular, can cause an avulsion fracture of the **calcaneocuboid** or **calcaneonavicular process.** Treatment is ice, elevation, and weight bearing as tolerated. Extraarticular fractures of the **calcaneal body** are rare. Nondisplaced fractures can be treated with a Jones compression dressing.

(3) **Sustentaculum tali.** A fracture to the sustentaculum tali usually presents following an inversion injury to the ankle with axial compression on the heel. Swelling to the medial heel is present below the malleolus. This injury is easily mistaken for an ankle sprain. The fracture can be seen on the axial view of the calcaneal radiographs. Since the flexor hallucis longus courses under the sustentaculum tali, extension of the great toe exacerbates the pain. Treatment is immobilization with a compression dressing, rest, elevation, and ice for 1 to 2 days, with orthopaedic follow-up. Subsequent treatment is casting with avoidance of weight bearing for 8 weeks.

Fractures of the hindfoot will usually require hospitalization after immediate orthopaedic consultation to facilitate definitive care as well as to treat associated injuries. A short leg posterior splint, elevation, ice, and pain control are appropriate in the acute phase.

2. **Dislocation.** Subtalar dislocation, also known as peritalar dislocation, involves dislocation of the talocalcaneal and talonavicular joints with intact tibiotalar and calcaneocuboid joints. These injuries are caused by substantial forces such as occur in automobile accidents or falls from heights but also in athletics. They are often accompanied by fractures of the talus or malleoli. The resultant deformity and skin tenting are impressive. The most informative x-ray view is the AP, which shows the talonavicular dislocation. The majority of subtalar dislocations can be reduced by closed methods. Prompt reduction before swelling can occur is aimed at minimizing further cartilaginous injury from forceful or repeated attempts. Flexing the knee to relax the pull of the gastrocnemius on the calcaneus facilitates reduction. General anesthesia is often required.

   a. **Medial.** Medial dislocations are the most common. Inversion, adduction, and supination forces cause the head of the talus to be dislocated laterally and the distal foot to be displaced medially. Lateral pressure from the dislocated talar head will often compromise the vascular supply to the overlying skin. Reduction can be accomplished using longitudinal traction on the heel with a downward force on the talar head and a combination of abduction and pronation of the foot.

   b. **Lateral.** Lateral dislocations are caused by eversion forces. These dislocations are reduced by longitudinal traction and adduction of the foot.

   c. **Open.** Open talar dislocations need irrigation, broad-spectrum antibiotics, and operative reduction.

B. **Midfoot**

   1. **Fractures.** The midfoot is the least mobile part of the foot and is rarely fractured. Midfoot fractures usually result from crush injury. Isolated midfoot fractures are rare. Cuboid and cuneiform fractures usually occur in combination and have associated subluxations or dislocations. Physical examination reveals tenderness and swelling over the fractured bone. Treatment for most nondisplaced fractures is a short leg cast. Isolated fractures of the navicular, cuboid, or cuneiforms are best immobilized in a short leg posterior splint, with prompt orthopaedic attention. As in all foot fractures, elevation and ice to prevent excessive swelling are important. Multiple fractures or open injuries resulting from violent trauma may necessitate hospitalization.

    a. **Navicular.** Fracture of the navicular is the most common isolated midfoot fracture. A small percentage of the population has an accessory navicular bone called the **os tibiale externum** which is often confused with a fracture.

      (1) **Cortical avulsion.** A cortical avulsion fracture occurs when ligamentous tension results in an avulsion of the dorsal articular element of the navicular. Small fractures are treated with immobilization for 4 to 6 weeks. Larger fractures may require fixation.

      (2) **Tuberosity.** Fractures of the navicular tuberosity are caused by eversion. They are treated with a walking cast for 4 weeks. These fractures may be complicated by nonunion.

      (3) **Body.** Fractures of the navicular body are rare and may be difficult to see on radiographs. Treatment for nondisplaced fractures is a walking cast for 6 to 8 weeks.

    b. **Cuboid.** The cuboid is the most lateral midfoot bone. Cuboid fractures occur by direct crush or inversion injuries. They are often associated with calcaneal fractures. Undisplaced fractures may be seen only in the oblique view. Treatment is immobilization with a short leg walking cast for 6 weeks.

    c. **Cuneiforms.** Fractures of the cuneiforms involve blunt trauma to the dorsum of the foot. Associated injuries are often present. Care

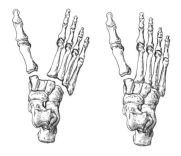

Fig. 4. Lisfranc dislocations.

must be taken in reviewing foot radiographs for cuneiform fractures. The navicular should overlap all three cuneiforms equally on the AP view and the gap between the metatarsal shafts should be equal. Treatment is immobilization with a short leg walking cast for 6 weeks.

C. **Tarsometatarsal dislocations**

1. **Lisfranc.** A Lisfranc fracture/dislocation is a rare but commonly missed injury. The recessed base of the **second metatarsal** is the locking keystone of the joint and is held in place by an oblique ligament between the medial cuneiform and the second metatarsal. Transverse ligaments connect the bases of the second to fifth metatarsals but not the first metatarsal. During injury, there is dislocation at the site of lowest resistance, usually the dorsal aspect of Lisfranc's joint at the base of the second metatarsal. There is typically an accompanying fracture of the proximal second metatarsal. The usual mechanism of action is an axial load. It may result from auto accidents when the foot is braced against the floorboard in extreme plantarflexion. Direct crushing blows can also cause this injury.

a. **Physical examination.** Physical examination reveals extreme swelling and tenderness over Lisfranc's joint. Paresthesias may be described overlying the midfoot. Because of the extreme forces involved in these injuries, open wounds with associated tissue damage and vascular impairment are typical. In a **homolateral** dislocation, all five metatarsals are displaced transversely. In an **isolated** dislocation, one or two metatarsals are displaced from the others. In a **divergent** dislocation, there is transverse but opposite displacement of the metatarsals (Fig. 4).

b. **Radiography.** Radiographic diagnosis can be difficult. The injury may be seen only on an oblique view. On an AP film, the medial margin of the second metatarsal should be aligned with the medial margin of the second cuneiform. On an oblique film, the medial aspect of the fourth metatarsal should be aligned with the medial aspect of the cuboid. A separation between the base of the first and second metatarsal bases is a reliable sign of injury. A fracture of the base of the second metatarsal should be assumed to be part of a Lisfranc dislocation until proven otherwise.

  c. **Treatment.** Treatment usually consists of hospitalization and immediate orthopaedic consultation for reduction and fixation under anesthesia. Complications such as acute vascular compromise from pedal artery compression or spasm as well as residual pain and osteoarthritis can occur.

D. Forefoot
  1. Fractures
   a. **Metatarsal.** Most metatarsal fractures are **transverse** fractures resulting from direct trauma as when a heavy object falls on the foot. Nondisplaced **neck** and **shaft** fractures should be placed in a short leg splint with neurovascular and skin checks and orthopaedic follow-up. Frequently, there is more than one metatarsal fracture. Although fractures are best seen on the AP and oblique views, the lateral view is the best for assessing the typically sagittal displacement. **Spiral** fractures are the result of twisting of the foot when the forefoot is fixed. Physical exam reveals swelling and tenderness over the dorsal midfoot. Axial compression of the metatarsal will exacerbate pain. It is important to document the presence of a dorsalis pedis pulse. Significant swelling can occur if the foot is not elevated. Nondisplaced **neck** and **shaft** fractures should be placed in a short leg splint with neurovascular and skin checks and orthopaedic follow-up. Subsequent treatment is often a short leg cast. Displaced fractures require reduction.

    (1) **March fractures.** The second and third metatarsals are the sites of maximum load bearing during push-off; consequently they are susceptible to stress or march fractures. Patients complain of insidious, progressive, poorly localized pain with minimal swelling or ecchymosis. A history of chronic or increased physical activity, as in joggers or basketball players, is common. Initial radiographs are often unremarkable. A bone

scan that shows increased activity in areas of stress may allow for an early diagnosis. Cessation of the activity that contributed to the injury for 4 to 6 weeks is curative. Patients may benefit from an initial period of partial weight bearing to protect the injury.

(2) **Base of the fifth metatarsal.** The base of the fifth metatarsal is commonly fractured in an inversion injury. With plantarflexion and inversion, the peroneus brevis tendon avulses the tuberosity of the base of the fifth metatarsal in a longitudinal fashion. Patients present to the emergency department complaining of a sprained ankle. There may be minimal tenderness over the base of the fifth metatarsal, and this injury may be missed by an unsuspecting examiner. The fracture is usually obvious on x-ray, although an accessory bone, the **os vesalianum,** is sometimes located near the base of the fifth metatarsal and can be confused with a fracture fragment. The injury is treated with a compression dressing and weight bearing as tolerated. Fracture of the tuberosity should not be confused with the more serious **Jones fracture**—a transverse fracture at the proximal diaphysis of the fifth metatarsal. These patients require plaster immobilization, crutches, and prompt orthopaedic referral. Jones fractures are treated with a short leg walking cast and have a high incidence of nonunion.

b. **Phalangeal and sesamoid**

1. **Toes.** Fractures of the toes usually occur with direct trauma or forced hyperextension. The fifth toe is often angulated laterally. Physical exam reveals swelling and ecchymosis. Subungual hematomas may also be present. Most second to fifth nondisplaced phalangeal fractures can be treated with dynamic splinting, such as **buddy taping** (Fig. 5). In buddy taping, it is important to insert padding between the toes to prevent skin maceration. Comminuted fractures of the great toe may require a walking cast. Fractures with angulation should be reduced using a digital block. Open fractures require irrigation, suturing, antibiotics, and prompt orthopaedic referral.

c. **Sesamoid.** Two sesamoid bones are located within the flexor hallucis brevis tendon and

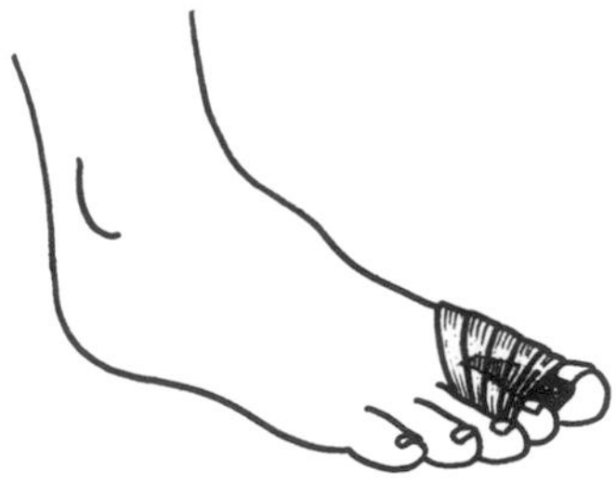

Fig. 5.   Buddy taping.

are occasionally fractured by direct trauma or chronic repetitive stress. Medial sesamoid fractures are more common than lateral ones. Physical exam reveals tenderness over the plantar aspect of the first metatarsal head and pain is increased on extension of the great toe. Bipartite sesamoids can make the diagnosis of a fracture difficult. **Sesamoiditis** is a clinical diagnosis and includes symptomatic bipartite sesamoids, tendinitis of the flexor hallucis longus at the site of the sesamoids, and synovitis of the first metatarsophalangeal joint. Sesamoid fractures should be treated with arch supports or a short leg cast if pain is severe. They are occasionally complicated by nonunion and may require surgical excision.

2. **Dislocations** of the metatarsophalangeal and interphalangeal joints are caused by dorsiflexion and compression of the phalanges.

a. **Metatarsophalangeal (MP) joint.** Dislocations of the MP joint are usually dorsal, although medial and lateral MP dislocations also occur. Physical exam reveals swelling, tenderness, painful ambulation, and a visible deformity. Most commonly, the toe is hyperextended dorsally on the metatarsal head. Reduction is performed by using hyperextension and traction. The patient is discharged to orthopaedic follow-up with crutches and a dorsal splint to prevent further hyperextension for 2 to 5 weeks. Unsuccessful closed reduction requires referral for open reduction.

b. **Interphalangeal (IP) joint.** Stable dislocations of the IP joint are treated with closed reduction and buddy splinting to the adjacent toe. Unstable dislocations require referral for internal fixation.

E. **Soft tissue injuries**

1. **Tarsal tunnel syndrome.** Tarsal tunnel syndrome is similar to carpal tunnel syndrome of the

upper extremity. It is an entrapment neuropathy in which branches of the posterior tibial nerve are compressed beneath the flexor retinaculum. Symptoms include paresthesias and pain at the medial malleolus with radiation to the heel and calf, frequently most prominent at night. Physical examination may reveal loss of two-point discrimination over the plantar aspect of the foot. Treatment is rest, antiinflammatory medications, and orthotic shoes. Definitive treatment by surgical release of the flexor retinaculum is sometimes indicated.

2. **Compartment syndrome.** Compartment syndrome occurs when excessive tissue pressures cause nerve and muscle ischemia. It occurs in the foot with severe crush injuries that result in multiple midfoot fractures or dislocations. Diagnosis is made on clinical grounds: pain, paresthesias, loss of two-point discrimination, tense skin, and massive swelling. Loss of pulse and pain with passive range of motion of the toes are unreliable indicators. Therefore, heightened clinical suspicion is necessary with excessive foot swelling. Treatment consists of emergency fasciotomy.

3. **Achilles tendon.** Patients with an Achilles tendon **rupture** describe an intense pain after extreme dorsiflexion injury or with a violent push-off. It is most common in males after the age of 30 as a result of rigorous recreational activities. Patients may describe a distinct "pop" followed by inability to plantarflex the foot. With complete disruption, there is a palpable defect in the tendon and the patient has a positive **Thompson test.** The test is performed with the patient in a prone position, the knees flexed. Failure of the foot to plantarflex when the gastrocnemius and soleus muscles in the calf are squeezed constitutes a positive test. Active individuals may benefit from operative repair, but those who are less active may have adequate healing with closed treatment. The patient may be discharged in a non-weight-bearing splint in passive equinus with orthopaedic referral for definitive treatment. Achilles **tendinitis** is common in sports. Patients present with pain, swelling, crepitus, erythema, and tenderness to palpation. Treatment is rest, ice, and nonsteroidal antiinflammatory drugs (NSAIDs).

4. **Plantar fasciitis** is an overuse syndrome causing inflammation of the plantar fascia. It typically occurs in athletes who do not stretch appropriately. Patients often complain of pain at the arch or heel of the foot. Physical exam reveals tenderness on the medial edge of the fascia at its insertion on the anterior calcaneus, which is fur-

ther exacerbated by dorsiflexing the toes. Radiographs may show a calcaneal spur. Treatment is rest, cold applications, and NSAIDs. Occasionally, this injury is treated with steroid injections.

BIBLIOGRAPHY

Hoppenfeld S. *Physical examination of the spine and extremities.* Norwalk, CT: Appleton-Century-Crofts, 1976.

Rockwood C, Green D. *Fractures in adults,* 3rd ed. Philadelphia: Lippincott, 1991.

Rosen P, Barkin RM, et al. *Emergency medicine concepts and clinical practice,* 3rd ed. St Louis: Mosby, 1992.

Rosen P, Doris P, et al. *Diagnostic radiology in emergency medicine.* St Louis: Mosby, 1992.

Ruiz E, Cicero J. *Emergency management of skeletal injuries.* St Louis: Mosby, 1995.

Simon R, Koenigsknecht S. *Orthopaedics in emergency medicine: the extremities,* 3rd ed. Norwalk, CT: Appleton-Century-Crofts, 1995.

Tintanelli J, Krome R, Ruiz E. *Emergency medicine: a comprehensive study guide,* 4th ed. New York: McGraw-Hill, 1996.

IV

Spine

23

Cervical Spine Injuries

Neil B. Jasani, Melinda S. Jasani,
and Robert E. O'Connor

Injuries to the cervical spine may involve damage to the musculoskeletal system, the nervous system, or both. Approximately one-third to one-half of all cervical spine fractures and dislocations have a concomitant neurological injury. The damage may be to the spinal cord and/or nerve roots, and the neurological deficit may be complete or partial and permanent or transient. The potentially devastating nature of these injuries makes appropriate assessment and management of potential cervical spine injury one of the most important and challenging tasks performed in the evaluation of a trauma patient. In fact, evaluation of the cervical spine is superseded in importance only by evaluation of the airway, breathing, and circulation.

This chapter addresses the clinical and radiological assessment of potential cervical spine injuries. Since many such injuries can be unstable on initial presentation, techniques used for cervical spine immobilization are discussed first.

I. **Cervical spine immobilization (Fig. 1).** The neck must be completely immobilized until it can be clinically or radiographically determined to be free of injury.

A. **Head.** The head must be held in the neutral position. This can be accomplished with Velcro blocks, which come with the backboard, or similar objects such as rolled towels or sandbags. Be certain the cervical collar is applied correctly. In addition, to further ensure that the head stays in a fixed position, it is taped to the board. It is important to maintain this alignment when performing cervical in-line stabilization during oral intubations.

B. **Body.** After the head and neck are immobilized, strap the trunk and extremities down on the backboard so that the torso does not move.

II. **Physical examination of the cervical spine.** Physical examination of the neck is important for assessing the degree of injury, although by necessity it is limited in the patient who has sustained significant trauma. These patients are often in full body immobilization with head blocks in place. The examination is accomplished with the patient in the supine position while still fully immobilized.

In clinically appropriate patients, the cervical collar is held in place with one hand while the strap is loosened with the other. Gently palpate the posterior part of the cervical spine, starting at the occiput and working your way toward the thoracic spine. Begin at the inion, which is a dome-shaped bump that lies in the occipital region on the midline and marks the center of the superior nuchal line. From the inion, move laterally to palpate the supe-

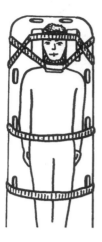

Fig. 1.   Backboard immobilization.

rior nuchal line, which is a small transverse ridge extending out on both sides of the inion. As you palpate laterally you will feel the mastoid process of the skull.

The spinous processes of the cervical vertebrae lie along the posterior midline of the cervical spine. To palpate them, slide around the side of the neck and probe the middle with your fingertips. Since no muscle crosses the midline, it feels indented. The lateral soft tissue bulges that outline the indentation are composed of deep paraspinal muscles and the superficial trapezius. Begin the palpation at the base of the skull; the C2 spinous process is the first one that is palpable (the C1 spinous process is a small tubercle and lies deep). As you palpate the spinous processes from C2 to T1, note if there is the normal lordosis of the cervical spine. From the spinous process of C2, move your hand laterally about 1 in. in either direction to palpate the joints of the vertebral facets that lie between the cervical vertebrae. These joints often cause symptoms of pain in the neck region. The joints feel like small domes and lie deep beneath the trapezius muscle. Take note of any tenderness elicited and palpate the joints bilaterally at each articulation until you reach the articulation between C7 and T1.

On some patients you may be able to palpate bifid C3-5 spinous processes (divided, and consisting of two small excrescences of bone). The C7 and T1 spinous processes are larger than those above them. The processes are normally in line with each other; a shift in their normal alignment may be due to a unilateral facet dislocation or to a fracture of the spinous process following trauma. The facet joints between C5 and C6 are most often osteoarthritic and therefore most often tender and possibly slightly enlarged. If the vertebral level of any one joint is uncertain, its level can be

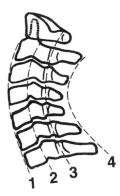

Fig. 2. Contour lines for alignment of the cervical spine, the lateral view.

estimated by lining up the vertebrae in question with the anterior structures of the neck. The hyoid bone is at the level of C3, the thyroid cartilage at C4 and C5, and the first cricoid ring at the level of C6.

One can clear the cervical spine clinically only if *all* of the following conditions are met:
1. No cervical pain or tenderness is present.
2. No paresthesias or neurological deficits exist.
3. Normal mental status is observed (the patient must be fully conscious and free of intoxicants or head injury).
4. No distracting source of pain is present.
5. The patient is at least 4 years old.
6. There is no history of loss of consciousness.

III. **Imaging studies**
  A. **Radiographs.** In many cases, the cervical spine cannot be cleared clinically and evaluation of radiographic studies takes on a high priority. The routine radiographic views consist of a lateral anteroposterior (AP), an open-mouth, and two (right and left) oblique views. A single cross-table lateral radiograph is only 80% to 90% sensitive in detecting injury and must not be relied upon as the only means of ruling out injury. A three-view radiographic series (lateral, AP, and odontoid) offers >95% sensitivity in detecting injuries and is routinely obtained at many institutions. The most important of these three views is the lateral view, as it will reveal the majority of unstable injuries and dislocations.
    1. **Lateral view.** Every lateral cervical spine film must be checked for key radiographic relationships. The following checklist should be used for every review (use the mnemonic **ABCS**).
      a. **Alignment.** There are four lines to be evaluated in the lateral view (Fig. 2).
        (1) **Anterior contour line.** Formed by the anterior margins of the vertebral bodies.

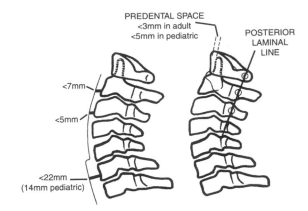

PREDENTAL SPACE
<3mm in adult
<5mm in pediatric

POSTERIOR
LAMINAL
LINE

<7mm

<5mm

<22mm
(14mm pediatric)

Fig. 3.   **Prevertebral space of the cervical spine, lateral view.**

These should line up within 1 mm of each other. However, pseudosubluxation of up to 3 mm is often seen in children at C2 on C3 and at C3 on C4.

(2) **Posterior contour line.** Formed by the posterior margins of the vertebral bodies. These should also line up within 1 mm of each other.

(3) **Spinolaminal line.** Formed by the bases of the spinous processes. These should match and follow the anterior and posterior contour lines.

(4) **Posterior aspects of spinous processes.** The posterior laminal line between C1 and C3 should line up within 2 mm of the base of the C2 spinous process.

b. **Bone.** Check the general integrity of the following bony areas: vertebral bodies, facet joints, posterior spinous processes, and odontoid process (otherwise known as the dens). In addition, check the predental space (the distance between the posterior aspect of C1 and the anterior aspect of the odontoid process). This space should be <3 mm in the adult and <5 mm in the child (Fig. 3).

c. **Cartilage.** Check the intervertebral disk space for uniform height.

d. **Soft tissue.** Note any swelling in the prevertebral space, so that the normal configuration is assured. The prevertebral space should run parallel to the anterior vertebrae from C2 to C4 (Fig. 3). Swelling occurs in approximately

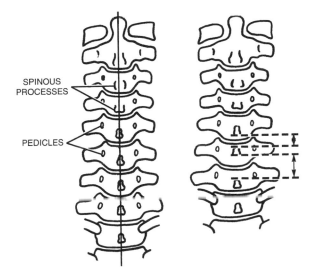

SPINOUS
PROCESSES

PEDICLES

Fig. 4. Prevertebral space of the cervical spine, anteroposterior view.

50% of bony injuries. One must investigate for ligamentous injuries if soft tissue swelling is present without any evident bony injuries.

(1) **Standard widths for adults:**
    (a) At C2, it should be less than 7 mm.
    (b) At C3-C4, it should be less than 5 mm.
    (c) At C6, it should be less than 22 mm.

(2) **Standard widths for children:**
    (a) At C3-C4, it should be less than two-thirds the width of the body of C2.
    (b) At C6, it should be less than 14 mm.

2. **Anteroposterior (AP) view**
  a. Inspect spinous processes such that they are viewed to be in a straight line. Malalignment may indicate a unilateral facet dislocation. A single spinous process out of alignment may indicate a fracture.
  b. Check the distances between the intraspinous processes such that they are noted to be equal. No single space should be 50% wider than the one immediately above or below it (Fig. 4). Abnormal widening of an intraspinous space is indicative of an anterior cervical dislocation. Malalignment occurs with fractures and bilateral facet dislocations. Furthermore,

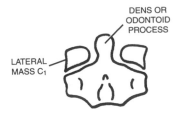

Fig. 5. Cervical spine, dens view.

one must check the pedicles to make sure that they appear as upright ovals, and these must be viewed for any evidence of fractures. You must also look at the intervertebral disk spaces to make sure that they are equal. As a final check, look at the vertebral bodies for any evidence of fractures or of rib fractures or pneumothoraces in the upper chest regions.

3. **Odontoid (open-mouth) view.** Check that lateral margins of C1 align with lateral margins of C2 (Fig. 5). Space on each side of the odontoid should be equal. Slight rotation of the neck may cause the spaces to appear unequal. The lateral margins of C1 and C2 should remain normally aligned if the injury is due to rotation. Inspect the odontoid and the rest of C2 for fractures. Overlying shadows may cause artifact due to superimposition of the arch of C1, incisor teeth, occiput, or soft tissue at the nape of the neck.

4. **Oblique views.** Standard oblique views require motion of the neck and are therefore contraindicated in trauma patients. They must, however, be considered in trauma patients when the three-view series suggests possible fractures or locked facets. Check for the "shingles on the roof" appearance of overlapping laminae and for any signs of disruption in this pattern that would be suggestive of a facet dislocation (Fig. 6). The laminae should appear as intact ellipses posteriorly, and this area must be scrutinized for any fractures. The interlaminar distance should be equal, and any increase in this distance is highly suggestive of a subluxation.

5. **Flexion-extension views.** These views are undertaken when plain radiographs are normal but there is a high index of suspicion for ligamentous injuries. In addition, if there is any focal posterior midline cervical tenderness or severe cervical pain, these views must also be entertained. In order to accomplish these views, the patient must be sober, cooperative, neurologically intact, and be able to move the neck independently. Neck motion should be performed actively by the patient

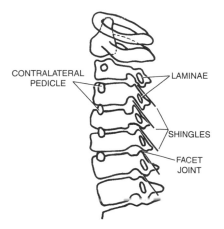

CONTRALATERAL PEDICLE

LAMINAE

SHINGLES

FACET JOINT

Fig. 6. Cervical spine, oblique view.

and should cease immediately if increased pain, parethesias, or neurological signs develop. Some of these flexion-extension views are performed under fluoroscopy with neurosurgical supervision. These views are checked for interruption of contour lines or widening of the interspinous spaces on the lateral view.

B. **Computed tomography (CT)**
1. **General principles.** Order 2- to 3-mm cuts above and below the area of interest. Contrast is not necessary.
2. **Indications**
   a. Fractures seen or suspected on plain radiographs should be followed up by CT for better definition.
   b. If the plain radiographs are inadequate or if you cannot visualize all the cervical vertebrae or the C7-T1 articulation on the lateral radiograph and there is a high clinical suspicion of an injury despite normal plain films, then CT scan of the affected area is warranted.
3. **Advantages and disadvantages.** The advantages of CT are that it produces excellent images of complex bony anatomy and the patient can remain in spinal immobilization while the spinal cord and canal are fully evaluated. These studies are of limited utility, however, in evaluating ligamentous disruptions, and there is poor visualization of horizontally oriented fractures on axial reconstruction.

C. **Magnetic resonance imaging (MRI)** is the imaging modality of choice for detecting neurological injury.

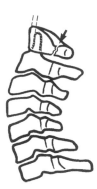

Fig. 7.   Jefferson fracture of
the cervical spine, lateral view.

1. **Advantage.** There is direct visualization of intra- and extramedullary spinal abnormalities.
2. **Disadvantages**
   a. Is incompatible with life-support equipment.
   b. Lacks high resolution for bony anatomy.
   c. Is often not readily available.
   d. Is time-consuming.
3. **Contraindications.** Metallic foreign bodies (pacemaker, cerebral aneurysm clips, prosthetic joints, etc.).

IV. **Cervical spine injuries**
  A. **Cervical strain.** Neck pain, stiffness, and the absence of positive findings on radiographic evaluation are usually due to paravertebral muscle spasm. If there is associated arm pain, the possibility of cervical disk protrusion or nerve root compression must be entertained. These are nonemergency problems for which the patient needs symptomatic relief of pain, a cervical collar, rest, mild analgesics, and the appropriate follow-up.
  B. **"Whiplash"** is a hyperextension injury usually caused by "rear-end" motor vehicle accidents. This injury has become much less frequent with the advent of high seat backs and head rests that block hyperextension of the neck. The injury is to the soft tissues of the neck and the appropriate treatment is symptomatic. Radiographs in both of these situations are usually normal, although one may see straightening of the normal lordosis, which is a nonspecific finding.

V. **Types of fractures**
  A. **Jefferson fracture (Fig. 7).** A break in the osseous ring of C1.
    1. **Prevalence.** Accounts for 2% to 13% of cervical spine fractures.
    2. **Mechanism.** This fracture is the result of indirect force, usually due to a blow to the vertex or a fall on the head. The weakest part in the arch of

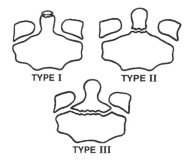

Fig. 8. Classification of odontoid
fractures of the cervical spine, dens view.

C1 is the posterior segment. It usually fractures
with the neck in slight extension. Flexion favors
fracture of the anterior arch.

3. **Presentation.** The patient presents with a stiff
neck, inability to nod or rotate the head, and sits
as if holding a weight on the head, refusing to
move it. In a patient with pain localized to this
area, the index of suspicion for a cervical spine injury should be very high. Neurological deficits are
rare in nonfatal injuries.

4. **Radiographic evaluation.** Lateral and open-
mouth views are essential. The lateral film may
reveal an increase in the retropharyngeal soft tissue space. The open-mouth view may reveal a
spread in the lateral masses, which, if greater
than 7 mm, is indicative of instability.

5. **Complications.** One-third of the patients have
associated odontoid or other cervical spine fractures. A high index of suspicion warrants a search
for these associated injuries.

6. **Treatment.** This fracture requires immobilization with a skeletal fixation device such as the
"halo" or Gardner-Wells tongs.

B. **Odontoid fractures** (Fig. 8). A fracture through the
odontoid process that does not involve the body of C2.

1. **Classification.** There are basically three types
of odontoid fracture; these can help in predicting
prognosis, healing, and stability.

   a. **Type I.** Avulsion of the apex of the odontoid.
   This is a very rare injury.

   b. **Type II.** A fracture at the base of the odontoid without involvement of the body of C2.
   This is unstable and has the highest rate of
   nonunion.

   c. **Type III.** A fracture of the body of C2. This is
   more stable than type II.

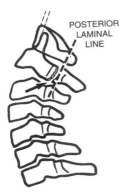

**Fig. 9.   Hangman's
fracture of the cervical spine.**

2. **Mechanism.** The etiology of odontoid fractures
   usually involves a combination of hyperextension
   and horizontal translation.
3. **Presentation.** The patient may complain of a
   feeling of impending doom and often presents
   with hands supporting the chin and occiput as if
   to prevent the head from "falling off." Pain may be
   localized to the occipital and suboccipital areas
   and is often accompanied by neck stiffness and
   spasm. Rarely is there an associated neurological
   deficit.
4. **Radiographic evaluation.** The open-mouth
   view often reveals the fracture. The lateral view
   is helpful to confirm any displacement of the fracture. If the index of suspicion is high and the routine cervical spine films are negative, tomography and/or CT scan of the affected area is then
   indicated.
5. **Treatment.** Type I fractures (rare) may be
   treated with a Philadelphia hard collar. For type
   II and III fractures, skeletal immobilization as
   quickly as possible is recommended.
C. **Hangman's fracture (Fig. 9).** A bilateral neural
   arch fracture of the axis (C2) without an odontoid
   fracture.
   1. **Mechanism.** Although the description correctly
      suggests the etiology of the fracture (i.e., a hang-
      ing), this injury is now commonly due to high-
      speed automobile accidents in which a combina-
      tion of hyperextension and axial compression is
      responsible for the injury.
   2. **Presentation.** The patient complains of neck
      stiffness and refuses to move the neck. Further
      history may elicit a compressive blow to the ver-
      tex. Neurological injury is uncommon because of
      the wide diameter of the spinal canal at this level.

3. **Radiographic evaluation.** AP and lateral films will reveal the fracture of the neural arch and whether or not subluxation is present. Subluxation is indicative of injury to the anterior or posterior longitudinal ligaments.
4. **Complications.** The fracture is unstable but heals readily with adequate immobilization. Associated fractures may be present in the lower cervical spine.
5. **Treatment.** Skeletal immobilization.

D. **"Burst" fracture.** This lesion involves a "bursting" or shattering of the vertebral body with fragments that may or may not impinge into the spinal canal.
1. **Mechanism.** Direct axial compression with the head in slight extension produces a bursting of the vertebral body. The most common level of the injury is C5.
2. **Presentation.** The patient often presents with a neurological deficit as a result of posterior protrusion of the bone or disk material into the spinal canal. A high incidence of neurological complications requires that the patient be carefully evaluated by either an orthopaedist or neurosurgeon to document the extent of the injury and also to initiate skeletal immobilization.
3. **Radiographic evaluation.** AP, lateral, and oblique films will demonstrate the fracture. An avulsion of the anteroinferior surface has been characteristically called a "teardrop" fracture. This is, in fact, a type of burst fracture. The serious problem associated with these fractures is caused by bone and/or disk material protruding into the spinal canal, causing cord compression. Although these injuries may appear relatively harmless, they can have very serious sequelae, including quadriplegia.
4. **Complications.** Neurological injury is quite variable, depending on the position and the amount of protruded material. Concomitant fractures of the cervical spine as well as closed head injury may also be present.
5. **Treatment.** In the presence of neurological deficit, immediate evaluation by an orthopaedist or neurosurgeon is recommended. Skeletal immobilization is mandatory.

E. **"Clay-shoveler's" fracture** (Fig. 10). This injury involves an avulsion of one or more of the lower cervical or upper thoracic spinous processes.
1. **Mechanism.** The fracture is due to forceful contracture of the muscles attaching to the posterior spinous processes, most commonly at C7.
2. **Presentation.** The patient presents with pain, stiffness in the neck, and tenderness that may be localized to the level of the avulsion fracture.

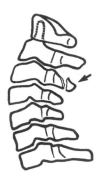

Fig. 10.   Clay-shoveler's
fracture of the cervical spine.

3. **Radiographic evaluation.** Lateral films of the cervical spine are the best to view the avulsion of the spinous process. It is a relatively stable fracture.
4. **Treatment.** Treatment is symptomatic, with analgesics and a soft collar.
F. **Atlantooccipital (C1) instability.** A complete atlantooccipital dislocation is usually fatal.
   1. **Mechanism.** A violent, twisting force of the head is usually the mechanism of injury. The degree of ligamentous injury determines the degree of instability of this joint.
   2. **Presentation.** The patient may present with pain and swelling in the neck and there may be no neurological deficit.
   3. **Radiographic evaluation.** Lateral films are necessary to evaluate this injury. The lateral films may reveal an increase in the retropharyngeal soft tissue space. The basion-odontoid relationship must be evaluated. Clinical instability is suggested if there is a horizontal translation of the odontoid below the basion greater than 1 mm or if there is a vertical distance between the odontoid and basion of greater than 5 mm. Flexion-extension views, if deemed necessary, should be obtained by the neurosurgeon or the orthopaedic surgeon and not the emergency physician.
   4. **Complications.** Owing to the highly unstable nature of this injury, treatment with skeletal traction may actually increase the displacement. Concomitant trauma of the cervical spine may also be present, as well as closed head injury.
   5. **Treatment.** Skeletal immobilization with careful application of traction is the treatment of choice. Radiographs must be taken once traction is applied to evaluate the distraction force on the injury.

G. **Atlantoaxial instability (C1-2).** This is an injury to the transverse ligament leading to instability of the C1-2 articulations.
  1. **Mechanisms.** Four different mechanisms, each causing a different injury, have been identified:
      a. **Anterior dislocation.** This injury is usually fatal because the cord is severely injured by compression between the neural arch posteriorly and an intact odontoid process anteriorly.
      b. **Anterior dislocation and odontoid fracture.** Here the neurological damage is variable, depending upon the extent of the injury.
      c. **Posterior dislocation.** This rare injury is due to a sudden extension of the head or a blow to the submental area. The atlas is dislocated posterior to the odontoid.
      d. **Rotatory subluxation.** This facet injury may produce irreducible torticollis if unilateral (it can be fatal if it is bilateral). The severity of these lesions can be related to the extent of the ligamentous injury.
  2. **Presentation.** Clinical presentation is variable owing to the nature of the injury and the different mechanisms involved. Pain and swelling of the neck are present with any type of movement.
  3. **Radiographic evaluation.** The lateral film is the most important, but it should not be relied on exclusively. On this film, careful measurements must be made to ascertain the relationship of the posterior arch of C1 to the anterior surface of the odontoid. The normal distance between C1 and C2 is 0 to 3 mm. This implies that the transverse ligaments are intact. A subluxation of 3 to 5 mm is indicative of rupture of the transverse ligament. Subluxation greater than 5 mm correlates with rupture of both the transverse and alar ligaments. This situation represents an unstable spine.
  4. **Complications.** Fracture of the lower cervical spine and closed head injuries may also be present.
  5. **Treatment.** Reduction of the subluxation and skeletal immobilization are needed as emergency treatment.
H. **Flexion "teardrop" fracture (Fig. 11).** A triangular fracture of the anteroinferior corner of the vertebral body. The involved vertebrae may be displaced and rotated.
  1. **Presentation.** Teardrop fractures are commonly seen after diving accidents. This can be an extremely unstable fracture/injury. It usually results from severe hyperflexion, causing disruption of all ligaments and facet joints. It is common to see the symptoms of anterior cord syndrome.

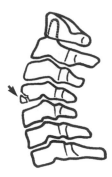

Fig. 11.   Flexion "teardrop"
fracture of the cervical spine.

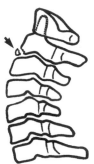

Fig. 12.   Extension "teardrop"
fracture of the cervical spine.

2. **Radiographic evaluation.** Besides plain films, a CT or MRI of the involved area may be helpful to assess the severity of the underlying injuries.
3. **Treatment** is based on the underlying injuries. Neurosurgical input is paramount for determining the final treatment plan.

I. **Extension "teardrop" fracture (Fig. 12).** This injury involves a triangular fragment that is avulsed from the anteroinferior vertebral body; it is best seen on the lateral radiograph. Note that radiographically, flexion and extension teardrop fractures are similar. It is the underlying mechanism of injury that differs and hence affects the prognosis. The most commonly involved area is C2, followed by C5-7.

1. **Presentation.** This injury is most commonly seen in older patients who fall, striking their chins. It is often associated with central cord syndrome.
2. **Radiographic evaluation.** As above for flexion teardrop fracture.
3. **Treatment.** As above for flexion teardrop fracture.

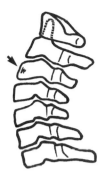

Fig. 13. Anterior wedge fracture of the cervical spine.

J. **Anterior wedge fracture (Fig. 13).** Radiographically, there is the appearance of a compressed anterior vertebral body. These anterior compressive forces are sometimes sufficient to cause impaction of one vertebra by adjacent vertebrae.
   1. **Presentation.** This lesion is most commonly seen in patients who have undergone a hyperflexion type of injury. Patients will often present with localized cervical spine pain.
   2. **Radiographic evaluation.** In most cases, plain films are sufficient. If there is concern about the extent of the injury, then tomography or CT scan can be performed.
   3. **Treatment.** This is generally a stable injury. Symptomatic treatment is usually all that is warranted.
K. **Lower cervical spine subluxation and dislocation.** The combination of hyperflexion and rotation is a common mechanism for dislocation or subluxation in the lower cervical spine.
   1. **Presentation.** The neck may be stiff and painful. Unilateral facet dislocation may be accompanied by symptoms of nerve root compression. There is usually no sign of cord injury, although in rare cases the Brown-Séquard syndrome may be present. Bilateral facet dislocation may be present, with symptoms of cord compression; this is frequently accompanied by quadriplegia.
   2. **Radiographic evaluation.** AP and lateral films are essential to evaluate the degree of subluxation. Oblique films are often helpful to better detect a facet fracture and loss of the normal facet articulations. Occasionally, tomograms are necessary. The essential evaluation is to be made on the lateral films. A subluxation of 25% of one vertebral body on the other is seen with a unilateral facet dislocation; this is an unstable injury. In association with facet dislocation one may see an

angular deformity of the vertebral bodies. This may be due to either a facet fracture or ligamentous injury. Lateral extension films may be necessary to elucidate this condition.

3. **Complications.** Neurological deficit may range from no injury to quadriplegia. In bilateral facet dislocation, stability is inversely proportional to the ease of reduction (i.e., the easier the reduction, the less stable the fracture and the greater the need for fixation).

4. **Treatment.** Reduction of the dislocation is essential. The unilateral facet dislocation is usually stable once reduced. Often, bilateral facet dislocations are unstable and require additional fixation.

BIBLIOGRAPHY

DeBehnke DJ, Havel CJ. Utility of prevertebral soft tissue measurements in identifying patients with cervical spine fractures. *Ann Emerg Med* 1994;24:1119–1124.

Hoppenfeld S. *Physical examination of the spine and extremities.* East Norwalk, CT: Appleton-Century-Crofts, 1976.

Macnab I, McCulloch J: *Neck ache and shoulder pain.* Baltimore. Williams & Wilkins, 1994.

Neviaser RJ, Eisenfeld LS, Wiesel SW, Lewis RJ. *Emergency orthopaedic radiology.* New York: Churchill Livingstone, 1985.

Rubinstein D, Escott EJ, Mestek MF. Computed tomographic scans of minimally displaced type II odontoid fractures. *J Trauma* 1996;40:204–210.

Scaletta TA, Schaider JJ. *Emergent management of trauma.* New York: McGraw-Hill, 1996.

Turetsky DB, Vines FS, Clayman DA, Northup HM. Technique and use of supine oblique views in acute cervical spine trauma. *Ann Emerg Med* 1993;22:685–689.

Lumbar Spine Injuries

Angelo Grillo and Robert E. O'Connor

The evaluation and management of lumbar spine injuries in emergency medicine requires a systematic and thorough approach. Historical aspects predict the type and degree of injury, while the physical examination refines the area of concern and details the degree of neurological involvement. Ancillary tests help confirm the diagnosis and guide consultation and referral. This chapter details the historical and physical components of the evaluation of lumbar injuries. Normal anatomy, physiology, and radiology are described, followed by an overview of pathophysiological mechanisms and treatment. The discussion then focuses on some of the more likely specific injuries.

I. **Normal anatomy and physiology.** A description of the normal anatomical and physiological characteristics of the lumbar spine aids in the evaluation and defines specific injuries.

   A. **General.** A lordotic curvature exists at the level of the lumbar vertebrae, allowing for the dissipation of axial loads away from the vertebral bodies and to the disks and musculature. As a result, disk and soft tissue injuries are more common than fractures.

      1. **Twelfth thoracic through the second lumbar vertebrae.** This portion of the thoracolumbar spine is most prone to injury.

         a. This is where the transition from thoracic kyphosis to lumbar lordosis occurs.

         b. This is also the area of transition between the relatively fixed thoracic spine, which is buttressed by the ribs, and the free lumbar spine.

      2. The spine can be considered to be formed by two columns: **anterior** and **posterior.** The anterior column is formed by the vertebral bodies, disks, and longitudinal ligaments. The posterior column consists of the vertebral arch, its processes, and the accessory ligaments that connect them. Disruption in both columns causes instability and constitutes a high risk for neurological injury. Isolated disruption of either one may not disrupt mechanical stability, thereby reducing the likelihood of cord injury.

      3. The renal pedicles lie at the level of the second lumbar vertebra, the third and fourth lumbar vertebrae generally meet at the level of the umbilicus, and the fourth lumbar vertebra is at the level of the top of the iliac crest.

      4. The number of lumbar vertebrae may vary. These are some of the commonly seen variants:

   a. The twelfth thoracic vertebra may have no
       associated ribs and resemble the lumbar
       vertebrae.
   b. The first lumbar vertebra may have ribs and
       thus resemble the thoracic vertebrae.
   c. The fifth lumbar vertebra may be com-
       pletely or partially fused with the sacrum.

B. Skeletal

1. The **vertebral body** (anterior) is the major
    weight-bearing structure. It is limited superi-
    orly and inferiorly by end plates with epiphyseal
    rings of Schmorl. Congenital defects in these
    end plates, where the disk protrudes into the
    body of the vertebra, are known as **Schmorl's
    nodes.** These usually result from trauma and
    are not congenital.

2. The **vertebral arch** (posterior) arises from the
    posterolateral aspects of the body bilaterally
    and consists of:
    a. Two **pedicles,** which arise from the pos-
        terior, superior aspect of the vertebral bod-
        ies.
    b. Two **laminae,** which meet in the midline
        posteriorly, where they join and give rise to
        the **spinous process,** directed posteriorly.
    c. Two **transverse processes,** which arise at
        the union of the pedicle with the lamina and
        are directed laterally.
    d. **Articular processes,** which arise at the
        union of the pedicle with the lamina and
        consist of two **superior** articular processes
        and two **inferior** articular processes.

C. Foramen

1. The **vertebral foramen** is a cavity formed by
    the union of the body and arch. Stacked foram-
    ina form the vertebral canal, through which
    passes the spinal cord and its coverings.

2. **Intervertebral foramina** are directed later-
    ally. They are bordered:
    a. Superiorly and posteriorly by a notch in the
        pedicle of the vertebra above.
    b. Inferiorly and posteriorly by the anterior
        surface of the superior articular process.
    c. Anteriorly, the superior aspect is bordered
        by the body of the vertebra and the inferior
        aspect by the intervertebral disk.

3. Conveys the spinal nerve and blood vessels.

D. Muscular

1. Anteriorly, the **psoas** muscles sit in the angle
    formed by the bodies and transverse processes.

2. Posteriorly, the **erector spinatus** fills the space
    between the spinous and transverse processes.

3. The abdominal musculature works in conjunc-
    tion with the lumbar spine to provide truncal

support in the region between the thorax and the pelvis.

E. **Joints**
1. **Facets.** The anterolateral surface of the inferior articular process of one vertebra fits with the posteromedial surface of the superior articular process of the vertebra below, meeting in the sagittal plane. The facets form a synovial **facet joint,** which provides for flexion and some extension in the lumbar region but limits rotation and lateral bending.
2. **Intervertebral disks**
   a. Fibrocartilaginous structures separating successive vertebral bodies.
   b. Act to allow flexion in any direction between vertebrae.
   c. Act to absorb and dissipate axial truncal loading by compressing and bending.
   d. Relatively avascular structures that depend on diffusion for their nutrition. The disk between the fifth lumbar and first sacral vertebrae is the largest avascular structure in the body, which contributes to its propensity to undergo degenerative changes. It is composed of
      (1) Superior and inferior **cartilaginous plates** that abut and adhere to the bony end plates of the vertebrae above and below, respectively.
      (2) The **annulus fibrosus**
         (a) At its superior and inferior borders join the cartilaginous plates.
         (b) Anterolaterally blends into and is bordered by the anterior longitudinal ligament.
         (c) Posteriorly is bordered by and merges with the posterior longitudinal ligament, forming the weakest portion of the annulus.
         (d) The relative size difference between the thicker anterior portion and the thinner posterior portion gives the lumbar disks a wedge shape and provides for the lumbar lordosis.
      (3) **Nucleus pulposus**
         (a) The semiliquid central mass of the disk, which, with aging, undergoes fibrotic changes and dehydration.
         (b) It is encapsulated by the annulus fibrosus and cartilaginous plates.

F. **Ligaments** act to unite the bony elements and stabilize the entire column.
   1. **Longitudinal ligaments**

  a. The **anterior longitudinal ligament** is a thick, broad band that runs down the anterior surface of the vertebral bodies. It blends with and attaches to the anterior portion of the intervertebral disks.

  b. The **posterior longitudinal ligament** is a less substantial structure present on the dorsal surfaces of the vertebral bodies. It, too, blends with and attaches to the intervertebral disks.

2. **Accessory ligaments**

  a. The **supraspinous ligament** runs dorsally over the tips of the spinous processes.

  b. The supraspinous ligament blends ventrally with the **interspinous ligaments,** which connect adjacent spinous processes.

  c. The **ligamentum flavum** interconnects adjacent laminae laterally. The void between is taken up by a venous plexus.

  d. The **intertransverse ligaments** lie between adjacent transverse processes in the lumbar region only.

G. **Neurological**

1. The **spinal medulla (cord)** passes through the lumbar spinal canal to the level of the first (second in early life) lumbar vertebra, where it terminates as the **conus medullaris,** which is tethered to the coccyx by a fibrous band—the **filum terminale.**

  a. From this point, lumbar and sacral nerve roots proceed caudally as the **cauda equina.**

  b. It occupies only one-third of the space of the spinal canal in the lumbar region.

2. The cord is ensheathed by the **spinal meninges.**

  a. **Dura mater**

    (1) The outermost meningeal layer running to the level of the upper sacrum.

    (2) The epidural space between the dura and the periosteum of the bony canal contains fat and a rich, valveless venous plexus.

  b. The **arachnoid** closely approximates the inner surface of the dura.

  c. **Pia mater**

    (1) The pia mater is a thick white membrane that adheres closely to the surface of the spinal medulla.

    (2) The **ligamentum denticulatum** passes from the pia through the arachnoid and attaches to the dura, allowing for support of the medulla.

    (3) Cerebrospinal fluid circulates in the subarachnoid space between the arachnoid and the pia mater.

3. The cord gives rise to bilateral paired nerve roots: the **anterior (motor) root** and the **posterior (sensory) root.** The roots join in the intervertebral canal to form the segmental nerve.

4. **Spinal nerves** pass out of the intervertebral canal through its superior aspect, where they split into the

a. **Dorsal rami,** which pass posteriorly, supplying the back with motor and sensory innervation.

b. **Ventral rami**, which pass into the psoas muscles.

(1) The first four ventral lumbar rami form the **lumbar plexus** and innervate the psoas and quadratus muscles; they form the femoral, obturator, and lateral cutaneous nerves of the thigh.

(2) The fourth and fifth lumbar rami contribute to the **lumbosacral plexus,** which passes through the greater sciatic foramen and enters the gluteal region as the **sciatic nerve** and further divides to provide innervation to the leg.

5. Several important **innervations** that will aid in examination are outlined below.

a. **Motor**

(1) L2 and L3 innervate hip flexors.

(2) L3 and L4 innervate knee extensors.

(3) L4 and L5 innervate ankle dorsiflexors.

(4) L5 and S1 innervate ankle plantarflexors.

(5) S2 and S4 innervate the rectal sphincter.

b. **Sensory**

(1) L2 innervates the lateral thigh.

(2) L3 innervates the medial thigh.

(3) L4 innervates the medial calf.

(4) L5 innervates the anterolateral calf.

(5) S1 innervates the lateral foot.

(6) S2 and S4 innervate the perianal area.

c. **Reflex arcs**

(1) L2, L3, and L4 mediate the knee jerk (patellar).

(2) S1 mediates the ankle jerk (Achilles).

H. **Vascular**

1. **Arterial.** Lumbar arteries from the aorta provide branches that track along the ventral and dorsal roots of the spinal nerves to form the **ventral** and **dorsal radicular arteries,** respectively.

a. The dorsal radicular arteries anastomose to form the **posterior spinal arteries** and feed the posterior portion of the spinal cord.

b. The ventral arteries anastomose to form the **anterior spinal arteries** and supply the anterior, motor portion of the spinal cord. Many of these anastomoses regress as development proceeds; thus one ventral radicular artery, termed the **anterior artery of Adamkiewicz,** may supply many segments.

2. **Venous.** Anterior and posterior median channels lie adjacent to their respective portions of the spinal cord and are connected by valveless intersegmental veins.

II. **Evaluation of the lumbar spine.** The multiply or severely injured patient should be approached in a systematic fashion. An initial survey should be performed with attention to **airway, breathing, circulation** (the ABCs) and neurological **disability.** During this assessment, attention should be given to resuscitation and life- and limb-threatening injuries. Examination of the lumbar spine should be performed during the secondary survey. If there is potential for any spinal injuries, the patient's spine should be maintained in a neutral and rigid position. For transfers, a rigid backboard is indicated with securing straps at the levels of the head, shoulder girdle, and pelvis.

A. **History.** Certain mechanisms are associated with specific injuries.

1. **Falls**
   a. Height of fall
   b. Position at impact
   c. Surface impacted

2. **Vehicle and vehicle/pedestrian collisions**
   a. Presence of lap belt, shoulder harness, and air bag
   b. Speed, angle of impact, vehicular damage
   c. Location and number of impacts

3. **Penetrating injuries**
   a. Gunshot wounds
      (1) Caliber
      (2) Number of shots fired
      (3) Distance fired from
   b. Stab wounds
      (1) Length and type of implement
      (2) Number of wounds

4. **Timing of presentation**
   a. acute
   b. subacute
   c. nonacute

5. **Pain**
   a. **Timing.** Pain that is worst at onset is more commonly associated with bony injury. Pain that becomes more severe with time is more likely to be from a muscular injury.
   b. **Location.** Midline pain is associated with bony pathology.
   c. **Radiation** down the leg implies radicular involvement.

6. **Neurological deficit.** Is there dysethesia, paresthesia, or anesthesia? Is there weakness or paralysis? Are any of these symptoms transiently present?
7. **Preexisting conditions** such as arthritis or neurological deficits
8. **Comorbid factors** such as intoxicants or head injury
9. **Immunization status**
10. **Medications**
11. **Allergies**

B. **Examination**
   1. Inspect the abdomen for hematomas and open wounds. Males should be checked for priapism.
   2. Palpate the pelvis for evidence of fracture. Evidence of pelvic fracture should prompt radiological evaluation for lumbar injuries, owing to their frequent coexistence.
   3. Perform a brief focused neurological examination, including reflexes, rectal tone, touch, movement, and proprioception of the lower extremities. Any abnormality should prompt complete and repeated neurological examination.
   4. Turn the patient to inspect and palpate the back.
      a. The spine should be maintained in a neutral position. This is achieved by "log rolling." One examiner controls the cervical spine and directs all movement. Other examiners are spaced along the body to provide sufficient support so the entire patient is rolled as a unit. The patient is a passive participant.
      b. The back is observed for evidence of penetration, malalignment, hematoma, and erythema. The spine is palpated and percussed over the spinous processes and any tenderness is noted.
      c. Persistent, localized tenderness has been associated with up to a 30% incidence of fracture despite normal radiological evaluation.
      d. Costovertebral angles and paraspinal muscles should be palpated for tenderness and spasm.
      e. A rectal exam should be performed, noting tone and sensation.
      f. The patient should be returned to the supine position by the log-rolling technique.

C. **Radiographic examination.** If the patient has intact neurological status and a normal neurological exam, is not intoxicated or distracted by other injury, and the evaluation specified above is unremarkable, the lumbar spine exam can be considered clinically normal. An important caveat is that many findings in the multiply injured trauma patient are revealed only on serial examinations. Patients with a normal lumbar spine exam and without high-risk injuries (pelvic fracture or other spinal fractures) do not require radiological evaluation of the lumbar spine.

If the above criteria are not met, radiological evaluation is indicated. Begin with lateral and anteroposterior (AP) views of the lumbar spine. If evaluation of these radiographs is normal (as described below) and there is no neurological impairment, the series may be completed, allowing the patient to move more freely.

The presence of persistent or transient neurological deficit should prompt aggressive evaluation, computed tomography (CT), and/or magnetic resonance imaging (MRI) despite normal initial radiographs.

1. **Plain radiographs.** In general, radiographs should be assessed for **adequacy, alignment, bony integrity, cartilage and joints,** and **soft tissue.** Evidence of any spinal fracture mandates a complete radiographic spinal series owing to the high likelihood (up to 30%) of noncontiguous vertebral fracture.

   a. **Anteroposterior (frontal)**
      (1) **Adequacy**
         (a) The film cassette is positioned to include the superior aspects of the pelvis and lower thoracic vertebrae with ribs.
         (b) Adequate penetration should delineate all bony structures but allow for soft tissue to be seen as well.
      (2) **Alignment**
         (a) Spinous processes should proceed cephalad to caudad in the centers of the vertebral bodies with good alignment and without break or step-off.
         (b) The pedicles should appear as sclerotic ovals within the bodies of the vertebrae and should be aligned cephalad to caudad.
         (c) The spinal canal should appear as a relatively translucent column through the center of the bodies, with smooth margins.
      (3) **Bones**
         (a) Each body should appear rectangular, with aligned concave lateral borders and parallel linear end plates. In patients with increased lumbar lordosis, the fifth lumbar vertebra will overlap the upper sacrum.

    (b) Transverse processes should appear symmetrical with smooth, uninterrupted borders. The slightly cephalad orientation of the fourth lumbar vertebra's transverse processes aids in identifying location.

    (c) Visible portions of the pelvis, sacrum, sacroiliac joints, lower ribs, and lower thoracic vertebrae should be examined for abnormality.

(4) Cartilage and ligaments. Disks should appear symmetrical in height.

(5) Soft tissue shadows of the spleen, liver, kidneys, and psoas muscles should be evaluated.

b. Lateral

  (1) Adequacy

    (a) The beam is focused just above the umbilicus at the level of the third lumbar vertebra.

    (b) Thoracic vertebrae, five lumbar vertebrae, and the sacrum should all be visible.

  (2) Alignment

    (a) Smooth lines of curvature should be formed by the anterior and posterior borders of the vertebral bodies as well as the tips of the spinous processes.

    (b) Each succeeding inferior articular process should overlap the preceding superior articular process.

  (3) Bones

    (a) Each body should appear rectangular, with aligned concave anterior and posterior borders and parallel linear end plates. A small break in the midposterior cortex of the body can be recognized as a penetrating vein. Otherwise, any break in the cortex should be considered a fracture.

    (b) The paired pedicles should be attached to the posterosuperior aspect of the vertebral body.

    (c) The spinous process should have a smooth, uninterrupted margin.

    (d) The intervertebral foramen should appear spacious, with smooth borders.

(4) Cartilage and joints. Disk spaces should be symmetrical and bordered by parallel adjacent end plates.

    c. **Oblique.** This view provides unilateral evaluation of interfacet joints, pedicles (pars interarticularis), articular processes, and intervertebral foramen. This requires patient motion and should be reserved for the patient with stable injuries.

    d. A **lumbosacral,** L5-S1, lateral coned-down view has the radiation beam centered at the level of the fifth lumbar disk to provide evaluation of disk height.

    e. **Flexion** and **extension** views can be performed to assess ligamentous stability.

2. **Tomography**

    a. **Plain** tomography has been largely supplanted by computed tomography and magnetic resonance imaging, but it can provide useful information about longitudinally oriented bony injuries.

    b. **Computed tomography** (CT) is the study of choice for bony vertebral injuries.

    c. **Magnetic resonance imaging** (MRI) is ideal for assessing soft tissue injuries—i.e., ligamentous and neurological.

    d. **Radionucleotide imaging (bone scanning)** helps differentiate acute from nonacute injuries and to identify occult injuries. Such scans may remain abnormal for up to 18 months after injury.

    e. **Myelography** has been replaced by MRI.

III. **Traumatic injuries**

A. **Mechanism of injury.** Spine injuries are categorized according to the mechanism of injury. Certain mechanisms produce characteristic injuries to the spinal column and cord. The twelfth thoracic vertebra is included in evaluating lumbar injuries because of its propensity for injury along with and in a manner similar to that of the upper lumbar vertebrae. Two-thirds of lumbar injuries occur in the thoracolumbar region. Fifteen percent of thoracolumbar fractures are associated with neurological injury. Neurogenic shock with bradycardic hypotension has been associated with thoracolumbar injuries.

1. **Hyperflexion**

    a. Most common mechanism of lumbar spine injury.

    b. Caused by axial loading—commonly a fall onto the feet or buttocks.

    c. Occurs most frequently in the upper lumbar region.

    d. Posterior elements are distracted while anterior ones are compressed.

    e. Results in wedged compression fractures of the vertebral body, spinous process fracture, or both.

2. **Compression**
   a. Caused by axial loading from falls onto the feet or buttocks.
   b. Results in burst fractures of the vertebral body or rupture of the intervertebral disk.

3. **Flexion/rotation**
   a. Most common mechanism of fracture associated with dislocation.
   b. Commonly occurs in the unrestrained motor vehicle occupant.
   c. May result in pure dislocation injury.

4. **Hyperextension**
   a. Occurs through axial loading of an extended lumbar spine.
   b. Typical patients are movers, weight lifters, and football players.
   c. Results in traumatic spondylolisthesis.

5. **Hyperextension/shear**
   a. Occurs commonly with falls and in pedestrians struck by motor vehicles.
   b. Translational (shear forces) are applied to one portion of the spine with sudden acceleration (or deceleration) while the remainder of the spine is hyperextended about the point of impact.
   c. Results in fracture/dislocation injuries.

6. **Flexion/distraction**
   a. Accounts for less than 10% of lumbar fractures.
   b. Occurs with sudden forward acceleration about a fixed fulcrum—typically when a motor vehicle occupant, wearing only a lap belt, undergoes sudden deceleration in a head-on collision and flexes about the belt—or in a fall from a height. The "seat-belt sign" is a harbinger of this injury when ecchymosis across the abdominal wall is present.
   c. May result in a **Chance fracture.**
   d. There is a high incidence of intraabdominal injury and aggressive workup for solid and hollow organ injuries must be pursued.

7. **Lateral bending**
   a. Occurs in lateral-impact motor vehicle accidents and falls onto the side.
   b. Results in unilateral compression fracture toward the side of flexion or transverse process fracture away from the side of flexion.

8. **Penetrating injuries**
   a. Usually the result of gunshots.
   b. Typically produce stable injuries.
   c. Surgical intervention should be pursued in the same manner as for blunt traumatic injuries. Debridement can be done when the patient is stable.

9. **Neurological injuries**
    a. Both peripheral (nerve) as well as central (spinal cord) injuries result from one of three mechanisms.
        (1) **Traction.** Routinely poor prognosis.
        (2) **Compression.** Recovery is dependent upon the degree and duration of compression.
        (3) **Shock.** Lack of required nutrients resulting in cell death. Unlike the case with traction and compression, shock is usually a secondary injury that can be prevented or limited with proper attention to oxygenation and hemodynamics.
    b. Presence of paralysis associated with intact deep tendon reflexes defines a central (spinal cord) lesion, while paralysis without reflexes defines a peripheral (nerve) lesion.
    c. **Types of incomplete injuries**
        (1) **Anterior cord syndrome.** Motor, pain, and temperature deficits with preservation of proprioception and vibration, associated with flexion mechanisms.
        (2) **Brown-Séquard syndrome.** Ipsilateral motor loss with contralateral pain and temperature loss, associated with penetrating injuries.
        (3) **Conus medullaris syndrome.** Terminal cord injury with areflexic bowel, bladder, and lower extremities. Sacral sparing—perianal sensation, rectal tone, or toe flexion indicating a partial cord lesion—is occasionally present.
        (4) **Cauda equina syndrome.** Lumbosacral nerve root (peripheral) injury with areflexic bowel, bladder, and lower extremities. Injury occurs below the level of spinal cord termination (L2). This is commonly a complete injury. Deficits are usually irreversible.
        (5) **"Spinal shock"** mimics a complete lesion initially with recovery of some upper motor neuron spinal cord activity.
            (a) Typically resolves in 24 hours.
            (b) Its resolution is heralded by return of the bulbocavernosus reflex; compression of the penis (or traction on a Foley catheter) produces contraction of the anal sphincter.
            (c) Any neurological deficit present at the time of recovery from spinal shock is likely to be permanent.

B. **Neurological status.** In evaluating an injury to the spine, it is of prime importance to assess neurological status completely and repeatedly.

1. Any evidence of neurological disability indicates mechanical instability.

2. Evidence of an incomplete spinal cord lesion provides for the possibility of significant recovery and mandates a search for surgically correctable lesions (decompression).

3. Evidence of progressive neurological deterioration or ascending levels of disability should prompt treatment as for a partial lesion and be pursued aggressively.

4. Evidence of a complete spinal cord lesion—no distal cord activity—indicates a poor prognosis for any neurological recovery. It may dictate delayed or no surgical intervention.

C. **Treatment.** The treatment of these injuries assumes that other potentially life-threatening injuries have been addressed and a detailed investigation for other injuries has been done. As mentioned in Sec. II, it is important to prevent further injury through immobilization on a rigid backboard, with the patient secured above and below the site of potential injury until stability is assured.

1. **Goals of therapy**
   a. To achieve reduction
   b. To provide stability
   c. To allow for any possible peripheral nerve recovery
   d. To prevent further morbidity
   e. To promote early mobilization and rehabilitation.

2. **General principles**
   a. All fractures should be referred to a spinal surgeon experienced in the treatment of traumatic injuries. Consideration should be given to admission for a period of observation to exclude neurological deterioration and occult cord injury.
   b. Once patients are stable, they should be treated in regional spinal centers whenever possible.
   c. Stable fractures without neurological injury can be managed with an initial period of bed rest, followed by physical therapy and 4 to 6 months of external bracing.
   d. Intestinal ileus has been known to accompany lumbar fractures and should be accounted for in the management and disposition of these patients.
   e. The use of **systemic steroids** has been reported to be of incremental benefit in improving the outcome of patients with spinal

cord injury. It should be initiated within 8 hours of injury to be of any benefit. Initially a bolus of 30 mg/kg of methylprednisolone is given, followed by 5.4 mg/kg per hour for 23 hours.

3. Postural reduction

a. The patient is maintained in a neutral position (zero degrees of flexion, extension, and bending) while being log-rolled periodically to prevent pressure injuries.

b. May be used for fractures with complete neurological injury.

c. Must be closely followed radiologically and clinically to reassess fracture stability.

d. Requires prolonged bed rest and may hinder rehabilitation.

e. Poor results as compared with surgery in most series.

4. Surgery. The surgical management of the patient with lumbar spinal injury is controversial. If surgery is to be effective, it should be accomplished early (under 4 hours from onset of injury).

a. **Indications**

(1) Emergent surgery is clearly indicated in patients with progressive neurological deterioration and those with open fractures. Remember tetanus and antibiotics.

(2) Emergent surgery is thought by many to be indicated for patients with partial cord lesions. It has been shown to improve neurological recovery in animal models but not in humans.

(3) Patients with complete cord injuries or those with mechanically unstable injuries without neurological insult can undergo delayed surgical intervention.

(4) Surgical repair generally decreases the rate of complications, length of hospitalization and rehabilitation, and cost.

b. **Techniques**

(1) Routine laminectomy is generally ineffective for relieving neural compression.

(2) Neural compression from fracture/dislocations can be approached via an anterior technique, a posterior technique, or a combination of both.

(3) Fixation is accomplished via rodding, wiring, or both.

(a) Harrington distraction rods mounted in the recess formed by the lateral masses and spinous processes.

Through bilateral distraction on the lateral masses stabilization and reduction of the fracture is achieved.

(b) Harrington contraction rods are mounted similarly to distraction rods except that contractive forces are applied to the lateral masses, resulting in reduction and straightening.

c. **Complications**

(1) Neurological deterioration from inadvertent cord trauma can occur in the perioperative period

(2) Hardware dislodgment resulting in neurological deterioration, loss of correction, or both

(3) Bony nonunion, which is common

IV. **Specific injuries**

A. **Wedge fractures** account for 60% of all spinal injuries.

1. **Generally stable** owing to intact posterior elements. In acute traumatic wedge fractures, it is important to prove that the posterior elements are intact, usually through the use of CT. If there is greater than 50% loss in vertebral height, there is the potential for the fracture to be unstable.

2. **Mechanism of injury.** Results from forcing of the posterior fragments into the canal, with marked angulation and narrowing of the canal. Both should be radiographically evident.

3. **Radiographs.** Loss of anterior height, disruption of the superior end plate, and an intact posterior cortical margin are seen.

a. A discrepancy of 2 mm or more in the height of the anterior and posterior cortical lines of the bodies of L2 through L5 indicates a fracture.

b. Generally, angulation of less than 10 degrees is present.

4. **Treatment**

a. Bed rest for 3 to 5 days followed by crutch walking for another week and physical therapy. Healing is complete in 4 to 6 months.

b. May require compression rods and fusion.

c. If left untreated, may result in marked kyphosis, pain, and neurological impairment.

B. **Multiple acute wedge fractures**

1. **Potentially unstable** and should be addressed in a manner similar to that of the single severe wedge fracture.

2. **Radiographs.** The age of these fractures cannot be determined radiographically. Therapy should be based on clinical findings.
3. **Treatment.** Those associated with osteoporosis generally require no intervention other than symptomatic relief.
4. Association with malignancy must be considered.
5. In the osteoporotic patient, little or no trauma is required to cause these injuries.

C. **Burst fractures** typically occur in upper lumbar vertebrae and are often associated with laminar fracture.
1. **Most are unstable.** Neurological impairment is caused by protrusion of posterior elements into the canal, impinging on the spinal cord. This has been reported in up to 50% of lumbar burst fractures.
2. **Radiographs**
   a. The frontal projection reveals biconcave disruption of the end plates and lateral displacement of body fragments. Widening of the interpedicular distance occurs.
   b. Laterally the appearance is similar, with ventral and dorsal displacement of body fragments.
   c. Loss of height is noted in both projections.
   d. CT is required to assess the degree of spinal canal encroachment and associated injuries.
3. **Treatment.** These injuries require surgical repair.

D. **Fracture/dislocations**
1. **Unstable.** They often result in neurological injuries.
2. **Mechanism of injury.** Flexion with rotation is the most common cause of fracture/dislocation.
   a. Seen as fracture of the superior aspect of the body associated with facet fracture or dislocation and rupture of the posterior ligaments.
   b. Most commonly occurs in the T12-to-L2 transition zone.
3. **Treatment.** Often requires open reduction for stabilization. Amenable to the application of distraction rods if the anterior longitudinal ligament is intact; otherwise compression rods are necessary.
4. **Specific injuries**
   a. **Hyperextension with shear** commonly causes fracture of the inferior aspect of the body, associated with pedicle disruption. Commonly the superior elements will be seen to be posteriorly displaced with respect to the inferior elements. Management with

fixation or rod stabilization is dependent upon the degree of instability.

b. **Traumatic spondylolisthesis with pedicle fracture** is a stable injury without neurological impairment. Managed symptomatically and with a body cast for 4 to 6 weeks followed by physical therapy.

c. **Hyperflexion with distraction** causes fracture through the body, laminae, pedicles, and spinous processes with ligamentous disruption—the Chance fracture. Classically, the injury is limited to one vertebra. Multiple variations occur through distribution of the fracture across multiple vertebrae. Radiographs show separation of the posterior elements in the lateral view and lateral angulation of the spine in the frontal view. There is a high incidence of associated intraperitoneal injury. Treatment is open fixation.

d. **Fracture/dislocations at the lumbosacral junction,** unlike the thoracolumbar junction, are rare injuries resulting from significant distraction with or without rotation.

E. **Transverse process fracture**
  1. **Stable** injuries without neurological implications.
  2. **Mechanism of injury.** Usually muscular contraction, but may result from direct trauma.
  3. Most of these fractures involve L2, L3, and L4.
  4. Fracture of the L2 transverse process, resulting from direct trauma, can be associated with renal pedicle injury.
  5. **Treatment.** Managed with symptomatic medications, several days of bed rest, and then physical therapy with lumbar support.

F. **Spinous process fracture**
  1. **Stable** injuries without neurological implications.
  2. **Treatment.** Managed as transverse process fractures.

G. **Dislocations**
  1. Associated with ligamentous injury and should be considered **unstable.**
  2. **Mechanism of injury.** Result from flexion/rotation, hyperflexion/distraction, or hyperextension/shear mechanisms.
  3. **Radiographs.** Recognized by bony misalignment without evidence of fracture.
  4. **Treatment.** May be reduced with postural reduction but generally require open reduction and fixation.
  5. **Bilateral interfacet dislocation** (BID) is a rare injury occurring via the hyperflexion/distraction mechanism and is thus known as a soft

tissue Chance injury. It is demonstrated radiographically by spinous process misalignment in the frontal projection and widening of the disk space posteriorly, with subluxation on the lateral projection.

H. Spinal cord injury without radiological abnormality (SCIWORA)
   1. Reported in the preadolescent age group.
   2. Neurological injury may present months after initial trauma.
   3. **Mechanism of injury.** The lesion results from dislocation with ligamentous disruption that has spontaneously reduced.
   4. **Radiographs.** This injury, which presents without radiologic abnormality, should be suspected in the patient without radiologically identifiable injury and neurological deficit or in the patient who has had transient neurological deficit. Investigation should involve tests aimed at soft tissue evaluation—i.e., flexion/extension views and MRI.
   5. **Treatment** is like that for dislocations.

I. Intervertebral disks
   1. **Mechanism of injury.** Disks are subject to the same forces as the vertebral bodies, resulting in
      a. **Protrusion.** The disk protrudes posteriorly without rupture of the annulus fibrosus.
      b. **Prolapse,** with partial disruption of the annulus.
      c. **Extrusion,** with perforation of the annulus and extrusion of the nucleus pulposus into the epidural space.
      d. **Sequestration,** with annulus and nucleus trapped in the epidural space.
   2. **Treatment.** The acute management of these injuries is, as are all other spinal injuries, based on the presence of neurological impairment and the stability of the spine as a whole.

J. Vascular injury
   1. Isolated vascular injury is uncommon.
   2. The accumulation of an epidural hematoma can cause progressive neurological deficit and requires immediate decompression.
   3. **Diagnosis.** Discovered through the use of serial neurological examinations. Best demonstrated through the use of MRI.
   4. Injury to the dominant anterior spinal artery may cause deficits many segments cephalad to the actual level of injury.
   5. Secondary vascular injury from relative hypoxia and ischemia is a preventable injury by maintaining adequate oxygenation and perfusion.

V. Summary. Management of the patient with a potential lumbar injury should proceed in an organized fashion. The goal is primarily to prevent neurological injury and secondarily to reduce or reverse musculoskeletal morbidity. Attention to acute, life-threatening injuries should precede spinal evaluation, with maintenance of spinal immobilization to prevent further injury. Initial evaluation should include an injury-specific history and a physical examination with attention to the neurological exam. Radiological evaluation should be used liberally to help define the injury. Emergent surgical consultation should be obtained for progressive neurological lesions, open fractures, and incomplete spinal cord lesions. Mechanically unstable injuries require appropriate splinting, urgent consultation, and repeated examination. All injuries should be referred owing to the potential for further progression and morbidity.

BIBLIOGRAPHY

Braken MB, Shephard MJ, Hellenbrand KG, et al. A randomized controlled trial of methylprednisolone or naloxone in the treatment of spinal cord injury: results of the second national acute spinal cord injury study. *N Engl J Med* 1990;332:1405–1411.

Browner BD, Jupiter JB, Levine AM, Trafton DG. Lumbar and sacral spine trauma. In: *Skeletal trauma.* Philadelphia: WB Saunders, 1992:805–847.

Chapman JR, Anderson PA. Thoracolumbar spine fractures with neurologic deficit. *Orthop Clin North Am* 1994;25:595–612.

Connolly JF, ed. *Depalma's the Management of fractures and dislocations: an atlas,* 3rd ed. Philadelphia: WB Saunders, 1981:400–458.

Dee R, et al. *Principles of orthopaedic practice.* New York: McGraw-Hill, 1989:922–931.

Driscoll PA, Nicholson DA, Ross R. ABC of emergency radiology. *BMJ* 1993;307:1552–1557.

Harris JH, Harris HH, Novelline RA. *The radiology of emergency medicine,* 3rd ed. Baltimore: Williams & Wilkins, 1993: 239–282.

Huelke DF, et al. Vertebral column injuries and lap-shoulder belts. *J Trauma* 1995;38:547–556.

Magee DJ. *Orthopaedic physical assessment.* Philadelphia: WB Saunders. 1987;170–217.

Resnick D, Niwayama G. *The diagnosis of bone and joint disorders,* 2nd ed. Philadelphia: WB Saunders, 1988:23–34.

Romanes GJ, ed. *Cunningham's textbook of anatomy,* 12th ed. New York: Oxford University Press, 1981:89–98.

Rosen P. *Emergency medicine concepts and clinical practice,* 3rd ed. St Louis: Mosby–Year Book, 1992:268–287.

Van Savage JG, et al. Fracture-dislocation of the lumbosacral spine: case report and review of the literature. *J Trauma* 1992;33:779–784.

Pediatric Orthopaedics

25

General Pediatric Orthopaedics

Timothy James Rittenberry and John T. Piotrowski

Up to one-third of emergency department visits involve pediatric patients. Some 10% to 15% of all childhood injuries are skeletal. Although orthopaedic injuries seldom contribute to mortality, they are a major cause of disability among seriously injured children. The emergency physician must therefore have a solid knowledge base in pediatric orthopaedics. Many aspects of general orthopaedics can be applied to the pediatric population; however, children are *not* just "little adults" in this respect, and the indiscriminate application of adult orthopaedic principles may have devastating long-term sequelae. An understanding of the dynamic nature of the developing pediatric skeleton and the implications for injury patterns as well as treatment modalities will reduce complications.

I. **Anatomy.** The anatomy of the pediatric skeleton constantly changes as the child grows and matures. The relative strength and vulnerabilities of the different skeletal components vary with maturation. This **chronobiological variation** as well as a child's ever-increasing level of activity and associated mechanisms of injury lead to unique patterns of skeletal failure. A knowledge of pediatric skeletal anatomy not only ensures that the physician will anticipate and better diagnose specific injuries but is also critical to effective communication with orthopaedic consultants (Fig. 1).

   A. The **diaphysis** is the central shaft of a long bone. It is composed of more mature lamellar bone.

   B. The **metaphysis** is the area of bone widening that extends from the diaphysis and terminates in the radiolucent physis or growth plate. This bone is trabecular and relatively immature, leaving the area particularly susceptible to torus fractures.

   C. The **physis** or epiphyseal plate is the endochondral growth plate. Here the cartilaginous germinal cells responsible for both longitudinal and latitudinal growth are located. The presence of a physis is the single most important difference between adult and pediatric orthopaedics. This area of newly calcifying cartilage is weaker than calcified bone or nearby ligamentous structures and is the most vulnerable component of the pediatric skeleton. The physis is frequently injured; this can damage the germinal cells and lead to devastating growth aberrancy or arrest. The physis is radiolucent.

   D. The **epiphysis**, the end of the long bone, is composed of both bone and cartilage. Fractures through this area are frequently intraarticular and typically disrupt the physis. The epiphysis is radiodense.

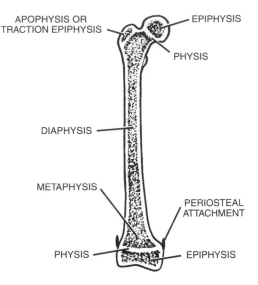

APOPHYSIS OR
TRACTION EPIPHYSIS

EPIPHYSIS

PHYSIS

DIAPHYSIS

METAPHYSIS

PERIOSTEAL
ATTACHMENT

PHYSIS

EPIPHYSIS

Fig. 1.   Pediatric long bone anatomy.

    E. An **apophysis** or traction epiphysis is an area of
tendon attachment to bone. This area is especially
prone to avulsion injuries in children, where tendon
is frequently stronger than bone.

  II. **Epidemiology.** Fractures in childhood are common.
Many factors affect the incidence of fractures, including
gender, age, and season. The incidence of fractures for
both boys and girls increases linearly until about age
12, at which time the incidence for males increases in a
steep linear fashion while the incidence for females
drops precipitously. This is in great part due to the increasing physical play and sport activities of boys cou-
pled with the earlier bone maturation and physeal fusion of girls. Of children sustaining at least one fracture
by age 16, 42% are male and 27% are female. Fractures
occur more frequently during summer months, as
warmer and longer days afford children more time to
play outside, increasing the chance of mishap. The rate
at which a sport increases the risk of fracture depends
on the nature of the activity. Football is typically the
riskiest, followed in descending order by basketball,
gymnastics, soccer, and baseball.

 III. **History.** Historical data in the evaluation of pediatric
orthopaedic injuries are often problematic. The history
may be limited or erroneous. Falls and accidents are frequently unwitnessed, and the child may occasionally be
deceptive in recounting the injury. The very young or es-

pecially apprehensive child will not be able to afford much information. When abuse is involved, the history may be inconsistent. Lack of accurate historical data indicating mechanism of injury makes physical examination and radiological assessment extremely important.

IV. **Physical examination.** Unfortunately, the physical exam can be particularly challenging in the very young patient. Direct observation may give no clues as to the exact site or nature of the injury, and performing informative palpation or range-of-motion testing in the crying child may be difficult at best. Time spent building rapport with a young child will usually allow examination of those areas thought *not* to be involved, before proceeding to a gentle but adequate exam of the most likely site of injury. This will help hone the differential diagnosis and narrow the focus for radiological assessment while eliciting the greatest cooperation from the child.

V. **Radiography.** Radiographs are more difficult to interpret in children than in adults. Fractures may be subtle, while those that involve the radiolucent physis may remain inapparent. Secondary ossification centers add further to the confusion. Comparison views of the unaffected extremity will facilitate interpretation whenever pathology may be confused with normal anatomy and are especially useful in evaluating the pediatric elbow.

VI. **Ligamentous injury.** Due to the relative weakness of the physis and the strength and resilience of associated ligamentous structures, direct and indirect trauma to joints is more likely to result in physeal failure than in ligamentous injury. Although sprains occur in children or young adults, it is more likely that a fracture involving the physis has occurred (see Sec. VIII.B, "The Salter-Harris classification"). This relative physeal weakness and ligamentous strength also leads to a lower incidence of frank joint dislocations. As skeletal maturity approaches, adult sprain and dislocation patterns begin to prevail.

VII. **Healing.** Fractures heal more quickly in children than in adults, and children are capable of remarkable corrective remodeling in fracture union. Even angulated fractures may remodel with little or no resultant deformity. This is especially true when the fracture's angulation exists in the same plane as the movement of a nearby hinge joint. Rotational malposition, however, will *not* undergo remodeling, and all rotational deformities must be corrected. Because of a child's ability to heal and remodel, open reduction and internal fixation (ORIF) is necessary less frequently than in adults. Rapid healing in children also requires prompt orthopaedic referral, within days rather than weeks, as callus formation may hinder attempts at reduction. Although pediatric injuries result in a lower incidence of delayed or nonunion, they may lead to growth aberration or growth arrest, particularly when the physis is involved.

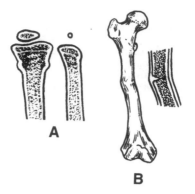

Fig. 2.   **Pediatric fracture patterns.**
A: Torus fracture. B: Greenstick fracture.

VIII.   Fracture patterns
A.   Greenstick and torus fractures. The resilience
and plasticity of the pediatric skeleton is remarkable owing to fewer lamellar components and
greater porosity overall. This limits fracture propa-
gation and lends itself to unique configurations of
bony failure. Comminuted fractures are uncommon
in the pediatric population. A greenstick fracture
may occur when stress is applied to a long bone
(Fig. 2). As an area of cortical bone fails in distraction, the opposite cortex undergoes plastic deformity without radiographically apparent fracture.
This plastic deformity may persist, and in severe
cases, completion of the fracture through the "bent"
cortex may be necessary to obtain adequate reduction. The torus or buckle fracture represents another fracture pattern unique to pediatric bone and
is typically noted in the metaphyseal area (Fig. 2).
As the metaphyseal bone fails with axial loading,
an area of cortex "buckles" without apparent fracture. This actually represents a localized compression fracture.
B.   The **Salter-Harris classification.** Many fractures
involving the physis have long been known to result
in injury to the osteogenic cells responsible for bone
lengthening, adversely affecting growth. The first
attempt to classify these fractures occurred in
1863. One hundred years later, Salter and Harris
proposed a classification system based on radiographic appearance; this has prevailed as the
means of recognizing, understanding, and commu-
nicating about these injuries. Familiarity with the
Salter-Harris classification is integral to understanding pediatric orthopaedics. Because these

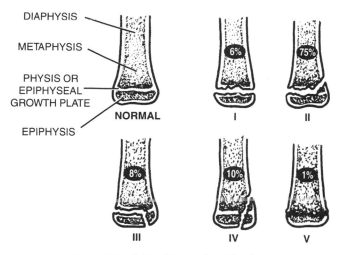

DIAPHYSIS

METAPHYSIS

PHYSIS OR
EPIPHYSEAL
GROWTH PLATE

EPIPHYSIS

NORMAL   I   II

6%   75%

III   IV   V

8%   10%   1%

Fig. 3.   The Salter-Harris classification.

physeal injuries result in a 10% to 15% incidence of growth aberration or growth arrest, diagnosis should be accompanied by parental education regarding this possible future complication (Fig. 3).

1. **Salter I.** The fracture line extends through the radiolucent physis only. The diagnosis is obvious if the epiphysis is displaced. If it is not, the radiograph will appear normal. When this is the case yet there is a suspect mechanism of injury and associated tenderness about the epiphyseal plate, the diagnosis of an undisplaced Salter I fracture is made. *This is a clinical diagnosis.* Salter I injuries are most common in the very young. Since the physis is not disrupted, healing is typically uncomplicated and growth complications are rare.

2. **Salter II.** The fracture line propagates along the physis and exits the metaphysis. The metaphyseal fragment is radiographically apparent although often subtle. This is the most frequently encountered Salter injury and is most often found after the age of 10.

3. **Salter III.** The fracture line propagates through the physis and exits through the epiphysis. This is a more severe injury because it is intraarticular and it disrupts the continuity of the osteogenic cells of the physis, greatly increasing the risk of a growth aberrancy. Some orthopaedists consider this an absolute indication for ORIF, since exact restoration of the

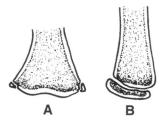

A   **B**

Fig. 4.   Metaphyseal lesions. A: Corner fracture. B: Bucket-handle fracture.

anatomy is necessary for optimal function and growth.

4.   **Salter IV.** The fracture line involves the metaphysis and the epiphysis, crossing the physis. As in Salter III fractures, the physis is injured and the fracture is intraarticular. ORIF is likely and the incidence of growth aberration is significant.

5.   **Salter V.** The physis is crushed due to a compressing axial load. This is a rare injury and is virtually impossible to diagnose acutely. It is more likely that the initial diagnosis of a nondisplaced Salter I fracture will be made and only with growth complication will the true nature of the injury reveal itself.

6.   **Salter VI.** This classification was coined by Rang and describes an injury to the perichondral ring *surrounding* the physis, as may result from a direct blow, burn, or local infection. Although the physis is uninjured, the inflammatory process may lead to bone formation, which bridges the epiphyseal-metaphyseal junction, effectively tethering growth in a single area of the physis and resulting in a progressive growth deformity.

IX.   **Child abuse.** Studies in some centers suggest that up to 25% of all fractures in children under 3 years of age may be due to abuse. The battered child tends to be young, with approximately two-thirds being under 3 years and one-third less than 6 months of age. Child abuse is unfortunately endemic in today's society, requiring physicians to maintain a high index of suspicion. Delay in seeking treatment, inconsistent history, and lack of parental concern are red flags that should alert the physician to the possibility of abuse. Diaphyseal injuries are twice as common as metaphyseal injuries although the latter are pathognomonic for child abuse. As bending and traction forces cause deformation of long bones, the periosteum is pulled from its attachments near the physis, resulting in metaphyseal "corner" or "bucket-handle" fractures (Fig. 4). It is interesting to note that injuries to the physis are rare. The most

Table 1. Fractures associated with child abuse

Highly specific
  Metaphyseal lesions
    Corner fractures
    Bucket-handle fractures
  Rib fractures
  Scapular fractures
  Spinous process fractures
  Sternal fractures
Moderately specific
  Multiple fractures
  Bilateral fractures
  Fractures of differing age
  Digital fractures
  Vertebral fractures

commonly fractured bones in the battered child are the ribs, humerus, femur, tibia, and skull. The presence of multiple fractures in differing stages of repair is highly suspicious for abuse. Other, less common fractures that are more specific for abuse include metaphyseal injuries, posterior rib fractures, and fractures of the sternum, scapula, or spinous processes (Table 1). If abuse is suspected, admission followed by a complete skeletal survey to search for multiple fractures in various stages of repair, periosteal reactions, and metaphyseal fractures is indicated. Nonosseous injuries should be actively sought, as the incidence of concomitant head and abdominal injuries is high. All cases of suspected abuse should be reported to the appropriate agencies.

BIBLIOGRAPHY

Connolly JF. *Fractures and dislocations: closed management.* Philadelphia: WB Saunders, 1995.

Kleinman PK. *Diagnostic imaging of child abuse.* Baltimore: Williams & Wilkins, 1987.

Ogden JA. *Skeletal injury in the child,* 2nd ed. Philadelphia: WB Saunders, 1990.

Rittenberry TJ. *Pediatric orthopaedics.* Core Curriculum Lecture Series, University of Illinois Residency in Emergency Medicine. Chicago: University of Illinois, 1996.

Rockwood CA, Wilkins KE, Beaty JH. *Fractures in children.* Philadelphia: Lippincott-Raven, 1996.

Salter RB, Harris WR. Injuries involving the epiphyseal plate. *J Bone Joint Surg* 1963;45A:587.

Pediatric Orthopaedics: The Upper Extremity

Timothy James Rittenberry and David A. Townes

Upper extremity injuries account for approximately 70% of all childhood fractures. The majority of these injuries are related to falls, sports, and motor vehicle accidents. The distal forearm leads the elbow in the overall incidence of fractures.

I. **Shoulder and humerus**
  A. **Clavicular fractures.** The clavicle is the most frequently fractured bone in children less than 10 years of age. It is the most common birth injury and is often unrecognized initially.
    1. **Classification.** Clavicular fractures may be divided into fractures of the middle, distal, and medial thirds. The majority of fractures occur between the middle and distal thirds of the clavicle. In younger children, these tend to be greenstick fractures. In the older child, complete fracture with or without displacement is more common. Physeal injuries of the medial clavicle can occur as late as the early twenties, as the medial clavicular epiphysis is the last growth plate in the body to close (Fig. 1).
    2. **Mechanism of injury.** The clavicle may be injured from either direct trauma or indirectly as forces are transferred from the shoulder or outstretched arm in a fall. Fractures from birth trauma are likely due to compression on the anterior shoulder by the symphysis pubis.
    3. **Physical examination.** The presentation of a child with a clavicular injury may be quite varied. The infant may be asymptomatic, with no initial evidence of injury, and diagnosis may be delayed until callus formation gives visual and palpable evidence. More commonly, a child may complain of neck or arm pain and have ecchymosis, local tenderness, swelling, or crepitus over the site of injury accompanied by an obvious deformity. Movement of the arm may be unaffected or may be restricted, with the child holding the injured arm close to the body and supporting it with the other hand. In the case of infants with birth trauma, the child may present with transient pseudoparalysis (an apparent Erb's palsy).
    4. **Radiography.** Radiography of the clavicle is necessary to confirm the diagnosis, as well as the presence of associated injuries. Routine anteroposterior (AP) views demonstrate most fractures, although an apical-lordotic view may be neces-

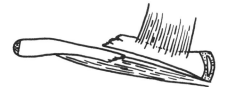

Fig. 1. Midshaft clavicular fracture.

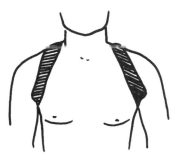

Fig. 2. Clavicular strap.

sary to demonstrate undisplaced fractures of the medial shaft of the clavicle.

5. **Treatment.** Fortunately, clavicular fractures in children tend to heal well, with minimal complication. The child is placed in a figure-of-eight splint, which he or she wears day and night for the first 2 weeks and by day for 2 more weeks. If the fracture involves the distal clavicle or the proximal clavicle with epiphyseal displacement, immobilization with a sling and swathe is appropriate. Fractures in children older than 6 years that have significant displacement require reduction. Rarely, surgical treatment is necessary when subluxation and vascular compromise occur. As with all orthopaedic immobilization, the neurovascular status of the involved extremity should be noted prior to discharge (Fig. 2).

6. **Complications.** Complications are uncommon in pediatric clavicular fractures. Owing to the extensive remodeling that occurs in children, malunion is rare. Excessive callus formation may lead to deformity in the area of injury.

7. **Disposition.** The child with an uncomplicated clavicular fracture may be discharged home from the emergency department to follow up with an orthopaedist or pediatrician.

B. **Acromioclavicular separation.** Injuries to the acromioclavicular (AC) joint are rare in children, as forces to this area in younger children often lead to a metaphyseal fracture rather than a ligamentous injury. Apparent AC separation in young children is more likely to represent a fracture involving the distal physis, although true AC separation becomes more common in adolescence.

1. **Classification.** Injuries to the AC joint are categorized by the degree of ligamentous disruption that exists. First-degree injuries involve a sprain or incomplete rupture of the acromioclavicular ligament. A second-degree injury implies a rupture of this ligament with a sprain of the coracoclavicular ligament. A third-degree injury indicates that both ligaments have been disrupted.

2. **Mechanism of injury.** The usual mechanism of injury is a direct force, such as a fall onto the shoulder.

3. **Physical examination.** Palpation will localize pain to the AC joint. In more severe injuries, there may be displacement of the clavicle superiorly with an obvious step-off deformity.

4. **Radiography.** Routine shoulder x-rays may be unremarkable, and AC views are often necessary. Radiographic findings may be subtle. Small fracture fragments at the distal end of the clavicle or a widened AC joint space may be seen. AC views with and without weights may demonstrate abnormalities. A first-degree sprain is diagnosed when no widening of the joint space is seen. Widening of the joint space by less than 1 cm indicates a second-degree sprain, and if the space is widened by more than 1 cm, the diagnosis of a third-degree sprain is made.

5. **Treatment.** First- and second-degree sprains may be treated with a sling and swathe. Third-degree sprains may require surgical repair, and orthopaedic consultation from the emergency department is advised.

6. **Complications.** There are no significant complications specific to an isolated AC joint injury, although AC instability may result in third-degree injuries.

7. **Disposition.** Patients with first- and second-degree sprains may be discharged from the department with analgesics and instructions to apply ice. Third-degree sprains should be discussed with an orthopaedic consultant prior to disposition.

C. **Shoulder injuries**

1. **Scapular fractures.** Fractures of the scapula are rare in children and when they occur are indicative of very high energy trauma directly to the scapula. They are typically associated with

other traumatic injuries of greater significance. In managing the scapular fracture itself, a sling and swathe worn for 4 weeks is sufficient.

2. **Brachial plexus injuries** are most commonly the result of birth trauma. It is a diagnosis that is often difficult to make in the emergency department. Parents may describe paralysis (Erb's palsy) of the arm, or an asymmetrical Moro reflex may be noted. Radiographs of the shoulder and clavicle should be obtained to rule out other injury. These patients should be referred to a pediatric neurologist.

3. **Rotator cuff injuries** occur in the pediatric population. These patients will have pain on abduction and external rotation of the shoulder as well as tenderness over the insertion of the rotator cuff muscles. Radiographs should be obtained to rule out a fracture. Minor rotator cuff injuries may be treated with sling immobilization, analgesics, and range-of-motion exercises. More severe injuries require orthopaedic evaluation.

4. **Dislocations.** These injuries are rare in infants and young children, increasing in frequency in adolescence, as bone maturity is reached.

   a. **Classification.** Shoulder dislocations are classified as anterior or posterior, depending on the relationship between the humeral head and the glenoid fossa. Anterior dislocations are more common.

   b. **Mechanism of injury.** These dislocations are caused by indirect trauma, with forceful abduction of the arm and extension of the shoulder. The mechanism of injury is essentially the same as in adults. Posterior dislocations tend to be the result of seizures or electrical injuries.

   c. **Physical examination.** Patients with shoulder dislocations will present with a flattened deltoid muscle and a prominent acromion. The humeral head may be palpable anterior, inferior, and medial to the glenoid in an anterior dislocation and posterior in a posterior dislocation. The physical exam should include a complete neurological assessment, including a sensory exam of the lateral portion of the shoulder and arm and a motor exam of the deltoid muscle to evaluate the axillary nerve. The distal vasculature should also be checked to rule out compromise. The range of motion of the shoulder will be greatly limited in these injuries.

   d. **Radiographs.** A lateral, anteroposterior, and transaxillary or Y view should be obtained to determine the location of the humeral head in relation to the glenoid fossa. Radiographs will also aid in determination of associated injuries such as fracture of the greater tuberosity of the humerus or a compression fracture of the posterolateral humeral head (the Hill-Sachs lesion). Postreduction radiographs should be obtained in both cases to ensure proper reduction.

  e. **Treatment.** Methods used to reduce a dislocated shoulder are the same as in adults (see Sec.I.C.4, "Dislocations"). Great care not to use undue force is paramount before bone maturity is reached and the proximal humerus physis remains open. Light sedation may be necessary, depending on the particular maneuver employed. Children may require operative intervention if rehabilitation to strengthen the shoulder muscles fails and recurrent dislocation occurs.

  f. **Complications.** Neurovascular or epiphyseal injury may complicate shoulder reductions but are greatly reduced with the use of proper technique. The axillary nerve is particularly vulnerable and its integrity should be checked and documented both before and after reduction.

  g. **Disposition.** After reduction, the arm should be placed in a sling and swathe, keeping the arm internally rotated, with prompt orthopaedic referral.

D. **Humeral shaft fractures.** Fractures of the humeral shaft make up to 5% of fractures in children.

 1. **Classification.** Fractures are named by the pattern of fracture (transverse, oblique, etc.) the location (proximal, middle, or distal third), and the alignment of the fragments. The proximal humerus is more commonly injured, with Salter I and II fractures much more common than Salter III, IV, or V. Interestingly, fractures of the proximal humeral metaphysis are more common than physeal injuries in this location between the ages of 5 and 11 (Fig. 3).

 2. **Mechanism of injury.** Fractures of the humerus result from direct or indirect trauma to the area. Chronic repetitive stress to the proximal physis, such as that incurred in a baseball pitcher, can cause fractures and slippage of the epiphysis, analogous to the slipped capital femoral epiphysis.

 3. **Physical examination.** The child with a humeral fracture will have tenderness over the area of injury. Swelling and deformity may be minimal. The child may resist attempts to move or manipulate the arm in any way. A complete neurovascular exam of the extremity is necessary, especially

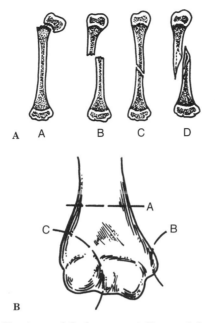

Fig. 3. (A) Fractures of the humerus. A: Transepiphyseal. B: Transverse. C: Oblique. D: Spiral. (B) Fractures of the distal humerus. A: Supracondylar fracture. B: Medial epicondylar fracture. C: Lateral condylar fracture.

to evaluate radial nerve disability, which occurs in 5% of cases.

4. **Radiography.** AP and lateral radiographs should be obtained. Fractures may be transverse, greenstick, torus, spiral, comminuted, or a combination of these. It may be difficult to identify a Salter I fracture of the proximal humerus unless displacement has occurred.

5. **Treatment.** The treatment will depend on the type, location, and severity of the fracture. Most fractures of the proximal metaphysis or epiphysis of the proximal humerus may be treated with a sling and swathe. Reduction is usually not indicated unless there is significant separation (>1 cm), angulation (>40 degrees), or rotation. In obvious fractures of the humeral shaft, immobilization in a sling and swathe with a "sugar-tong" coaptation splint can be applied prior to obtaining radiographs in order to minimize any neurovascular injury. In the case of midshaft fractures, angulation of up to 20 degrees and up to 2 cm of override are acceptable. In all fractures, any interposition of muscle, nerve, or vascular

structures requires immediate orthopaedic involvement and prompt reduction.

6. **Complications.** Injury to the axillary or circumflex nerve and entrapment of the radial nerve are among the possible complications of humeral shaft fractures. Longitudinal growth retardation is another concern.

7. **Disposition.** Any pediatric patient with an uncomplicated fracture of the humeral shaft should be adequately immobilized and may be discharged after orthopaedic consultation.

II. **Elbow.** The child with a swollen and/or painful elbow provides a considerable diagnostic challenge. Elbow injuries constitute about 10% of upper extremity injuries and range from the innocuous "nursemaid's elbow" to the potentially disastrous supracondylar fracture. While the peak incidence for physeal injuries is between 10 and 13 years of age, most physeal fractures of the elbow occur in the 5- to 8-year-old.

Fractures and dislocations that occur in the elbow are classified by the location of the injury. They are typically categorized as supracondylar fractures (which may also be thought of as fractures of the distal humeral metaphysis), fractures of the lateral and medial condyles, medial epicondylar fractures, intercondylar and transcondylar fractures, and fractures of the olecranon itself. Radial head subluxation or nursemaid's elbow is a special type of elbow injury seen in the pediatric population.

Routine x-rays include the AP and lateral view in 90 degrees of flexion. Radiographic interpretation in this area is difficult because of the chronobiological variation of secondary and epiphyseal ossification centers. The mnemonic CRITOE (Table 1) helps to confirm what one expects to see on x-ray. However, the liberal use of comparison films is necessary in assessing these injuries.

A. **Supracondylar fractures.** The age of the patient aids diagnosis, as this is an injury almost exclusive to those less than 10 years old, with about half of these elbow injuries occurring between the ages of 5 and 8. There is a 2:1 male-to-female ratio. Extension-type supracondylar fractures make up 98% of these injuries (Fig. 4).

Table 1.   Chronological appearance of the ossifications centers of the pediatric elbow

Capitellum	Age	2
Radial head	Age	4
Internal (medial) epicondyle	Age	6
Trochlea	Age	8
Olecranon	Age	10
External (lateral) epicondyle	Age	12

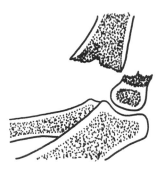

Fig. 4. Supracondylar fracture.

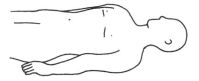

Fig. 5. The dinner-fork deformity of a displaced supracondylar fracture.

1. **Mechanism of injury.** These fractures occur when the elbow is hyperextended during a fall onto an outstretched hand.
2. **Physical examination.** The child will present with a painful elbow and local swelling. A severely displaced fracture may give an overt "dinner-fork" appearance (Fig. 5).
3. **Radiographs.** In a child presenting with an acutely swollen and painful elbow in whom supracondylar fracture is suspected, splinting the child *prior* to manipulation by radiography technicians is probably prudent. In the face of neurovascular compromise necessitating prompt reduction, immediate portable x-ray views will be useful, with immobilization and standard radiographs to follow. Radiographic appearance may range from an obvious transverse fracture to a grossly normal appearance of the bony anatomy. Overt extension-type fractures will exhibit anterior displacement of the proximal humeral fragment. In all radiographs of the elbow, one should look for subtle evidence of injury. The presence of a posterior fat pad or bulging anterior fat pad (the "sail sign") indicates that an occult fracture has occurred (Fig. 6). Evaluation of the anterior

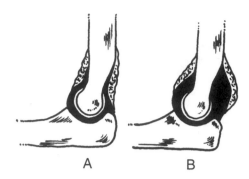

Fig. 6.   Fat-pad signs of the elbow. A: Normal. B: Displacement of anterior and posterior fat pads by hemarthrosis.

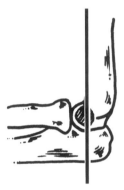

Fig. 7.   The anterior humeral line. The shaded capitellum is intersected in its middle third.

humeral line assesses posterior displacement. This longitudinal line, drawn along the anterior cortex of the humerus on the true lateral view, should intersect the middle third of the ossification center of the capitellum (Fig. 7). Failure to do so indicates an occult posteriorly displaced supracondylar fracture.

4.   **Treatment.** Any supracondylar fracture with obvious deformity and neurovascular compromise requires immediate reduction by applying forearm traction along the humeral axis with the elbow in slight flexion. Skin "puckering" in the antecubital fossa indicates that the anteriorly displaced anterior bone fragment has pierced the subcutaneous tissue, which will impair reduction. Supracondylar fractures are immobilized using a

long arm posterior mold with the elbow in approximately 70 degrees of flexion to allow for the progression of antecubital swelling, which can compromise arterial or venous flow. Care must be taken in applying circumferential cast padding or bandage to avoid undue compression of the forearm or antecubital fossa, as this may contribute to compartment syndrome.

5. **Complications.** The incidence of associated soft tissue injuries is high as the proximal bone fragment is thrust into the antecubital fossa. Some 7% of these fractures have accompanying nerve injuries, most frequently the radial and least often the ulnar nerve. Vascular compromise of the brachial artery either from direct trauma, spasm, or compression from soft tissue swelling may lead to forearm compartment syndrome and subsequent Volkmann's ischemic contracture in up to 1% of patients. Laceration of the brachial artery is uncommon. Thorough and ongoing distal neurovascular examination is critical in these injuries. Any forearm pain with passive movement of the wrist and fingers is indicative of compartment syndrome. Compartment syndromes and varus deformity have decreased dramatically in recent years, with percutaneous pinning overtaking hyperflexion to maintain anatomical reduction.

6. **Disposition.** The supracondylar fracture is a true orthopaedic emergency requiring immediate consultation. Although a select few patients who present many hours after injury with a nondisplaced fracture, minimal or no swelling, no evidence of neurovascular involvement, and able parents may occasionally be safely discharged to follow-up within 24 hours with the consulting orthopaedist, these are the exceptions. The vast majority will be admitted for neurovascular checks and definitive orthopaedic care.

B. **Lateral and medial condylar fractures.** Lateral condylar fractures account for 15% of pediatric elbow fractures, with a peak incidence between 5 and 6 years. Medial condylar fractures are rare but occur most frequently in the 6-to-10-year-old age group (Fig. 8).

1. **Mechanism of injury.** The usual mechanism of this injury is varus stress to the elbow with traction on the lateral condyle by the extensors of the forearm. This often results from a fall onto an outstretched arm.

2. **Physical examination.** The child with this injury will present with marked swelling and tenderness over the lateral elbow.

3. **Radiography.** As with all injuries to the elbow, a series of radiographs that includes AP and lateral

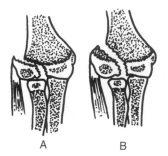

Fig. 8. Lateral condylar fractures.
A: Salter III fracture. B: Salter IV
fracture.

views should be obtained. Most of these appear as
Salter III or IV fractures. Radiographs tend to
underestimate displacement.

4. **Treatment.** If the fracture is nondisplaced, it
may be placed in a long arm cast with the elbow
at 90 degrees of flexion and the forearm in full
supination. Displaced fractures usually require
open reduction but may be treated with percutaneous pinning. These fractures often require surgical correction, and orthopaedic consultation
should be obtained.

5. **Complications.** Acute neurovascular compromise is uncommon. More often, complications are
delayed from weeks to years and include nonunion,
ulnar nerve palsy, and growth arrest with resultant elbow disability.

6. **Disposition.** These fractures are considered unstable and must immediately be referred to an orthopaedic surgeon.

C. **Medial epicondylar fractures.** Fractures of the
medial epicondyle constitute 10% of all elbow fractures, occuring most often in the 7- to 15-year age
group; they are rare under the age of 4 years and are
four times more common in males.

1. **Mechanism of injury.** The medial epicondyle is
a traction apophysis to which the flexors of the
forearm are attached. Valgus strain on these muscles causes avulsion and often displacement of the
medial epicondyle. These may also occur in association with a posterior elbow dislocation (about
50% of the time) or from a direct blow (Fig. 9).

2. **Physical examination.** A child with a fracture
to the medial epicondyle will present with the elbow partially flexed. The range of motion is decreased secondary to pain. Swelling is noted and
tenderness elicited over the medial aspect of the
elbow. A full neurovascular exam should be done,
with special attention to the ulnar nerve, which is
most susceptible to damage in this injury.

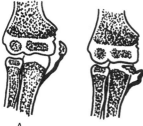

Fig. 9. **Medial epicondyle fracture. A: Displaced fracture. B: Intraarticular entrapment.**

3. **Radiography.** The radiographic findings may be subtle and comparison views are often needed for confirmation. Any displacement of the epicondyle is reflected in widening of the physis medially.

4. **Treatment.** Treatment is dependent on the degree of injury. In minimally displaced fractures, immobilization may constitute definitive care. Fractures that are significantly displaced and rotated or those with ulnar nerve dysfunction may require operative interventions, as will any fracture associated with intraarticular entrapment, as may be seen after reduction of a posterior elbow dislocation.

5. **Disposition.** Once the physician is certain that entrapment of the medial epicondyle has not occurred, the child may be sent home with close follow-up by an orthopaedic surgeon. A long arm posterior splint placing the elbow in moderate flexion and the forearm in pronation is used.

D. **"Little League elbow."** This is a special type of medial epicondylar injury. Referred to as **traction apophysitis,** this injury is a chronic, stress-induced injury of the medial epicondyle. It is often seen in young pitchers and causes tenderness and swelling at the medial epicondyle with mild loss of elbow extension. The treatment is the reduction of inciting activities.

E. **Dislocations.** The elbow is the most commonly dislocated joint in childhood; this injury makes up 5% of all elbow injuries. Its peak incidence is in adolescence. Pure dislocations are rare; the majority are associated with a fracture (Fig. 10).

1. **Mechanism of injury.** The most common mechanism of injury is a fall onto an outstretched arm.

2. **Physical examination.** The child with a dislocation at the elbow will have pain, swelling, deformity, and markedly decreased range of motion at the elbow. The elbow is held semiflexed, with a deformity similar in appearance to a displaced

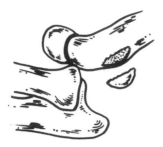

Fig. 10.   Posterior elbow dislocation with associated medial epicondylar fracture.

supracondylar fracture. A thorough neurovascular exam is essential because of the possibility of
injury to the brachial artery and of ulnar or median nerve entrapment.

3. **Radiography.** The arm should be immobilized
prior to obtaining radiographs when a displaced
supracondylar fracture remains a possibility. If
there is evidence of vascular compromise, immediate portable radiographs are of use to expedite
reduction, with immobilization and standard radiographs to follow. Radiographs should be examined not only for obvious dislocation but also for
associated fractures, with specific attention to the
location of the medial epicondyle. Many dislocations reduce spontaneously, and a fracture or fat
pad may be the only evidence of injury. Postreduction views must again ensure that the medial epicondyle has not been fractured and is not entrapped in the joint space.

4. **Treatment.** The dislocated elbow must be reduced promptly. Adequate sedation and analgesia
are essential. To achieve reduction, traction must
be applied along the axis of the humerus to overcome the muscular forces of the upper arm and
then along the axis of the forearm to bring the
coronoid process from posterior to the normal anterior position. Hypersupination of the forearm
during reduction may be helpful. Correction of
any lateral or medial displacement of the forearm
first will also assist reduction. A subsequent
neurovascular exam is required, followed by immobilization with the arm in as close to 90 degrees of flexion as swelling allows without vascular impairment. Another neurovascular check
should follow splinting. Inability to reduce a posterior elbow dislocation mandates open reduction.

5. **Complications.** Neurovascular injury is the
most important complication of posterior elbow
dislocation. Entrapment of the medial epicondyle

is associated with ulnar nerve injury. Median nerve injury is rare.

6. **Disposition.** Immediate orthopaedic consultation with admission to the hospital to monitor for the development of neurovascular compromise will be necessary.

F. **Radial head subluxation.** Also known as nursemaid's elbow or acute annular ligament interposition, this injury is most common in the 2- to 3-year age group. It is rare after the age of 7. In many cases the history alone is diagnostic.

1. **Mechanism of injury.** The mechanism of injury is abrupt traction on the pronated forearm. This allows the annular ligament to slide over the radial head and become interposed between the radial head and the capitellum. A tear of the annular ligament itself may or may not occur.

2. **Physical examination.** The arm is held in slight flexion and the forearm in pronation. The child may be in no apparent distress but may refuse to use the affected extremity while guarding it from motion or manipulation.

3. **Radiography.** An appropriate history and otherwise unremarkable physical exam preclude the need for radiographic evaluation. If the history or physical exam are in question, radiographs should be obtained to rule out a supracondylar fracture or other injury.

4. **Treatment.** Treatment of this injury in the emergency department is very simple and rewarding. Reduction is accomplished by first holding the child's elbow with the physician's thumb over the radial head. With the operator's other hand, the child's hand is pulled, extending the elbow. This is immediately followed by supination of the forearm and flexion of the elbow. The "click" of the reducing radial head is often felt under the physician's thumb. Normal function of the injured extremity is usually observed in less than 15 minutes.

5. **Complications.** There are no complications that are specific to this injury. The recurrence rate is estimated at about 30%.

6. **Disposition.** After reduction, children should be observed to ensure full use of the injured extremity prior to discharge. Caregivers should be instructed on the mechanism of injury and how to prevent it.

G. **Olecranon fractures.** Fractures of the olecranon and coronoid process are infrequent in children.

1. **Mechanism of injury.** Fractures of the olecranon in children are often the result of direct trauma rather than a fall onto an outstretched arm or avulsion forces at the triceps expansion.

In adolescents, chronic overuse, as seen with tennis, may lead to stress fractures.

2. **Physical examination.** The child with a fractured olecranon presents with pain, swelling, and decreased range of motion at the elbow.

3. **Radiography.** Interpretation of radiographs of the elbow is often difficult. Fractures of the physeal/metaphyseal junction are often poorly visualized, and the normal appearance of the ossification center of the olecranon may lead to false-positive readings. The normal distance between the olecranon metaphysis and the ossifying epiphysis may measure up to 5 mm on lateral views. Comparison view of the uninvolved elbow may be necessary.

4. **Treatment.** The severity of the injury will determine the type and extent of treatment. Fractures of the olecranon that are nondisplaced should be immobilized in a long arm splint or cast with the elbow at 90 degrees. Incomplete fractures may be treated with a sling, while displaced or complex fractures should be treated in immediate consultation with an orthopaedic surgeon; many require pin fixation.

5. **Complications.** Fractures of the olecranon do well. Nonunion, growth arrest, and functional loss are rare.

6. **Disposition.** After immobilization in a long arm posterior mold, these children may be sent home with prompt orthopaedic follow-up.

III. **Radius and ulna.** Some 45% of pediatric fractures occur in the radius. The majority of these are in the distal third. The mechanism of injury is typically a fall onto an outstretched hand with a hyperextended wrist. These fractures are also caused by direct trauma. In contrast to adult fractures of this type, the radial and ulnar shafts are often fractured at the same level. Fractures of the distal radius are typically Salter I or II physeal injuries, while metaphyseal fractures are often torus or greenstick. Diaphyseal injuries include bowing, greenstick fracture, and complete fracture of the ulna and radius. The most common of these injuries is a Salter II fracture of the distal radius. The adult Monteggia and Galeazzi patterns of fracture with dislocation of the proximal radial head or distal radioulnar joint, respectively, can occur. A Monteggia fracture must be ruled out whenever isolated fracture or bowing of the ulna is found.

A. **Classification.** Fractures of the radius and ulna are classified by type, severity, and location of the injury and by any associated injuries.

B. **Mechanism of injury.** While there is some variability, the most common mechanism of injury is either a fall onto an outstretched hand or direct trauma.

C. **Physical examination.** The child with fracture of the forearm will present with pain, tenderness, swelling, decreased range of motion, and variable deformity. In some displaced fractures, tenting of the skin may be noted. A full neurovascular exam is essential.

D. **Radiography.** These fractures are usually obvious radiographically. It is important to image the *entire* forearm, including the wrist and elbow joint, to rule out a Monteggia or Galeazzi fracture. The physician should pay special attention to the degree of angulation, displacement, and rotation. A line drawn axially through the center of the proximal radius should intersect the capitellum at its middle in all views of the elbow to rule out dislocation of the radial head.

E. **Treatment.** Fractures of the radius and ulna are largely managed by closed reduction and immobilization, with excellent functional results. The goal of therapy is to restore axial and rotational alignment while preserving the interosseous spacing, thus facilitating unhindered supination and pronation. As bone maturity nears, rates of open reduction and internal fixation (ORIF) approach those of adults.

F. **Complications,** The greatest risk of complication comes from inadequate correction of angulation or rotation. Neurovascular compromise and nonunion are rare.

G. **Disposition.** As in any Salter injury, growth arrest is a risk. Compartment syndrome and Volkmann's ischemia are most likely to occur when severe deformity and marked swelling are present in a forearm fracture. Clinicians experienced and comfortable with fracture reduction may wish to manipulate injuries with marked deformity. This should be done with orthopaedic consultation. Repeated attempts at reduction must be avoided because they can cause additional injury to associated tissues and may worsen forearm swelling in shaft fractures or increase physeal injury and growth aberration in Salter injuries. Although most injuries are safely immobilized in a long arm posterior splint and discharged to prompt orthopaedic follow-up, those injuries with marked forearm swelling and/or deformity may well require hospitalization for neurovascular checks and definitive treatment.

IV. **Injuries of the wrist and hand**

A. **Fractures.** Fractures about the hand are relatively uncommon in children, accounting for only 5% to 7% of all fractures. Most prevalent are **distal phalangeal crush injuries, Salter fractures of the proximal phalanx, metacarpal phalangeal joint dislocations,** and **scaphoid fractures.**

1. **Mechanism of injury.** In general, fractures of the carpal bones result from a fall onto an outstretched hand, while fractures of the metacarpal bones and phalanges result from direct trauma.

2. **Physical examination.** A high index of suspicion should be maintained, as an adequate and detailed hand examination may prove difficult at best. Skin integrity, soft tissue swelling, gross deformities, and any neurovascular deficits are noted. Angular and rotational deformities are best seen with the digits placed side by side in full flexion. In this posture the nail beds should be coplanar. A mallet deformity suggests damage to the extensor tendon or a displaced Salter injury at the distal interphalangeal (DIP) joint. A boutonnière deformity suggests damage to the extensor mechanism over the proximal interphalangeal (PIP) joint with volar subluxation of the lateral bands. Both of these may result from a blow to the hand. A fracture of the fifth proximal phalanx demonstrating severe ulnar angular deformity is seen frequently and is known as an "extra octave" fracture.

3. **Radiography.** AP, lateral, and oblique views of the digits and carpus should be done. However, accurate radiographic interpretation requires a knowledge of the age-specific morphology of the many ossification centers and is often difficult. Comparison views may be of use. Special views such as the carpal navicular may be necessary if injury is suspected. As in adults, repeat x-rays within 1 to 2 weeks to rule out occult navicular fracture are indicated.

4. **Treatment.** Any fracture that is open or that involves the joint space should be managed in direct consultation with an orthopaedist. In general, carpal bone fractures require immobilization for 6 to 10 weeks. Phalangeal and metacarpal bone fractures should be immobilized for 3 to 4 weeks. If a rotational deformity is present, ORIF may be necessary. Distal phalangeal crush injuries require meticulous cleaning and repair of associated soft tissue injury, with antibiotic coverage to decrease the incidence of osteomyelitis. The pediatric mallet finger equivalent is treated in much the same fashion as in the adult with full DIP extension.

5. **Complications.** Complications arise from a failure to recognize a fracture or to correct rotation or angulation and infection. Immobilization of the hand in small children is challenging. A bulky soft dressing may be necessary in infants. In older children, finger or gutter splints that incorporate an adjacent uninjured finger are applied, keeping the metacarpophalangeal (MCP) joints flexed from 70 to 90 degrees and both the interphalangeal joints in mild flexion. A thumb spica splint is necessary if navicular fracture is suspected. Once the finger is immobilized, prompt

follow-up with an orthopaedist or hand specialist is appropriate.

V. **Other injuries.** Ligamentous injuries and dislocations of the hand and fingers are rare in children; when they occur, they are managed as in adults.

VI. **Conclusion.** Orthopaedic injuries of the upper extremity are very common in the pediatric patient population. Any physician working in the emergency department should be familiar with their diagnosis and treatment. Many of the principles of adult orthopaedics apply to the pediatric population; however, some key differences between adults and children must be understood. It is an understanding of these differences and how they affect the treatment of the pediatric orthopaedic patient that will ensure the delivery of quality care to these special patients.

BIBLIOGRAPHY

Fleisher GR, Ludwig S. *Pediatric emergency medicine,* 3rd ed. Philadelphia: WB Saunders, 1993, chap 109

Ogden JA. *Skeletal injury in the child,* 2nd ed. Philadelphia: WB Saunders, 1990.

Rittenberry TJ. *Pediatric orthopaedics.* Core Lecture Series, University of Illinois Residency in Emergency Medicine. Chicago, University of Illinois, 1996.

Rockwood CA, Wilkens KE, Beaty JH. *Fractures in children,* 4th ed. Philadelphia: Lippincott-Raven, 1996.

Rosen P, Barkin RG, Danzl DF, et al. *Emergency medicine—concepts and clinical practice,* 3rd ed. St. Louis, Mosby, 1992, chaps 24–26.

Simon RR, Koenigsknecht SJ. *Emergency orthopaedics—the extremities,* 3rd ed., chaps 6–13, 32.

Strange GR, Ahrens W, Lelyveld S, Schafermeyer R. *Pediatric emergency medicine—a comprehensive study guide.* chaps 16–18.

Pediatric Orthopaedics: The Lower Extremity

Timothy James Rittenberry and Kenji Oyasu

In children, injury to the lower extremity is less common than injury to the upper. Several entities, such as slipped capital femoral epiphysis or Osgood-Schlatter disease, are unique to the pediatric population. While some lower extremity injuries and fractures will be obvious or easily diagnosed, the limping child remains one of the common diagnostic challenges in pediatric ambulatory care. Understanding the specific problems of the pediatric lower extremity is necessary in the day-to-day care of children.

I. **Pelvis and hip (Fig. 1)**
   A. **Pelvic fracture.** Pelvic fractures are uncommon in children; however, they are extremely serious injuries. Since the pediatric pelvis is pliable and resilient, the presence of pelvic fracture usually indicates extreme forces. Some 80% of pelvic fractures in children are caused by vehicular trauma. Pelvic fractures fall into three broad categories: **fractures of the pelvic ring, avulsion fractures,** and **acetabular fractures** (Fig. 2).
      1. **Mechanism.** Fractures of the pelvic ring are the result of the extreme forces typical of vehicular trauma or falls from a height. Avulsion fractures are infrequent in the very young, but avulsion of the iliac spine or ischium as the result of strenuous muscular traction is encountered in adolescent athletes. Acetabular fractures are associated with hip dislocation or direct pelvic trauma.
      2. **Physical examination.** Fracture of the pelvic ring is likely to accompany life-threatening injuries. Once the patient is stabilized, compression at the anterosuperior iliac spine may reveal instability or pain at the fracture site. Pain may be elicited on range of motion (ROM) of the hips in the inguinal region with a ramus fracture or in the hip itself with acetabular injury. A complete neurological exam of the lower extremity is essential, as impairment of sciatic, femoral, or obturator nerves as well as the lumbosacral plexus may occur. Localized swelling, tenderness, or ecchymosis may be noted at the site of avulsion injuries.
      3. **Radiography.** In the face of blunt trauma and suspected fracture of the pelvic ring or acetabulum, x-rays must be delayed until the patient is adequately stabilized and other injuries have been adequately addressed. Multiple views, including anteroposterior (AP), inlet, and outlet views, are

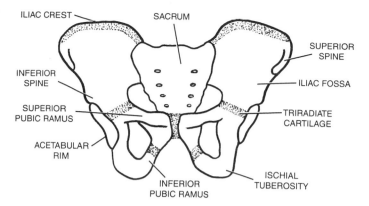

Fig. 1. The pediatric pelvis.

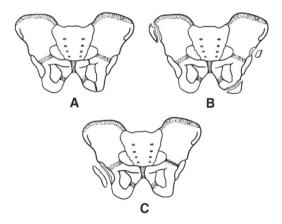

Fig. 2. Fractures of the pelvis. A: Disruption of the pelvic ring. B: Avulsion fracture. C: Acetabular fracture.

obtained *without* gonadal shielding. Computed tomography (CT) is typically necessary to define the fracture precisely and any associated hematoma. In suspected avulsion fractures, care is taken to compare the involved area with the contralateral area to avoid misinterpreting a normal-appearing apophysis as fracture.

4. **Treatment.** In fractures of the pelvic ring, a prioritized team approach to all associated life-threatening injuries supersedes specific care of the pelvic

injury. Because of the thick periosteum and robust cartilaginous and ligamentous support, pediatric pelvic fractures are often more stable than their adult counterparts. Young children more easily tolerate bed rest and heal more quickly than adults, making internal or external fixation less likely. Stable fracture may require only bed rest, while more displaced fractures may also require skeletal traction for reduction. As bone maturity nears, operative methods for reduction and stabilization prevail. In avulsion injuries, the patient should rest and be obliged to avoid weight bearing for several weeks to promote healing.

B. **Traumatic hip dislocation.** This uncommon injury in children and adolescents has a bimodal age distribution with increased frequency from ages of 4 to 7 and 11 to 15. The hip may be displaced anteriorly or posteriorly, depending on the mechanism of injury. Posterior dislocations make up approximately 80% of traumatic hip dislocations.

1. **Mechanism.** Because of increased joint laxity, hip dislocations in children under the age of 6 years can be due to such trivial trauma as minor falls or "doing the splits." In older children, severe trauma—such as motor vehicle accidents or significant falls—is involved, and the dislocation is often associated with acetabular fracture.

2. **Physical examination.** In posterior dislocation, the joint capsule is torn posteriorly by the head of the femur and the limb is held in flexion, adduction, and internal rotation. The femoral head can occasionally be felt in the gluteal region. The child will be in severe pain and will resist any passive or active motion at the hip. In anterior dislocation, the affected limb is normally abducted, externally rotated, and flexed. The femoral head is sometimes palpable in the groin.

3. **Radiography.** To define the dislocation and evaluate for associated acetabular or femoral fracture, AP and lateral views of the pelvis and femur are required. Gross displacement of the femoral head is usually visible on the AP view. A line drawn on the AP view from the anterosuperior iliac crest to the ischial tuberosity through the acetabulum helps determine the true position of dislocation. CT of the hip will demonstrate position and associated acetabular injury (Fig. 3).

4. **Treatment.** Prompt reduction is the recommended treatment for traumatic hip dislocation; it is ideally performed within 6 hours of injury and certainly within 12 hours. General anesthesia is recommended for closed reduction. Reduction techniques for posterior dislocation include pelvic stabilization and axial traction along the femur with the hip in flexion, as in the Allis or Stimson ma-

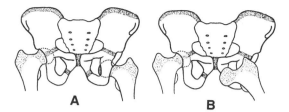

Fig. 3. Hip dislocations. A: Posterior ischial dislocation. B: Anterior obturator dislocation.

neuver (see Chapter 19, Hip and Femur, II, A, 1).
The majority of closed reductions are successful
and few require operative management.

5. **Disposition.** Once stabilized, children with hip
   dislocation require immediate orthopaedic consultation for admission and reduction. In the presence of isolated hip dislocation, closed reduction in
   the emergency department may be successful using conscious sedation techniques.

6. **Complications.** The major complications of traumatic hip dislocation are missed femoral fracture,
   aseptic necrosis, sciatic nerve palsy, and degenerative arthritis.

C. **Congenital hip dislocation.** At birth, the lack of development of both the acetabulum and the femur may
   lead to complete dislocation of the hip. There is loss of
   contact between the femoral head and the acetabulum, with the femoral head displaced laterally and superiorly. Females are affected six to eight times more
   often than males.

   1. **Mechanism.** These are congenital anomalies.
   2. **Physical examination.** In the neonatal period,
      diagnosis is made by demonstrating instability of
      the hip by one of two maneuvers. The Ortolani ma-
      neuver is performed with the relaxed child supine.
      With the examiner's fingers placed over the
      greater trochanter and the thumb over the in-
      ner thigh, both hips are flexed to 90 degrees and
      slowly abducted from the midline. With gentle for-
      ward pressure on the greater trochanter, a "click"
      or feeling of slippage indicates subluxation of the
      femoral head. Alternatively, the thumb may be
      used to apply slight pressure to the medial thigh
      as it is adducted, which causes the femoral head
      to sublux posteriorly. More subtle signs include
      redundant gluteal fat folds or unequal thigh
      length, best appreciated with the knees and hips
      in flexion.
   3. **Radiography.** Radiographs of the neonatal pelvis
      are notoriously unreliable. After 6 weeks of age,

lateral displacement of the femoral head is the
most reliable sign.

4. **Treatment.** If this condition is diagnosed in the
first few weeks of life, treatment consists of splinting with the hip maintained in flexion and abduction. Operative reduction may be necessary after
18 months of age.

5. **Disposition.** Orthopaedic consultation is necessary to plan for prompt definitive care.

6. **Complications.** Failure to diagnose congenital
hip displacement within the first year may result
in flexion contracture, marked lordosis, and a painless limp with a lurch to the affected side (Trendelenburg sign). Bilateral involvement will result in
a waddling gait. Excessive force used during reduction can result in avascular necrosis of the hip.

D. **Slipped capital femoral epiphysis (SCFE).** SCFE
is a transepiphyseal separation of the proximal
femoral epiphysis. The femoral epiphysis is usually
displaced posteriorly and medially relative to the
femoral neck. The condition occurs most frequently in
early adolescence and more commonly in overweight
male children. Bilateral involvement occurs in up to
25% of patients. Patients usually present with vague
symptoms of pain or progressing limp over a pro-
tracted period of time. The pain is often referred to the
groin, knee, or medial thigh.

1. **Mechanism.** The cause is not clear, although some
authorities have demonstrated decreased strength
in the perichondrial ring, which stabilizes the epiphyseal area in the adolescent years. The mechanical load to the obliquely oriented physis can produce a pathological fracture through the growth
plate. The condition occasionally presents acutely
after a fall or direct trauma, but this probably represents an acute slippage on the already present
condition; frank transepiphyseal fracture is rare.

2. **Physical examination.** A consistent finding on
examination is limitation of internal rotation of
the hip. The femur is held in slight flexion and external rotation and this may be associated with local tenderness about the hip.

3. **Radiography.** Radiographic evaluation should include the AP, lateral, and "frog-leg" (external rotation and abduction) views of the hips. The displacement of the femoral epiphysis may be subtle;
evaluation of Shenton's line on the AP pelvis and the
appearance of the "frog-leg" view of the hip help
identify the injury. The examination of Kline's line
will further improve diagnostic accuracy. Any asymmetry of the relationship of the femoral head to the
femoral neck should raise suspicion of SCFE (Fig. 4).

4. **Treatment.** Patients are admitted and kept non-
weight bearing until operative intervention, typically pinning, occurs. Severe separations with dis-

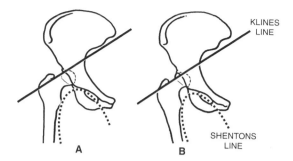

Fig. 4. Shenton's and Kline's lines. A: Slipped capital femoral epiphysis. B: Normal.

placement require closed reduction prior to pinning.

5. **Complications.** Avascular necrosis and growth arrest, which seem related to the degree of dislocation, may occur.

E. **Transient synovitis of the hip.** This occurs most commonly between the ages of 3 and 10 and is more frequent in boys. The diagnosis must be made with extreme caution, especially in children less than 18 months of age, in whom septic arthritis must be considered. Onset may be insidious or abrupt, manifesting as limp or pain in the hip, knee, or thigh.

   1. **Mechanism.** The cause of transient synovitis is not known. Allergy, viral infection, and trauma may all have a role.

   2. **Physical examination.** A well-appearing child has pain but allows passive range of motion of the hip with minimal pain or limitation.

   3. **Radiography.** Views of the hip and femur are typically unremarkable, although an increased joint space may indicate effusion.

   4. **Treatment.** Transient synovitis of the hip is a *diagnosis of exclusion*. Once other entities, most importantly septic arthritis, are ruled out, the child may be treated with rest and analgesics. Skeletal traction may be of use in the most severe cases.

   5. **Disposition.** Discharge with prompt orthopaedic follow-up is appropriate.

   6. **Complications.** Transient synovitis is benign and self-limited.

F. **Septic hip.** The hip is the most commonly infected joint in childhood.

   1. **Mechanism.** The joint is infected by direct spread from adjacent tissues or hematogenously. The most common pathogens are *Staphylococcus, Streptococcus,* gram-negative baccili, or *Haemophilus influenzae.*

2. **Physical examination.** Although the findings of septic hip in the neonate can be nonspecific, older children with pyogenic arthritis appear strikingly ill, with fever, malaise, vomiting, and severely restricted motion of the affected joint. Patients will not tolerate passive range of motion and the hip is usually held in flexion, abduction, and slight external rotation to maximize the available joint space. In infants, suspicion is aroused by decreased hip abduction with irritability and poor feeding. Infants may not have a significant fever. In addition to physical and x-ray findings, patients will typically have elevated erythrocyte sedimentation rates and leukocytosis. Fluoroscopically guided arthrocentesis confirms the diagnosis.

3. **Radiography.** Early in the course of septic hip, widening of the joint space may be discernible. Later changes include destruction of the joint space, resorption of epiphyseal cartilage, and erosion of adjacent bone. Evidence of osteomyelitis of the femoral metaphysis should alert the physician to the likelihood of joint infection.

4. **Treatment.** Pyogenic arthritis is best treated by arthrotomy for surgical drainage. Antibiotics are selected based on age, Gram stain, and culture of the aspirate. A reasonable empirical antibiotic therapy combines nafcillin and a third-generation cephalosporin. Three weeks of therapy is recommended for staphylococcal infection, while other organisms require 2 weeks. Oral therapy may begin when the patient is clinically improved. Intra-articular injections of antibiotics are not necessary.

5. **Disposition.** Children will need to be admitted for parenteral antibiotics and immediate diagnostic arthrocentesis and, if necessary, surgical drainage by an orthopedist.

6. **Complications.** If infection is present for more than 24 hours, dissolution of the proteoglycans of the articular cartilage will occur, with subsequent fibrosis of the joint.

G. **Avascular necrosis of the femoral head (Legg-Calvé-Perthes disease).** The highest incidence of avascular necrosis of the femoral head occurs between the ages of 3 and 10 with boys affected four times more often than girls. Although uncommon, this condition is included in the differential diagnoses of hip pain and limp.

1. **Mechanism.** Although the pathological and radiographic features are well known, the exact cause is not. Necrosis may follow trauma or infection, but idiopathic lesions may develop during periods of rapid bone growth. The common underlying pathology probably involves occlusion of the anterior, posterosuperior, and posteroinferior vessels pass-

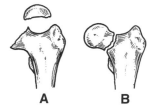

Fig. 5. Femoral neck fractures. A: Displaced transepiphyseal fracture. B: Nondisplaced transcervical fracture.

ing along the neck of the femur from either complete division of the vessels, kinking, or tamponade due to hemarthrosis.

2. **Physical examination.** Patients present with hip pain or antalgic gait of insidious progression over weeks to months. Persistent pain is the most common symptom and limited range of motion is usually the only physical finding.

3. **Radiography.** Radiographic findings correlate with the progression of necrosis. Joint effusion with slight widening of the joint space and periarticular swelling are the earliest findings. As replacement of the necrotic ossification centers occurs, there is rarefaction of the bone in a patchwork fashion, producing alternating areas of bone lucency and density that appear as fragmentation of the femoral epiphysis. There may be widening and flattening of the femoral head, termed coxa plana. If the growth center of the femoral neck becomes involved, a varus deformity will occur.

4. **Treatment.** Multiple treatment approaches exist, all of which employ protection of the femoral head within the acetabulum. Bracing is used to retain the hip in abduction, flexion, and internal rotation.

5. **Complications** include progressive joint stiffness and pain. The prognosis for complete restoration of the necrotic femoral head in children is excellent, but function will depend on the amount of deformity. Those in whom the disease manifests late in childhood and those who have complete involvement of the femoral head have a poorer prognosis.

H. **Proximal femoral fractures.** Pediatric hip fractures are extremely rare. They are more common in boys, with a male-to-female ratio of 3:2. Since considerable force is always involved, associated injuries are common. Pathological fractures may occur in disease states such as hypothyroidism, juvenile rheumatoid arthritis, renal osteodystrophy, pyogenic arthritis, and malignancy. Owing to the strength of the combined periosteal-perichondrial complex, fractures may be nondisplaced. Ischemic necrosis, a potential complication, can affect the epiphysis, metaphysis, or the physis individually or in any combination. Fractures may be transphyseal, transcervical (most common), or intertrochanteric (Fig. 5).

1. **Mechanism.** Proximal femoral fractures in children are usually the result of violent trauma. If a history of seemingly trivial trauma is elicited, the physician's suspicion for pathological fracture or abuse should be aroused. Stress fractures from chronic microtrauma may also occur.

2. **Physical examination.** The child is reluctant or unable to bear weight on the affected leg. The injured limb is noted to appear shortened and in external rotation. When the fracture is displaced, the patient will be unable to move the hip actively and will have marked restriction of passive range of motion.

3. **Radiography.** Diagnosis is confirmed by the AP and lateral views. The direction of the fracture line and the degree of displacement should be noted as well as whether the femoral head is retained within the acetabulum. Normal-appearing plain films in the face of clinical suspicion may be complemented by CT or nuclear magnetic resonance studies.

4. **Treatment.** A nondisplaced fracture of the proximal femur may be immobilized with a hip spica cast. Displaced fractures will require more aggressive treatment with closed reduction or open reduction and internal fixation (ORIF) under general anesthesia. Endoprosthetic replacement is not an option in the pediatric population.

5. **Disposition.** Admission and orthopaedic evaluation are mandatory once associated life-threatening injuries have been addressed.

6. **Complications.** There is a high incidence of complication regardless of therapeutic modality, including coxa vara deformity, avascular necrosis, nonunion, and leg-length discrepancy.

I. **Femoral shaft fractures.** Diaphyseal fractures of the femur make up approximately 2% of all pediatric fractures. The most frequent site of injury is the middle third, where normal anterolateral bowing is at its maximum. Greenstick fractures may occur, usually at the distal metaphysis. The incidence peaks from 2 to 5 years of age and is three times more frequent in boys than girls. Falls are the most common cause in children under age 3. As with all pediatric fractures, the possibility of abuse must be entertained. In older children with a stronger femoral shaft, fracture results from violent trauma, and care must be taken to identify and treat associated injuries. Although isolated femoral fractures rarely lead to hemodynamic instability, patients with associated injuries may require transfusion (Fig. 6).

1. **Mechanism.** Direct trauma from falls and motor vehicle accidents is the most common cause. The

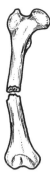

Fig. 6. Femoral shaft fracture.

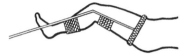

Fig. 7. Thomas splint.

severity of violence as well as strong muscular traction typically contribute to displacement with variable amounts of overriding.

2. **Physical examination.** The patient is examined gently to avoid unnecessary pain. Localized pain, swelling, inability to move the affected limb, deformity, shortening, and crepitus will be noted. The neurovascular status of the distal extremity should be serially assessed and documented. Femoral fractures are commonly associated with intraabdominal, pelvic, and genitourinary injuries, necessitating a thorough physical examination.

3. **Radiography.** AP and lateral radiographs of the femur easily define the location, the degree of displacement, and angulation of the fracture.

4. **Treatment.** Proper emergency department care includes gentle handling and adequate splinting, once other life-threatening injuries have been addressed, to prevent further soft tissue injury. The Thomas splint provides excellent immobilization of femoral fractures (Fig. 7). Definitive treatment varies. As anatomical reduction in the pediatric patient is not essential for adequate function, the simplest form of treatment is usually the best. Patients with uncomplicated fractures of the femoral shaft may be treated immediately with a spica cast or may require traction for several weeks, followed by casting. Recently, pediatric orthopaedists have

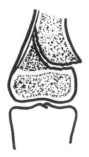

Fig. 8.   Fracture/separation
of the distal femoral physis.

employed internal and external fixation with greater frequency. Vascular compromise mandates ORIF.

5. **Disposition.** All patients with femoral fractures are admitted for treatment. Slow vascular leaks must be excluded with a period of observation. All associated injuries must be addressed and the possibility of abuse must be excluded.

6. **Complications.** Neurovascular compromise is the most alarming complication in the acute setting. Leg-length discrepancy, which can result from excessive overriding or from stimulation of linear growth, is the most frequent complication. Shaft fractures with angular deformities increase the possibility of slipped capital femoral epiphysis. Muscular atrophy due to prolonged immobilization typically requires rehabilitation to reestablish strength and gait.

J. **Fracture of the distal femoral epiphysis.** Distal femoral epiphyseal injuries are relatively common, constituting 5% of all physeal fractures. They most commonly present as Salter II fractures, although any Salter pattern may be seen. Because the distal femoral epiphyseal complex is a major contributor to leg length, these injuries can lead to serious long-term problems should any degree of growth arrest occur (Fig. 8).

1. **Mechanism.** Fracture of the distal physis is usually caused by indirect trauma, most commonly violent valgus, varus, or hyperextension stress at the knee. Typically, a football player is hit from the side at the knee while his cleated foot is fixed to the ground, thereby sustaining a compression force across the portion of the growth plate nearest the blow while generating tension stress on the opposite side. This results in separation of the epiphysis and metaphysis on the tension side and an oblique fracture through the metaphysis on the compression side. Separation due to direct trauma can also occur, as when the knee is crushed be-

tween two car bumpers. Less commonly, separation can result from birth trauma, particularly in breech presentations. Forced hyperextension may result in fracture-separation with the femoral metaphysis forced posteriorly, resulting in popliteal artery injury.

2. **Physical examination.** The patient is unable to ambulate or bear weight immediately after the injury. The knee may be held in flexion because of hamstring spasm and the patient complains of severe pain. If the separation is also displaced, the thigh may appear shortened. The presenting deformity will depend on the degree and direction of displacement. Swelling of the knee and soft tissue develops rapidly. Whenever the diagnosis of epiphyseal separation is suspected, careful distal neurovascular examination is mandatory.

3. **Radiography.** Standard plain films with AP and lateral views typically reveal the fracture. Oblique views of the distal femur may reveal occult fractures through the epiphysis or metaphysis. Stress films may be helpful if spontaneous reduction of a displaced Salter I injury is suspected or if multiple views are negative, yet strong clinical suspicion remains. Views of the contralateral extremity may be necessary when there is a question of narrowing of the lucent physeal line.

4. **Treatment.** Closed reduction with 4 to 6 weeks of immobilization in a long leg cast may suffice in nondisplaced, stable fractures. Inadequate closed reduction, instability, or Salter III or IV fractures require ORIF. In the acute setting, adequate analgesia and control of muscular spasm are of tantamount importance.

5. **Disposition.** All injuries of this type will require immediate orthopaedic referral and hospitalization. Appropriate surgical consultation should be obtained if there is neurovascular compromise. A posterior long leg splint should be applied.

6. **Complications.** Complications include popliteal artery damage, neurapraxia of the peroneal nerve, and recurrent displacement. Delayed complications include angular deformity, leg-length discrepancy, and joint stiffness.

II. **Knee**

A. **Separation of the proximal tibial epiphysis.** Although physeal injuries are relatively common during childhood, injury of the proximal tibial physis is rare and constitutes less than 1% of all physeal injuries. This is a result of the protection afforded the physis by the proximal fibula, the downward extension of the tibial tuberosity, and the medial collateral ligament (Fig. 9).

1. **Mechanism.** Fracture/separation of the proximal tibial epiphysis is the result of direct trauma, as

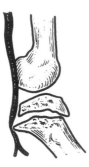

Fig. 9.   Fracture/separation
of the proximal tibial physis.

when a child's leg is pinned between two bumpers.
More often, however, the mechanism of injury is
indirect, as in femoral epiphyseal injuries.

2. **Physical examination.** Patients present with
   history of trauma and severe pain and swelling of
   the knee. Passive and active extension will be very
   limited due to hamstring spasm, tense hemarthrosis, and protective muscle splinting. Tenderness is
   present over the proximal tibial growth plate 1 to 2
   cm below the joint line. If there is posterior displacement of the proximal metaphysis, a step-off
   may be felt at the level of the tibial tubercle. If
   there is medial or lateral displacement, there will
   be associated valgus or varus deformity. Neurovascular examination may reveal arterial insufficiency from injury of the popliteal artery at the
   time of epiphyseal separation.

3. **Radiography.** Plain films of nondisplaced Salter I
   fractures will appear normal and a small metaphyseal fragment may be the only evidence of
   nondisplaced Salter II injury. An increased patellofemoral space on the lateral view is indicative of
   extensive hemarthrosis. Stress x-rays may be necessary to fully delineate the extent of injury. CT
   scanning is not done in the acute setting but may
   be useful in planning treatment of Salter III and
   IV injuries. Arteriography is indicated when vascular compromise is obvious and may be indicated
   if significant fracture/separation has occurred.

4. **Treatment.** A Salter I injury is treated with closed
   reduction. Salter III and IV fractures are likely to
   require ORIF.

5. **Disposition.** All injuries of this type will require
   immediate orthopaedic referral and hospitalization for definitive care. A posterior long leg splint
   is used to stabilize the injury.

6. **Complications.** Acutely, there is risk of popliteal
   artery injury and peroneal nerve impairment. Re-

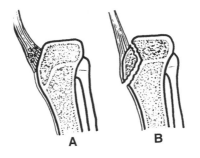

Fig. 10.   Tibial tuberosity lesions. A: Osgood-Schlatter
lesion. B: True avulsion of the tuberosity.

current deformity, leg-length discrepancy, and degenerative joint disease may occur in time.

B. **Avulsion of the tibial tubercle.** Acute avulsion of
the tibial tubercle is rare, representing about 1% of
physeal injuries. Osgood-Schlatter disease, which is
caused by chronic and repetitive pulling by the patellar tendon and resulting in small avulsions of the tubercle surface, is more commonly encountered. These
two conditions probably represent a spectrum of disease, from the innocuous Osgood-Schlatter lesion to
the more severe Salter-Harris type III avulsion fracture of the entire proximal tibial epiphysis. Osgood-
Schlatter disease is seen most commonly in adolescent
athletes between the ages of 11 and 14 years and is
found bilaterally in up to 25% of patients (Fig. 10).

1. **Mechanism.** Acute traumatic avulsion of the tibial tubercle may occur during sports or play activities when violent contraction of the quadriceps
muscle causes tension of the patellar ligament, exceeding the combined strength of the physis underlying the tubercle, the surrounding perichon-
drium, and the adjacent periosteum. Acute
avulsions occur more frequently in adolescents
with preexisting Osgood-Schlatter disease.

2. **Physical examination.** The Osgood-Schlatter
knee is insidious in onset. Young athletes present
with intermittent, activity-related knee pain located about a slightly swollen and very tender tibial tubercle. Patients will have at most partial disability with little restriction of movement due to
pain. Acute traumatic avulsions, however, will
result in immediate, marked pain and swelling.
Edema and tenderness are centered over the anterior aspect of the proximal tibia. There may be
joint effusion, even tense hemarthrosis, particularly in a type III fracture/separation. A freely mo-

bile triangular fragment may be palpable with crepitus, and the patella may be notably displaced cephalad. Knee extension against resistance will be severely limited.

3. **Radiography.** AP and lateral views of the knee or tibia are necessary in patients with unilateral disease or suspected acute avulsion. Soft tissue technique can further define the margins of the patellar ligament and the smaller irregular fragments of bone at its distal insertion, characteristic of Osgood-Schlatter disease. Acute avulsion of the tubercle will appear as a more obvious Salter III fracture/separation. When symptoms and findings are bilateral and consistent with Osgood-Schlatter disease, radiographic evaluation is not necessary. Unilateral disease should be x-rayed to rule out the possibility of osteomyelitis or bone tumor.

4. **Treatment.** Treatment for Osgood-Schlatter disease is symptomatic and supportive. The goal is to ease pain and swelling. Temporary restriction of vigorous activities and sports may be sufficient. If symptoms are severe enough to interfere with daily activities, a knee immobilizer or long leg cast may be indicated for up to 6 weeks. Operative treatment consists of simple excision and is reserved for symptomatic ununited ossicles after growth plate closure. Acute avulsion of the tibial tubercle with displacement will require ORIF.

5. **Disposition.** The overall prognosis for Osgood-Schlatter disease is good. After the symptoms resolve, the patient usually regains full function and may return to activities. Orthopaedic referral is recommended for follow-up.

   Acute avulsion of the tibial tubercle will require immediate referral and hospitalization. Immobilization with a long leg posterior splint is indicated.

6. **Complications.** Acute avulsion of the tibial tubercle may result in immediate compartment syndrome, partial growth arrest of the physis, and loss of knee flexion.

C. **Patellar injuries.** Patellar fractures in children are uncommon owing to the thick layer of cartilage that surrounds the osseous portion of the patella and acts as a cushion to direct trauma. In addition, the distracting force generated by a child's quadriceps musculature is much less than that of the adult. Traction forces can, however, cause a **sleeve fracture** of the patella as a large portion of the cartilaginous lower pole of the patella is avulsed (Fig. 11). Patellar **dislocation** may result in an osteochondral fracture of the medial margin of the patella. Abnormal knee architecture (genu valgum, patella alta, flattening of the lateral femoral condyle) alters the intrinsic biomechanics,

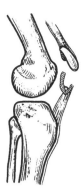

Fig. 11. Sleeve fracture of the patella. The small calcific avulsion on x-ray may be associated with a large cartilaginous separation.

allowing such lateral dislocation to occur, most frequently in obese females 16 to 20 years of age.

1. **Mechanism.** Fracture of the patella occurs by direct blow, sudden contraction of the extensor mechanism, or a combination of both. Direct trauma may cause a linear or comminuted fracture pattern and is usually the result of a fall. Avulsion of the distal pole of the patella has been known to occur because of such indirect stresses as jumping or propelling a skateboard. Preexisting abnormalities in the extensor mechanism may predispose the patient to avulsion fractures. Osseochrondral fractures of the medial patellar margin occur with dislocation of the patella as it strikes the lateral femoral condyle.

2. **Physical examination.** The injured knee is swollen and tender. There is often an associated tense hemarthrosis with limited ability to extend the knee fully, particularly against resistance. The patient may be unable to stand and bear weight on the injured extremity. A high-riding patella or a palpable gap may be noted. In avulsion of the distal pole, voluntary contraction of the quadriceps muscle draws the patella upward, but the patellar ligament remains lax. With a marginal fracture, straight leg raising is intact and tenderness may be elicited along the medial patella. A dislocated patella is clinically obvious. It is important to look for evidence that a patellar dislocation may have occurred with spontaneous reduction. Passive manipulation of the patella toward the lateral femoral condyle may reveal instability, increased pain, and patient apprehension.

3. **Radiography.** AP, lateral, and "sunrise" views of the patella are obtained. **Transverse** fractures

are best seen on the lateral view, as the major fragments may tilt toward one another with a wider gap anteriorly. The articular cartilage may remain intact even with a complete fracture through the bony portion of the patella. The extent of the fracture may be best illustrated with the knee flexed to 30 degrees. Careful examination may reveal a very small and innocuous-appearing fracture of the inferior patellar pole, indicating the possibility of a much more extensive sleeve fracture.

Longitudinal fractures are best seen on axial or skyline views. The amount of tilt, lateral subluxation, and lateral overhang of the patella relative to the femoral condyles are appreciated as well on this view. A **bipartite patella** is a normal variant that may be mistaken for a fracture and is best seen on the AP view. It appears as a crescent-shaped radiolucent line in the superior and lateral quadrants of the patella. If the patient is symptomatic, it is helpful to obtain contralateral x-rays to support the diagnosis.

4. **Treatment.** Closed therapy is recommended for nondisplaced fractures if active extension is possible at the time of presentation. Aspiration of the hemarthrosis may provide symptomatic relief. Patients will require long leg circumferential casting from groin to ankle with the knee flexed no more than 5 degrees for 4 to 6 weeks with full weight bearing allowed early. Operative treatment is reserved for displaced fractures with loss of active knee extension or open fractures with intraarticular involvement. An uncomplicated patellar dislocation is reduced easily with the patient seated on the gurney by placing the hip in full flexion and the knee in extension prior to manipulating the patella. A knee immobilizer or cylindrical cast is used for 2 to 3 weeks.

5. **Disposition.** Prognosis is good for nondisplaced fractures or a displaced fracture with adequate reduction and good apposition. Patients may be immobilized and discharged in a knee immobilizer or long leg posterior splint from the emergency department with close orthopaedic follow-up. Open fractures will require parenteral antibiotics and immediate orthopaedic referral.

6. **Complications** of an unreduced displaced fracture include patella alta, extensor lag, and quadriceps atrophy.

D. **Nonphyseal fractures of the tibia and fibula.** Fractures of the tibia and fibula are the most common injuries of the pediatric lower extremity and are the third most common long bone injury. They can be classified into three major categories based on the bones fractured: **isolated tibial fracture, isolated fibular fracture,** and **fracture of both tibia and fibula,**

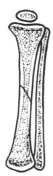

Fig. 12. Toddler fracture.

which occurs in about 30% of cases. Children less than 4 years of age are likely to sustain nondisplaced spiral fractures of the tibia. This is especially common in toddlers learning to walk and is known as a "toddler fracture." Between 5 and 10 years of age, transverse fractures of the tibia predominate (Fig. 12).

1. **Mechanism.** Tibial shaft and metaphyseal fractures are commonly caused by indirect trauma such as rotational or twisting forces and less commonly by direct trauma. Indirect trauma will result in an oblique or spiral fracture, while direct trauma usually results in a transverse or butterfly pattern. Common causes of these injuries include falls, sports, motor vehicle accidents, and bicycle spoke injuries. Isolated tibial fractures most commonly occur with outward rotation of the body over a fixed foot. With an intact fibula, there is usually no shortening of the limb, although varus angulation may develop. Up to age 6, torsion of the foot produces a spiral fracture of the tibia with no fibular fracture. Isolated fibular fractures are rare and usually result from a direct blow to the lateral aspect of the lower leg.

2. **Physical examination.** Signs and symptoms of a tibial or fibular fracture depend on the degree of injury and the age of the patient. In the very young child with a toddler fracture, the diagnosis is often based on parental information and clinical findings alone. Frequently a clear mechanism of injury is lacking. The child will complain of pain to a variable degree or not at all yet refuse to bear weight. There may be local tenderness at the fracture site but no obvious deformity. An isolated fracture of the fibular shaft may show only a minor degree of pain, while the pain of a transverse fracture of the tibial shaft in an older child will be severe. Incomplete fractures may not prevent weight bearing and the child may present with a limp. Neurovas-

cular impairment is uncommon but may occur especially with proximal injury. Careful evaluation of distal pulses and the ability to dorsiflex and plantarflex the toes and foot is important when the injury involves the proximal tibial metaphysis, as compartment syndrome may develop.

3. **Radiography.** AP and lateral views that include the knee and ankle joints must be taken. Incomplete and torus fractures are difficult to appreciate and may require contralateral films for comparison. Isolated spiral fractures of the tibia may be seen on only one view. A toddler fracture may not be apparent radiographically at the initial exam. The diagnosis may be confirmed when repeat films 10 to 14 days later reveal subperiosteal formation of new bone.

4. **Treatment.** Pediatric fractures of the tibial and fibular shafts are usually uncomplicated and can be treated with closed reduction and immobilization. The toddler fracture is immobilized in a long leg cast for 3 weeks, while older children may require 6 weeks of immobilization. Surgical fixation may be required in the adolescent with an open or unstable fracture.

5. **Disposition.** Isolated undisplaced fractures of the tibia require placement of a long leg posterior mold and are often treated on an outpatient basis after the immediate orthopaedic consultation. Patients with more complicated fractures and those involving the tibia and fibula are hospitalized. Owing to the proximity of the bifurcation of the popliteal artery, fractures of the proximal third of the tibia require great care and hospitalization for neurovascular monitoring.

6. **Complications.** Benign-appearing fractures of the proximal tibial metaphysis may result in vascular injury or significant valgus deformity. Compartment syndrome may follow vascular injury or fractures with extensive soft tissue injury. Open fractures are associated with a high incidence of delayed union, nonunion, and infection.

E. **Fractures of the distal tibial and fibular physes** comprise 4% of all ankle injuries. In young children, the ligaments are stronger than bone, and ligamentous injuries are unlikely. Severe forces usually result in disruption of the physis before they cause complete ligamentous disruption. The growth plates of the distal tibia and fibula are involved in 15% to 25% of all physeal injuries. A Salter I fracture should always be considered in the case of an ankle injury that results in pain or soft tissue swelling without radiographic evidence of fracture.

1. **Mechanism.** Most of the ankle injuries in children are caused by indirect mechanisms. The foot is usually fixed in a position such as inversion or

eversion while the leg rotates over the foot. Direct injuries such as axial compression are rare but can have serious sequelae. These injuries are responsible for a wide variety of Salter-Harris fractures of the distal tibia and fibula. Injuries can be classified into the following groupings:

   a. **Supination/external rotation**
   b. **Pronation/eversion/external rotation**
   c. **Supination/plantarflexion**
   d. **Supination/inversion**
   e. **Axial compression**
   f. **Juvenile Tillaux**
   g. **Triplane fracture**

2. **Physical examination.** Since ligamentous injuries are rare in children, the areas of maximal tenderness may be over the epiphysis, metaphysis, or physis. The clinical findings will vary with the degree of injury. Careful examination of the injured extremity will reveal areas of tenderness, swelling, and ecchymosis. There may be obvious deformity when a fracture/separation of the distal tibial physis is present. The neurovascular status should be assessed early and often during the treatment course. It is important to examine the whole limb, especially the lateral aspect of the leg and the entire fibula, since a proximal fibular fracture can occur in pronation/eversion/external rotation injuries.

3. **Radiography.** The radiographic evaluation should include AP, lateral, and oblique views. An x-ray that shows the entire tibia and fibula is important to rule out proximal fibular fracture. In assessing x-rays, particular attention should be paid to the direction of the physeal displacement, the type of physeal injury, and the location of the metaphyseal fragment. Soft tissue swelling may be the only evidence that a Salter I or minimally displaced distal fibular fracture is present. The juvenile Tillaux fracture of the distal tibial physis or the triplane fracture are seen in the presence of the partially fused tibial physis of the adolescent; these fracture patterns must be sought whenever this partial fusion is observed. The complex nature of the triplane fracture may require CT to fully delineate its extent and help plan for reduction.

4. **Treatment.** Injuries of the Salter I and II type can typically be managed conservatively, but if adequate reduction cannot be achieved, ORIF is necessary. Juvenile Tillaux fractures and triplane fractures are treated as injuries of the Salter III and IV type. If more than 2 mm of displacement is present after reduction, operative intervention is required. In patients under the age of 10, some displacement can be accepted, since bone remodeling will occur. Open reduction for displacement greater

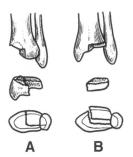

Fig. 13.   Distal tibial fracture. A: The triplane fracture. B: The tillaux fracture.

A   B

than 2 mm will reduce the incidence of premature asymmetrical growth arrest and subsequent growth aberrancy.

5. **Disposition.** Prognosis is good for nondisplaced fractures or a displaced fracture with adequate reduction and good apposition. Patients may be immobilized and discharged from the emergency department with close orthopaedic follow-up for isolated closed injury. Open fractures will require parenteral antibiotics and immediate orthopaedic referral. Total time of immobilization depends on the child's age and the type of fracture.

6. **Complications** include angular or rotational deformities, leg-length discrepancy, delayed union or nonunion, osteoarthritis, and avascular necrosis.

F. **Fracture of the talus.** Fracture of the talus occurs rarely in children. The most severe injuries resemble adult patterns but generally do not occur until skeletal maturity is approached.

1. **Mechanism of injury.** Forced dorsiflexion is the most common mechanism of injury, as the talar neck impinges upon the anterior lip of the tibia (Fig. 13).

2. **Physical examination.** Fractures with obvious deformity present little problem in evaluation, but nondisplaced fractures can be difficult to diagnose. Swelling and tenderness of the dorsal foot in the region of the talus, especially when a history of dorsiflexion injury is elicited, should alert the examiner to this possibility, but local swelling may be absent in nondisplaced fractures. Dorsiflexion of the ankle joint will exacerbate pain.

3. **X-ray.** Anterior, posterior, lateral, and oblique x-rays should be obtained, with the beam centered on the hindfoot. Transchondral fractures that occur at the cartilaginous surface of the talar dome can occur in children over age 10 and are difficult to diagnose. Careful examination of the mortise view, looking for irregularities, is very important.

4. **Treatment.** If the fracture is nondisplaced or minimally displaced, treatment consists of immobilization in a non-weight-bearing cast after resolution of soft tissue swelling. When the head of the talus is displaced, closed reduction with adequate anesthesia should be undertaken and the foot immobilized appropriately to avoid recurrence of the deformity. If the reduction is unstable, the child may require percutaneous pinning or open reduction. Most often, the foot is casted with the forefoot in 20 to 30 degrees of plantarflexion in a non-weight-bearing cast for 6 to 8 weeks.

5. **Disposition.** Prognosis is good for nondisplaced or adequately reduced displaced fractures. Patients may be immobilized and discharged from the emergency department with close orthopaedic follow-up for isolated closed, nondisplaced fractures. Open fractures require parenteral antibiotics and immediate orthopaedic referral. Total time of immobilization will depend upon the child's age and the type of fracture.

6. **Complications.** The most significant complication of talar injury is avascular necrosis. Development of the talus ossification center may be impaired, depending on the amount of ischemia. In children over the age of 10, ischemic necrosis becomes more common. Most cases become evident within 6 months following injury. Displaced fractures of the neck, crush injuries, and dislocations of the talus carry the highest risk, followed by ORIF.

G. **Calcaneal fractures.** Calcaneal fractures are uncommon in children. Occult fractures, however, have been found to be more common than previously thought. Fracture of the calcaneus should be considered in any limping toddler with or without a history of trauma. These injuries must be differentiated from infection, rheumatological disease, neurological conditions, occult soft tissue injury, or pathological fracture due to bone cyst. Three significant differences in pediatric calcaneal injuries as compared with those in adults should be kept in mind. First, Boehler's angle will not reliably detect fracture until the teenage years. In addition, intraarticular fractures are less likely to require operative intervention. Finally, associated axial loading injuries to the body, such as vertebral compression and renal pedicle injury, are extremely rare.

1. **Mechanism of injury.** Calcaneal fractures in adults usually result from a high-energy load. In children under the age of 10, fractures can result from falls of less than 1 m. In older children, the average height is 4 m. Fracture of the calcaneus in toddlers is typically a low-energy fracture with a compression mechanism that resembles the torus

fractures of the distal radius. Lawn-mower injuries are the most frequent cause of open calcaneal injuries in children. Calcaneal apophyseal fractures may occur as a result of the direct trauma or avulsion of the Achilles tendon.

2. **Physical examination.** A history of a fall and subsequent inability to walk, with localized pain, swelling, and tenderness, often make diagnosis simple. Careful palpation of the heel in a child refusing to walk may well provide the key to diagnosis.

3. **X-ray.** Standard AP, lateral, and axial views are used. If initial pain films are negative yet the diagnosis of occult calcaneal fracture remains in question, follow-up films may reveal an arc of sclerosis across the tuberosity of the calcaneus, which will confirm the diagnosis. Although a bone scan may confirm the diagnosis earlier, it does expose the child to more radiation and increase the cost of treating a self-limited condition that will heal completely with minimal treatment.

4. **Treatment.** The prognosis for calcaneal fractures in the pediatric age group after closed reduction and immobilization is excellent. Children will require non-weight-bearing long leg immobilization until the fracture is healed, usually 4 to 6 weeks. No complications have been reported in children following closed fractures of the calcaneus.

5. **Disposition.** Patients may be immobilized and discharged from the emergency department with close orthopaedic follow-up for isolated closed injury. Open fractures will require parenteral antibiotics and immediate orthopaedic referral. Total time of immobilization depends upon the child's age and the type of fracture.

6. **Complications.** Rarely, intraarticular injuries will require ORIF.

BIBLIOGRAPHY

Ciarallo L, Fleisher G. Femoral fractures: are children at risk for significant blood Loss? *Pediatr Emerg Care* 12:343–346.

Hughes MJ, D'Agostino J. Posterior hip dislocation in a five year old boy: a case report, review of the literature, and current recommendations. *J Emerg Med* 1996;14:585–590.

Ogden JA. *Skeletal injury in the child,* 2nd ed. Philadelphia: WB Saunders, 1990.

Reisdorf EJ, Roberts MR, Wiegenstein JG. *Pediatric emergency medicine.* Philadelphia: WB Saunders, 1993.

Rittenberry TJ. *Pediatric orthopaedics.* Core Lecture Series, University of Illinois Residency in Emergency Medicine. Chicago, University of Illinois, 1996.

Rockwood CA, Wilkins KE, Beaty JH. *Fractures in children,* 4th ed. Philadelphia: Lippincott-Raven, 1996.

Rosen P, Barkin RM, Danzl DF, et al. *Emergency medicine,* 3rd ed. St Louis: Mosby, 1992.

VI

Special Topics in Emergency Medicine

Foreign Bodies in Soft Tissues

Diana Rae Williams

Penetrating trauma may be accompanied by residual embedded foreign bodies (1–3). Retained foreign bodies are unusual; however, if they are not appropriately detected and managed, serious complications may ensue, including delayed healing, infection, pain, and loss of function (4). Furthermore, failure to diagnose foreign bodies is the second most common source of malpractice claims against emergency physicians (5). This chapter describes important historical factors, physical exam findings, appropriate imaging studies, and emergency department interventions for patients who have sustained penetrating trauma with the potential for retained foreign bodies.

I. **Mechanism of injury.** Mechanism of injury is the key historical factor in evaluating a patient with penetrating trauma. Other essential information includes the time the injury occurred and the environmental setting in which the injury was sustained.

Glass, which shatters on the skin, most commonly from windows or bottles, is a notorious etiology of foreign bodies. Retained glass is most commonly a result of a motor vehicle accident or stepping on glass (2). Those patients who have the perception that glass is present in the wounds are more likely to have retained glass than those patients without a sensation of retained glass (2).

Penetrating trauma from metallic sources occurs most frequently when nails are stepped on. Occasionally, all or part of the nail may remain in the wound (1). Low-velocity BBs and metal that is being hammered or chiseled may enter but lack sufficient force to exit a wound, while higher-velocity guns and industrial nail guns may enter, create a large path of destruction, and exit (6–8).

Wood and other organic substances such as thorns and cactus spines may break off in a wound. These substances are particularly challenging because they are difficult to detect radiographically, yet they are highly reactive and require removal (4,9,10).

High-pressure injectors and spray guns cause serious and debilitating soft tissue damage far beyond the point of entry. These devices are used to inject grease, paint, paint solvent, hydraulic fluid, diesel fuel, and water and may be powerful enough to cut concrete or metal (11). The onset of significant pain with these types of injury may be delayed until 1 to 3 days after the injury occurs (12).

II. **Diagnosis**
   A. **Physical examination.** Examination of an open wound after it has been aseptically cleaned and irrigated should include a visual examination of the wound, palpation for masses, and detailed sensory, motor, and vascular examinations. Particular atten-

tion should be given to open wounds of the head and foot and to puncture wounds (2).

The wound should be explored to its fullest extent. Bleeding that obscures viewing should be controlled with a tourniquet and anesthesia for appropriate pain management should be used. Blind palpation with a gloved finger should not be performed if it is known that sharp objects may be in the wound; an instrument should be used in these situations.

Exploration of puncture wounds is limited by the small skin opening. The margins of these wounds may be extended to enhance exploration if the index of suspicion for a foreign body warrants such measures. The site of plantar puncture wounds significantly affects the likelihood of infectious complications. Wounds in the weight-bearing forefoot region, where little soft tissue separates the plantar surface from the cartilaginous and bony structures, have the greatest likelihood of complications (13).

High-pressure injection injuries are unique in that the external evidence of injury, often a small puncture wound, may mislead an unsuspecting emergency physician into underestimating the extensive soft tissue damage that occurs beneath the skin (12).

B.   **Imaging studies.** If there is any suspicion that a foreign body remains following exploration of a wound, radiographic imaging should be performed. The most readily available and least expensive technique is plain radiography. However, some types of foreign bodies are not radiopaque. Alternative imaging techniques include ultrasonography, computed tomography, and magnetic resonance imaging.

1.   **Techniques**

a.   Plain radiography. If a foreign body is suspected but not visualized in an open wound, radiographs of the affected area should be taken. In one study of retained foreign bodies of the hand that were not diagnosed on initial presentation to a physician, 78% were radiopaque (4). Rarely, foreign bodies migrate from their point of entry; thus, when the emergency department evaluation does not occur in the immediate postinjury period, the emergency physician should consider radiographs of the area surrounding the point of entry and perhaps the adjacent joints (14–16). Radiographs should be taken prior to removal of a protruding, deeply embedded foreign object in order to maximize information about the depth and direction of the wound (17).

A foreign body usually has a density different from that of the tissue within which it is embedded. This density discrepancy affects the attenuation of an x-ray beam as it passes through the homogeneous soft tissue. A foreign body that is more dense than the surrounding soft tissues appears as a radiopacity, and a foreign body that is less dense than the surrounding tissues appears as a radiolucency. The detectability of a foreign body on a radiograph is dependent on its size, density, and orientation in relation to surrounding bone and soft tissues (18,19).

b. **Ultrasonography.** Ultrasonography detects foreign bodies in soft tissues by reflecting sound waves or casting acoustic shadows from the foreign bodies (10). It is most useful with superficial foreign bodies, and larger foreign bodies are more easily detected than small ones (20). Ultrasonography is most accurate in easily accessible sites, areas such as the web spaces between fingers are more challenging to evaluate for foreign bodies (21).

c. **Computed tomography.** Computed tomography (CT) may also be used for the detection of retained foreign bodies. By CT, multiple x-ray beams are passed through the same cross-sectional slice of tissue at different angles during different intervals of time; thus, much smaller differences in attenuation may be detected than with plain radiography (22). CT is more reliable than ultrasonography for detecting foreign bodies that are deeply embedded and those located behind bone. CT is very reliable for detecting glass and plastic foreign bodies but is less reliable for gravel and wooden foreign bodies. Freshly embedded (dry) wood is more likely to be detected than wood that is wet from having absorbed fluid from the surrounding tissues (23). CT is reliable in localizing and demonstrating the extent of hematomas and abscesses surrounding an occult foreign body (24,25).

d. **Magnetic resonance imaging.** Magnetic resonance imaging (MRI), while less available to the emergency physician and not likely to be used in the acute setting, may be used in a situation when a patient presents with complications from a foreign body that has been embedded for some time. MRI uses strong magnetic fields to excite hydrogen atoms, which then produce a radio signal. Tissues have hydrogen atoms, but foreign bodies except gravel lack free water and therefore produce a signal void (23). MRI is an excellent tool for detecting glass, plastic, and dry and wet wooden foreign bodies; it is more reliable than CT in detecting wood (23). The magnetic material in many types of gravel produces streak artifact that interferes with identification and localization of the foreign body (23). Obviously the magnetic field of the imager could displace metal; thus it would never be utilized to detect or localize embedded metallic foreign bodies. It is more reliable than CT in detecting the presence of edema, hemorrhage, and infection surrounding foreign bodies (25).

2. **Foreign body and radiographic technique**

The composition, size, and location of the suspected foreign body as well as the availability of the various imaging techniques determines which type of imaging study should be utilized to detect the presence of a foreign body in soft tissues.

a. **Glass.** Radiographic evaluation is indicated in all wounds caused by glass unless they are very superficial. Glass foreign bodies are frequently detected radiographically in lacerations in which the bottom to the wound is not visible and occasionally in those in which the bottom is visualized (3).

Glass in fragments as small as 2 mm in the presence of overlying bone and 0.5 mm in the absence of overlying bone is easily detected on plain radiographs (18). All varieties of glass are visible, and the presence of heavy metals such as lead is not necessary to detect the glass.

Radiographic detection of fragments of glass in the "limited detection" range of 0.5 to 2.0 mm is probably not enhanced by increasing the number of radiographic views from two to four (26). If glass is not visualized on radiographs but is highly suspected, an ultrasound should be performed. If the suspected foreign body is deeply embedded or located behind bone, ultrasonography is unreliable and CT should be performed. MRI may be utilized if a foreign body is suspected but cannot be visualized by ultrasonography or CT.

b. **Wood, thorns, spines.** Freshly embedded wood as small as 3 mm has been visualized on plain radiographs in an experimental model (19); however, wood foreign bodies that are retained in wounds are rarely radiopaque (4,10). Wood may be visualized as a radiolucency that contrasts with the greater density of the surrounding tissue (19), or the air surrounding the object may be visualized within the denser surrounding tissue (23). Visualization is decreased with denser wood such as mahogany, a painted surface, and absorption by the wood of fluid (19). Wood is usually visible by ultrasound, particularly when it is more than 5 mm in size (10,20,21). If wood is not detected sonographically, CT will usually detect dry as well as wet (more than 24 hours after being embedded) wood. MRI, while expensive and not readily available, accurately detects wooden foreign bodies (23).

Thorns and cactus spines are not visible on radiographs but may be detected ultrasonically (9,27,28). Sea urchin spines are sometimes radiopaque and may be detectable by ultrasound (29,30).

c. **Metal.** Metal except aluminum is readily visible on radiographs (4,31). Metal that escapes radiographic detection may be visualized by ultrasonography (20), although very small pieces (0.5- and 0.9-mm needles) are difficult to detect (32). CT is very reliable in detecting metallic foreign bodies (22). MRI should never be used for metallic foreign bodies, as the ferromagnetic forces may displace the foreign body, damaging nearby structures.

d. **Gravel.** Gravel may be radiopaque, depending on its composition. Homogeneous gravel such as marble, limestone, and slate is usually visible; however, heterogeneous substances such as granite, lava glass, lava stone, and cinders have a variable presentation on plain radiographs (23,33). Gravel that is radiolucent may be visualized by ultrasonography (27). All gravel is easily detected by CT (23,33). MRI has limited usefulness in localizing gravel, since it may contain magnetic material, which creates significant streak artifacts (23,33).

e. **Plastic.** Plastic foreign bodies are not usually visible on radiographs because their density is similar to that of the surrounding tissue (23,34). Plastic may be detected by ultrasonography (27,34) and is easily detected by CT and MRI (23).

f. **Injected materials.** Substances such as grease, oil, and paint may be detected on plain radiographs. Grease, which may have lead-based components, and lead-based paints may appear as a radiopacity; grease has also been detected as a radiolucency in contrast with the more dense surrounding tissue (12). Subcutaneous emphysema or a lacy calcification may be detected radiographically after injection of non-lead-based paints (12). The high pressure under which these substances are injected may force them far from the site of injection. Liberal use of radiography is recommended to evaluate the extent of injury (12,35).

III. Treatment

A. Removal. Once it has been determined that a wound contains a foreign body, the usual course of action is to attempt to remove it. Factors that increase the urgency with which a foreign body should be removed include high reactivity of the foreign body; actual or potential impairment of the functioning of vessels, tendons, or nerves; and infection.

While most foreign bodies should be removed in the emergency department at the earliest opportunity, in certain situations more harm may be caused by attempting removal. In these cases the foreign body should be left in place and removed by an appropriate consulting physician or removed immediately in the operating room.

Wounds should be thoroughly irrigated following removal of a foreign body. "Clean" wounds may be closed with sutures while wounds that are significantly contaminated should be left open (7). Repeat radiographs should be taken after the removal of radiopaque foreign bodies to make sure that no foreign bodies remain in the tissues.

1. **Glass, metal, plastic.** Glass, metal, and plastic foreign bodies that are accessible should be removed in the emergency department. Glass fragments retained in the hand have been known to migrate and cause delayed functional impairment of nerves or tendons (15,16). However, if one of these relatively inert foreign bodies is located in an inaccessible site and there is no pain, infection, or actual or potential impairment based on proximity of the foreign body to anatomical structures, the wound can be splinted. The patient can then be referred to a specialist who will assess the need for and timing of removal (36).

   Plantar puncture wounds are most commonly caused by nails (1). Contaminated wounds should be cleaned, irrigated, and debrided if necessary. The benefits to the patient of coring, probing, packing, and prophylactic antibiotics are controversial (1,17,37–39). There is no evidence that any of these interventions decreases the likelihood of wound complications; in fact, blind probing may force foreign bodies more deeply into the foot.

   Missiles fired from rifles, handguns, and industrial nail guns may cause tissue destruction that extends beyond the wound tract. Appropriate treatment of these injuries in the emergency department includes an accurate examination of vascular, sensory, and motor functioning; cleaning and irrigation; radiographs to assess the location of any retained missiles; and referral to surgical specialists (7,8).

2. **Wood, thorns, cactus spines.** Foreign bodies that incite tissue inflammation must be removed

as soon as possible. Organic material such as wood, thorns, and cactus spines cannot be digested by body enzymes and will provoke infection (36). Splinters disintegrate easily and should not be pulled out via the entrance wound. Rather, an incision should be made along the long axis of the wound or the wound should be completely excised (40).

Often, foreign bodies, in particular organic material, are contaminated with soil. Inorganic and organic components of the soil impair the ability of leukocytes to ingest and kill bacteria, increasing the likelihood of infection (41). Clay has a much greater percentage of "infection-potentiating factor" than does black topsoil, and sand is innocuous (42). Clay fractions are found in the subsoil rather than the topsoil and therefore are more likely to be present at excavation sites and in swampy or marshy environments (7).

Locally toxic foreign bodies may create complications when they are embedded in a wound. Sea urchin spines cause severe pain at the site of puncture. This pain is not a result of the puncture wound but rather of inorganic debris and calcareous materials introduced into the puncture wounds by the spines (29). Poisonous varieties of sea urchins also inject a heat-labile venom. Sea urchin spines should be removed if accessible. Those spines located near a tendon sheath or a nerve must be removed because of the possibility of synovitis and granuloma formation and neuropathy. If removal is not possible in the emergency department, the patient must be referred to a specialist (29,36).

3. **Mercury and lead.** Mercury and lead foreign bodies may have systemic effects. Metallic mercury from a broken thermometer has been reported to cause mercury emboli to the lungs, renal tubular necrosis, and myocarditis; surgical intervention with removal of the mercury is indicated (43). Lead foreign bodies, such as bullets, are rapidly encapsulated by fibrosis, which prevents lead intoxication. However, if the lead is exposed to circulating body fluid—for example, in a joint—the fluid serves as a solvent for the lead and it may enter the systemic circulation, causing lead intoxication (44).

4. **High-pressure injections.** High-pressure injected grease, paint, or solvent may track along tendon sheaths, neurovascular bundles, and fascial planes, compressing tissue and inciting tissue inflammation. These injuries require immediate surgical intervention; conservative treatment will likely result in the eventual amputation of the affected areas (35,36).

B. **Tetanus.** All patients with wounds containing foreign bodies must have received tetanus toxoid immunization within the previous 5 years. Those patients who were not previously immunized require tetanus immune globulin in addition to tetanus toxoid.

C. **Antibiotics.** Retained foreign bodies increase the chances that a wound will become infected. Antibiotics will not prevent the development of infection in the presence of a retained foreign body (1). The most effective treatment of an infected wound with a retained foreign body is removal of the foreign body (1,10).

   The role of antibiotics in reducing the likelihood of wound infection after removal of a foreign body or when removal of a foreign body is deferred to a specialist is controversial (6,17,31,38).

   The role of antibiotics in preventing infection in grossly contaminated wounds is not known and is controversial (7,17). Antibiotics may reduce the number of bacteria in these wounds; however, an overgrowth may occur of those bacteria that are not covered by the antibiotic selected.

   Antibiotics should be administered when there is evidence of infection (1,31,37,38).

   Wound infections of the hand are most commonly caused by *Staphylococcus aureus,* with group A β-hemolytic *Streptococcus* the second most commonly found bacterium (36). Treatment with antistaphylococcal antibiotics such as dicloxacillin or cephalexin should be initiated in uncomplicated cellulitis. Gram-negative coverage should be reserved for organisms whose presence has been proved by culture. Cellulitis resulting from puncture wounds of the foot is also most commonly caused by *Staphylococcus aureus* (1). An uncommon (approximately 1%) but serious complication of plantar puncture wounds is osteomyelitis-osteochondritis, most commonly (more than 90%) caused by *Pseudomonas aeruginosa* (1,17). *Pseudomonas aeruginosa* has been cultured from the foam-rubber material in the soles of tennis shoes (45). Ciprofloxacin provides gram-positive and gram-negative coverage, including *Pseudomonas.* However, there is no evidence that prophylactic antibiotic treatment with an antipseudomonal antibiotic in patients with plantar puncture wounds decreases the likelihood of developing osteomyelitis (17,37).

D. **Immobilization and elevation.** Patients with deferred removal of the foreign body who are referred to a specialist should have the joints near the wound site splinted to impair migration of the object (36). Patients with infected wounds, with or without a retained foreign body, should be encouraged to keep the affected area elevated (36,37). Patients with infected foot wounds should avoid weight bearing (37).

E. Follow-up. All patients, whether the foreign body is removed in the emergency department or by a specialist, should have follow-up within 48 hours.

REFERENCES

1. Fitzgerald RH, Cowan JDE. Puncture wounds of the foot. *Orthop Clin North Am* 1975;6:965–972.
2. Montano JB, Steele MT, Watson WA. Foreign body retention in glass-caused wounds. *Ann Emerg Med* 1992;21:1360–1363.
3. Avner JR, Baker MD. Lacerations involving glass. *Am J Dis Child* 1992;146:600–602.
4. Anderson MA, Newmeyer WL, Kilgore ES. Diagnosis and treatment of retained foreign bodies in the hand. *Am J Surg* 1982; 144:63–67.
5. Dunn JD. Risk management in emergency medicine. *Emerg Med Clin North Am* 1987;5:51–69.
6. Morgan WJ, Leopold T, Evans R. Foreign bodies in the hand. *J Hand Surg* 1984;9B:194–196.
7. Edlich RF, Rodeheaver GT, Morgan RF, et al. Principles of emergency wound management. *Ann Emerg Med* 1988;17:1284–1302.
8. Edlich RF, Silloway KA, Rodeheaver GT, et al. Industrial nail gun injuries. *Comp Ther* 1986;12:42–46.
9. Crawford R, Matheson AB. Clinical value of ultrasonography in the detection and removal of radiolucent foreign bodies. *Injury* 1989;20:341–343.
10. Rockett MS, Gentile SC, Gudas CJ, et al. The use of ultrasonography for the detection of retained wooden foreign bodies in the foot. *J Foot Ankle Surg* 1995;34:478–511.
11. Fialkov JV, Frieberg A. High pressure injection injuries: an overview. *J Emerg Med* 1991;9:367–371.
12. O'Reilly RJ, Blatt G. Accidental high-pressure injection gun injuries of the hand. *J Trauma* 1975;15:24–31.
13. Patzakis MJ, Wilkins J, Brien WW, et al. Wound site as a predictor of complications following deep nail punctures to the foot. *West J Med* 1989;150:545–547.
14. Chow J, Schenck RR. Foreign body migration in the hand (letter). *J Hand Surg* 1982;13:462.
15. Browett JT, Fiddian NJ. Delayed median nerve injury due to retained glass fragments. *J Bone Joint Surg* 1985;67B:382–384.
16. Jablon M, Rabin SF. Late flexor pollicis longus tendon rupture due to retained glass fragments. *J Hand Surg* 1988;13A:713–716.
17. Inaba AS, Zukin DD, Perro M. An update on the evaluation and management of plantar puncture wounds and *Pseudomonas* osteomyelitis. *Pediatr Emerg Care* 1992;8:38–44.
18. Tandberg D. Glass in the hand and foot. *JAMA* 1982;248:1872–1874.
19. Mucci B, Stenhouse G. Soft tissue radiographs for wooden foreign bodies—a worthwhile exercise? *Injury* 1985;16:402–404.
20. Bray PW, Mahoney JL, Campbell JP. Sensitivity and specificity of ultrasound in the diagnosis of foreign bodies in the hand. *J Hand Surg* 1995;20A:661–666.

21. Gilbert FJ, Campbell RSD, Bayliss AP. The role of ultrasound in the detection of non-radiopaque foreign bodies. *Clin Radiol* 1990;41:109–112.

22. Kirks DR, Harwood-Nash DCF. Computed tomography in pediatric radiology. *Pediatr Ann* 1980;9:53–69.

23. Russell RC, Williamson DA, Sullivan JW, et al. Detection of foreign bodies in the hand. *J Hand Surg* 1991;16A:2–11.

24. Bauer AR, Yutani D. Computed tomographic localization of wooden foreign bodies in children's extremities. *Arch Surg* 1983;118:1084–1086.

25. Bodne D, Quinn SF, Cochran CF. Imaging foreign glass and wooden bodies of the extremities with CT and MRI. *J Comput Assist Tomogr* 1988;12:608–611.

26. Courter BJ. Radiographic screening for glass foreign bodies— what does a "negative" foreign body series really mean? *Ann Emerg Med* 1990;19:997–1000.

27. Manthey DE, Storrow AB, Milbourn JM, Wagner BJ. Ultrasound versus radiography in the detection of soft-tissue foreign bodies. *Ann Emerg Med* 1996;28:7–9.

28. Failla JM, van Holsbeeck M, Vanderschueren G. Detection of a 0.5-mm-thick thorn using ultrasound: a case report. *J Hand Surg* 1995;20A:456–457.

29. Strauss MB, MacDonald RI. Hand injuries from sea urchin spines. *Clin Orthop* 1976;114:216–218.

30. De Flaviis L, Scaglione P, Del Bo P, Nessi R. Detection of foreign bodies in soft tissues: experimental comparison of ultrasonography and xeroadiography. *J Trauma* 1988;28:400–404.

31. Lammers RL. Soft tissue foreign bodies. *Ann Emerg Med* 1988;17:1336–1347.

32. Little CM, Parker MG, Callowich MC, Sartori JC. The ultrasonic detection of soft tissue foreign bodies. *Invest Radiol* 1986; 21:275–277.

33. Oikarien KS, Nieminen TM, Makarainen H, Pyhtinen J. Visibility of foreign bodies in soft tissue in plain radiographs, computed tomography, magnetic resonance imaging, and ultrasound. *Int J Oral Maxillofac Surg* 1993;22:119–124.

34. De Lacey G, Evans R, Sandin B. Penetrating injuries: how easy is it to see glass (and plastic) on radiographs? *Br J Radiol* 1985; 58:27–30.

35. Sirio CA, Smith JS, Graham WP. High-pressure injection injuries of the hand. *Am Surg* 1989;55:714–718.

36. Smoot EC, Robson MC. Acute management of foreign body injuries of the hand. *Ann Emerg Med* 1983;12:434–437.

37. Chisholm CD, Schlesser JF. Plantar puncture wounds: controversies and treatment recommendations. *Ann Emerg Med* 1989; 18:1352–1357.

38. Verdile VP, Freed HA, Gerard J. Puncture wounds to the foot. *J Emerg Med* 1989;7:193–199.

39. Brook JW. Management of pedal puncture wounds. *J Foot Ankle Surg* 1994;33:463–466.

40. Stein F. Foreign body injuries of the hand. *Emerg Med Clin North Am* 1985;3:383–390.

41. Haury B, Rodeheaver GT, Pettry D, et al. Inhibition of nonspecific defenses by soil infection potentiating factors. *Surg Gynecol Obstet* 1977;144:19–24.

42. Rodeheaver G, Pettry D, Turnbull V, et al. Identification of the wound infection-potentiating factors in soil. *Am J Surg* 1974; 128:8–14.
43. Rachman R. Soft tissue injury by mercury from a broken thermometer. *Am J Clin Pathol* 1974;61:296–300.
44. Windler EC, Smith RB, Bryan WJ, Woods GW. Lead intoxication and traumatic arthritis of the hip secondary to retained bullet fragments. *J Bone Joint Surg* 1978;60A:254–255.
45. Fisher MC, Goldsmith JF, Gilligan PH. Sneakers as a source of *Pseudomonas aeruginosa* in children with osteomyelitis following puncture wounds. *J Pediatr* 1985;106:607–609.

Sports Medicine

Paul J. Donovan

Over 70 million Americans are involved in recreational and/or organized sports. Injury due to sport is common and may result from an acute traumatic event or an overuse (inflammatory) condition. The majority of sports-related injuries seen in the emergency department are of the traumatic type. Although the overall emergency evaluation and care of the injured athlete is similar to that of the nonathlete, differences exist with regard to specific clinical conditions and the rehabilitative care phase of treatment.

I. **Types of injuries**
    A. **Soft tissue injury.** Orthopaedic soft tissue injuries are common in sports. These include **ligamentous, joint capsule,** and **musculotendinous** injuries. **Grading** the severity of these injuries can have important therapeutic and rehabilitative implications and will affect the timing of the athlete's return to sport. Ligamentous and musculotendinous injuries are graded I to III **sprains** or **strains**, respectively.
        1. **Grade I** injury is a stretch of the involved structures.
        2. **Grade II** injury is a partial tear.
        3. **Grade III** is complete tearing of the involved ligaments or musculotendinous unit.

            Most musculotendinous partial tears involve the musculotendinous junction. Common examples of these are the hamstring and quadriceps muscles. Tendon rupture and avulsion of a tendon from its bony attachment can also occur. Common examples are patellar and Achilles tendon ruptures. Clinically, as the severity of the injury increases, the amount of the patient's pain, physical findings, disability, and joint instability will increase. Patients with grade I and II sprains and strains will generally return to sport within 1 to 3 weeks, whereas those with grade III (complete tears) will often take 6 to 8 weeks to heal and surgical repair is often necessary.

            Contusions to large muscle groups, such as the quadriceps, is also common, especially in contact sports such as football and soccer. These are also graded according to the severity of injury. Injury can vary from a minimal disruption of the muscle fibers, to partial disruption of the muscle, to complete disruption. Although it is easy to minimize these types of injuries, they can lead to significant long-term disability if the initial emergency management is not appropriate. The principles of RICE (rest, ice, compression dressing, and elevation) apply. A special emphasis on maintaining range of motion (ROM) early on is important. Serious complications—such as myositis ossificans, compartment syndrome, and fascial herniations—can occur if contusions are not treated appropriately.

B. **Avulsion fractures**

1. **Avulsion fractures about a joint,** though generally small, can lead to significant ligamentous joint instability if they are not recognized during emergency evaluation of the injured athlete.

   a. The **Bankart lesion** that sometimes accompanies anterior shoulder dislocation is an avulsion fracture of the glenoid rim. It often complicates the rehabilitative process and leads to increased risk of redislocation in these individuals; its presence in an athletic individual is often an indication for surgery.

   b. The **gamekeeper's (or skier's) thumb,** an injury to the ulnar collateral ligament at the metacarpophalangeal joint of the thumb, if associated with a large intraarticular fragment, often associated with persistent instability and is an indication for surgical repair.

   c. Knee injuries are common in sports and **avulsion fractures about the knee** can be an indication of significant knee instability. A **Segond fracture,** an avulsion fracture of the lateral proximal tibia, results from an avulsion of the associated joint capsule. These can be associated with medial collateral and/or anterior cruciate ligament (ACL) injury. An **avulsion of the tibial spine,** which is the tibial attachment of the ACL, is a serious injury, since this usually results in an ACL-deficient knee. These require appropriate immobilization and early orthopaedic follow-up.

2. **Avulsion fractures about the ankle,** especially when they involve the dome of the talus, are often undetected on initial emergency evaluation and lead to persistent pain, swelling, and disability. If, during initial emergency evaluation such an injury exists, splinting and early orthopaedic follow-up is necessary.

3. **Avulsion fractures of the base of the fifth metatarsal** due to a peroneal tendon avulsion needs to be distinguished from the more serious **Jones fracture**, which is a fracture through the base of the fifth metatarsal. The presence of an avulsion requires protected immobilization, whereas a Jones fracture often requires operative repair, and (or) cast immobilization.

C. **Stress fractures.** Stress fractures or fatigue fractures occur because of repetitive loading of a specific area of bone. They most commonly occur in runners. Frequently the patient will complain of ongoing pain without an acute traumatic event. Because the plain x-rays are often negative, the emergency physician must have a high index of suspicion for such injury given the clinical history. Common sites of stress fractures of the lower extremity involve the metatarsals, tibia, fibula, and occasionally the femur. Clinically, tenderness over the bony area with the appropriate history points to a stress fracture until proven otherwise. Diagnostically a bone scan becomes positive earlier in the disease process than plain radiographs. Avoidance of weight bearing and orthopaedic follow-up would be indicated as emergency measures.

II. **Injuries of the upper extremity**

A. **Shoulder.** The majority of shoulder problems seen in the emergency department are thoroughly covered in Chapter 10. Although contact sports such as football, hockey, and skiing have a high incidence of fracture(s) and dislocations of the acromioclavicular and glenohumeral joints, overuse or inflammatory conditions such as tendinitis and bursitis predominate in baseball, volleyball, swimming, weight lifting, and racquet sports. Some knowledge of the technical and biomechanical factors of sports is useful in elucidating the patient's problem. For example, the throwing mechanism in baseball is composed of several phases: cocking, windup, acceleration, release, and deceleration. For athletes who have shoulder pain with throwing, the phase of throwing that exacerbates the pain is often a clue to diagnosis.

1. **Tendinitis and bursitis.** Rotator cuff tendinitis is a common cause of shoulder pain and impingement in athletes. Often the patient will present with a history of repetitive use of the shoulder with gradually worsening pain or an acute exacerbation of pain on a chronically symptomatic shoulder. As a rule the pain is generalized, often dull and aching, primarily with overhead activity. Activities at less than 90 degrees of abduction are usually pain-free.

a. **Examination.** There is usually tenderness over the lateral and anterior aspect of the shoulder, often over the supraspinatus tendon at its proximal insertion on the greater tuberosity of the humerus. Frequently there is a painful arc on abduction between 80 and 150 degrees that worsens with external and/or internal rotation. **Jobe's testing**, which is done with the arm at 30 degrees of forward flexion and 90 degrees of abduction with the arms extended at the elbows, will often cause pain with resisted abduction consistent with supraspinatus tendinitis. Pain with external rotation is consistent with teres minor and infraspinatus tendinitis. Associated weakness may be due to either pain and/or partial rotator cuff tear. Because tendinitis and bursitis often represent a continuum of the inflammatory process, subacromial bursitis, which is the most common type of shoulder bursitis, will generally accompany these conditions.

b. **Radiographs.** Radiographs are typically normal in these conditions. However in chronic tendinitis, calcification can occur in the rotator cuff tendons, most often in the supraspinatus tendons. Calcification can be seen radiographically on the anteroposterior (AP) externally rotated view. Magnetic resonance imaging (MRI) or ultrasound can be done for suspected partial or complete rotator cuff tears.

c. **Treatment.** Initial emergency treatment is rest, ice, and nonsteroidal antiinflammatory drugs (NSAIDs). In the severely symptomatic patient, injection of a local anesthetic and cortisone may be added.

d. **Complications.** Potential complications of rotator cuff tendinitis include partial or complete rotator cuff tears. The patient will often have persistent pain and weakness. Surgery is indicated for chronic symptomatic partial tears and also complete rotator cuff tears. Follow-up and rehabilitation includes assessing glenohumeral instability, associated muscle weakness, and/or biomechanical or training errors. Specific rotator cuff strengthening exercises are usually begun when the acute painful symptoms have resolved.

2. **Tendinitis and rupture of the long head of the biceps tendon** occurs especially with weight lifting and racquet sports.

a. **Examination.** The patient often presents with anterior shoulder pain with bicipital tendinitis. Tenderness is usually elicited on palpation over the bicipital groove located on the anterosuperior aspect of the humeral head and neck. **Speed's test**—which involves resisted flexion, adduction, and supination with the elbows extended—will usually be positive.

If the patient presents with a sudden onset of a popping or tearing sensation in the anterior shoulder, with noted weakness, this can be due to rupture of the long head of the biceps tendon. Diagnosis is made on physical exam by palpating the retracted muscle belly in the mass of the biceps and also noting an asymmetrical enlargment on abduction of the shoulder to 90 degrees with the elbows flexed. Comparison with the normal arm is always necessary.

b. **Radiographs.** Usually normal.

c. **Treatment.** Treatment is conservative with rest, ice, and NSAIDs; occasionally a local anesthetic and cortisone can be injected along the sheath of the tendon on either side of the bicipital groove. For rupture of the long head of the biceps, loss in strength of 15% to 20% can occur. In the competitive athlete, surgical repair is indicated. In the recreational athlete, conservative management may be appropriate.

d. **Complications.** Tendinitis may predispose to rupture.

3. **"Little League" shoulder.** Little League shoulder is a stress injury to the epiphyseal plate of the proximal humerus. It is often seen in young throwers and less often in young tennis players.

a. **Examination.** The patient often presents with pain and tenderness over the proximal shoulder in the region of the lateral aspect of the humeral head and neck.

b. **Radiographs.** May be normal or demonstrate widening of the epiphyseal line. Bone scan is a more sensitive test with noted increased activity in this region. Radiographs in 3 to 4 weeks can show evidence of new bone formation regardless of the initial x-ray finding.

c. **Treatment.** Conservative with rest, ice, NSAIDs, and a sling, with orthopaedic follow-up and gradual return to sport.

d. **Complications.** Permanent growth plate injury or complete epiphyseal separation can occur.

B. **Elbow**

1. **Lateral and medial epicondylitis.** Also known as "tennis elbow" and "golfer's elbow," respectively, this is an overuse condition affecting the tendinous origin of the wrist extensors and wrist flexors at the distal humeral epicondyle.

a. **Examination.** These common overuse syndromes present with the patient complaining of pain about the elbow and a history consistent with repetitive motion. Physical examination demonstrating local tenderness over the common origin of the wrist extensors at the lateral epicondyle that is worsened with resisted extension at the wrist is consistent with tennis elbow. Tenderness elicited over the medial epicondyle at the origin of the flexors that is worsened with resisted wrist flexion is consistent with golfer's elbow. When the adolescent or teenage baseball player presents with medial elbow pain, it is often due to a traction apophysitis of the medial epicondyle or, given a history of acute onset of pain while throwing, occasionally an avulsion of the medial epicondyle. This is known as "Little League" elbow.

   b. **Radiographs.** Plain radiographs in these conditions may be normal; however, attention should be paid to the presence of possible loose bodies with degenerative changes. With the skeletally immature, epicondylar separation can occur with avulsion injuries.

   c. **Treatment.** Treatment is conservative with rest, ice, and NSAIDs. A widely displaced avulsion fragment on x-ray may require surgical reattachment. Definitive care for these injuries involves proper conditioning and attention to any training errors. Often some sort of compression device (i.e., tennis or golfer's elbow strap) is useful for decompression of either the extensor or flexor stresses on the elbow. Physical and manual therapy is indicated for refractory symptoms. Local steroid injections may also be useful.

   d. **Complications.** Usually the patient with a history of chronic elbow pain will present with acute exacerbation of the pain. In some cases of tennis or golfer's elbow, the respective extensor or flexor origin can be avulsed or "lysis" can occur during a forceful forearm or wrist motion. Chronic epicondylitis may be an indication for surgical tenolysis.

2. **Rupture of the distal biceps tendon.** This is a rare injury, since 97% of biceps injuries affect the proximal biceps. However, tears do occur as a result of degeneration or in the weight-training athlete. The mechanism is usually an abrupt hyperextension of a flexed biceps. The patient complains of acute onset of pain with an associated pop or tearing sensation in the flexor aspect of the elbow, followed by abrupt weakness.

   a. **Examination.** Physical examination is remarkable for weakness on flexion and supination of the involved elbow, with a palpable defect over the distal biceps tendon and radial tuberosity. Associated swelling due to hemorrhage may often obscure the diagnosis.

b. **Radiographs.** These are typically normal. Occasionally there will be a small avulsed fragment of the distal aspect of the tendon. MRI is useful in further evaluation.

c. **Treatment.** Emergency management consists of ice, sling, and NSAIDs with close orthopaedic follow-up for surgical repair.

d. **Complications.** Use of anabolic steroids should be suspected in the weight-training athlete with this injury.

C. Hand

1. **Ulnar collateral ligament (UCL) injuries (skier's thumb).** Although initially described as an overuse injury by Campbell in 1955, UCL injuries are most common in the skier falling with a pole in his or her hand who undergoes a valgus stress to the thumb. Injuries to hockey and football players have also been described. The ulnar collateral ligament stabilizes the thumb at the metacarpophalangeal (MCP) joint.

a. **Examination.** The patient will have pain and tenderness over the ulnar aspect of the MCP joint of the thumb and on stressing the MCP joint on abduction (radial stress). This is done in both full extension and 15 to 20 degrees of flexion in order to stress the accessory and the UCL proper, respectively. The normal asymptomatic thumb should also be stressed for comparison.

b. **Radiographs.** These are often normal but may show an avulsed intraarticular fragment. While stress radiographs have been advocated, they are often difficult to obtain, painful for the patient, and—from an emergency standpoint—of little clinical value.

c. **Treatment.** Emergency treatment includes thumb spica immobilization, ice, and NSAIDs. For first-degree injuries with no detectable instability, definitive care often involves immobilization for 1 to 2 weeks. For complete tears in which surgery is not advised, immobilization for 3 to 6 weeks is definitive therapy. Small avulsions that are not intraarticular can be treated conservatively. Large intraarticular fragments or injuries with complete disruption as evidenced by significant joint instability require surgical repair for a more stable functional outcome.

d. **Complications.** A **Stenner** lesion results when the adductor aponeurosis is interposed between the torn UCL. Surgical repair is necessary. Failure to recognize this injury or undertreatment can result in chronic instability.

2. **Extensor tendon injury (baseball or mallet finger.** This is a common injury usually resulting from a forced flexion of a distal phalanx. Baseball, football, and basketball players are very susceptible to this injury.

   a. **Examination.** The patient often presents with an obvious flexion deformity of the distal interphalangeal (DIP) joint, often the index or middle finger, with an inability to extend the finger.

   b. **Radiographs.** These may be normal or most commonly demonstrate a small dorsal avulsion at the DIP joint. In the young individual, the avulsion often represents a Salter III fracture through the epiphysis and epiphyseal plate

   c. **Treatment.** This consists of splinting the DIP in a slight extension for a minimum of 6 to 8 weeks.

   d. **Complications.** Complications of chronic flexion deformity usually result from inadequate treatment. Occasionally a swan-neck deformity will result as the extensor tendon loses its connection to the distal phalanx. Occasionally, if the intraarticular avulsed fragment involves 25% or more of the articular surface and/or is unreduced in the extended position, surgical fixation is needed.

3. **Flexor digitorum profundus avulsion (Jersey finger).** This injury results from a sudden forced hyperextension at the DIP joint of the finger; it commonly occurs in football players.

   a. **Examination.** Often the patient will present complaining of pain and inability to flex the distal phalanx at the DIP.

   b. **Radiographs.** These may show an intraarticular avulsion on the volar aspect or may be normal.

   c. **Treatment.** Emergency treatment involves splinting in flexion at both the proximal and distal interphalangeal joints with early orthopaedic follow-up for surgical repair.

   d. **Complications.** Permanent inability to flex the DIP joint if improperly treated.

III. **Injuries to the lower extremities**

   A. **Hip and pelvis.** Hip injuries represent approximately 5% to 10% of all sports-related injuries; they are most commonly sustained in contact and running sports such as football, soccer, and track. Contusions to the bony prominences about the pelvis as well as inflammatory conditions and apophyseal avulsions in the skeletally immature athlete are fairly common conditions. Fortunately, serious injuries such as hip dislocations and pelvic fractures are rare; however, both are potential limb- and life-threatening injuries that require prompt emergency attention and similar treatment regardless of mechanism of injury.

1. **Apophyseal injuries.** Several apophyses located about the hip are subject to traction forces exerted by the associated tendinous attachments. These apophyses are subject to both inflammation (apophysitis) and avulsion injuries, and the athlete often presents with either an acute onset of pain or acute worsening of a chronically painful condition.

   a. **Examination.** The individual is often involved in a running sport. They may feel or hear a pop if there has been an avulsion. Typical areas of injury are the anterior superior iliac spine (ASIS), the origin of the sartorius muscle; the anterior inferior iliac spine (AIIS), the origin of the rectus femoris portion of the quadriceps; and the ischial apophysis, which is the origin of the hamstring tendons. Localized tenderness over the respective areas that worsens with active range of motion is diagnostic.

   b. **Radiographs.** Radiographs of the pelvis are often indicated when avulsion is strongly suspected. Often consultation with the radiologist is important for the correct (oblique) view to help delineate the injury further. Generally, greater than a 1 cm of widening of the apophysis is consistent with avulsion.

   c. **Treatment.** Avoidance of weight bearing followed by ice and NSAIDs. If an avulsion is present and widely separated (greater than 1 cm) in a young competitive athlete, surgical repair may be indicated.

   d. **Complications.** If the athlete resumes the sport too soon, the possibility of subsequent avulsion is increased. Chronic apophysitis can often lead to apophyseal fragmentation.

2. **Contusions.** Contusions to the bony prominences about the pelvis are common. The typical "**hip pointer**" often occurs in football. The athlete usually receives a helmeted blow to the iliac crest or the lateral aspect of the hip.

   a. **Examination.** The athlete usually complains of pain over the involved area with associated tenderness, swelling, and ecchymosis.

   b. **Radiographs.** Radiographs are usually unremarkable. MRI may demonstrate a "bone bruise."

   c. **Treatment.** Involves rest, ice, weight bearing as tolerated, and return to sport when pain-free, with adequate padding over the involved area.

3. **Soft tissue injuries.** Soft tissue injuries about the hip and pelvis are usually due to musculotendinous strains or capsular sprains of the hip. Areas of involvement frequently include the gluteal muscles, hamstrings, and quadriceps.

   a. **Examination.** The athlete often complains of pain, possibly a tearing sensation in the involved muscle group. Tenderness associated over the involved musculotendinous unit may be associated with swelling and ecchymosis. If a large area of hemorrhage is present, a complete musculotendinous tear should be suspected.

   b. **Radiographs.** Often normal.

   c. **Treatment.** Rest, ice, compression, elevation, and avoidance of weight bearing or weight bearing as tolerated.

   d. **Complications.** Myositis ossificans is a disabling complication of a significant quadriceps contusion. Compartment syndrome and fascial herniation, although rare, can also occur.

4. **Stress fractures.** The runner who presents to the emergency department complaining of vague hip pain should alert the examiner to a possible stress fracture of the hip. Common sites involve the femoral neck and, more rarely, the femoral shaft.

   a. **Examination.** The patient usually complains of rather vague hip pain escalating in its severity, especially at night or at rest. This would often be consistent with an alteration in training regimen, such as increased mileage, a change in terrain, or a change in footwear. Tenderness is often unaccompanied by swelling or ecchymosis.

   b. **Radiographs.** Plain radiographs may demonstrate an incomplete fracture or be normal initially. A bone scan and/or MRI will be more sensitive.

   c. **Treatment.** Avoidance of weight bearing as tolerated with ice and NSAIDs along with early orthopaedic follow-up. Generally this takes 6 to 8 weeks to heal.

   d. **Complications.** An undiagnosed stress fracture about the hip can, if unrecognized, lead to a complete fracture with displacement.

B. **Knee.** The knee is frequently involved in injuries of the lower extremity. This can be associated with considerable disability and loss of time from sports. Ligamentous and meniscal injuries result from twisting or pivoting motions, as in football, basketball, and downhill skiing. The **anterior** and **posterior cruciate ligaments** (ACL and PCL) are responsible for stabilizing the knee in the anterior and posterior directions, respectively. The **medial and lateral collateral ligaments** (MCL and LCL) are responsible for stabilizing the knee medially and laterally. The menisci are shock-absorbing structures and are also important in joint lubrication. Patellar subluxation or dislocation can occur. Osgood-Schlatter's disease or apophysitis of the tibial tubercle is a common cause of chronic anterior knee pain in the young athlete.

1. **Ligamentous injuries.** Of greatest concern to the athlete with an injured knee is a tear of the **ACL.** These injuries may occur in isolation or typically in combination with **MCL** and/or meniscal injuries. The athlete often presents with a history of an audible pop, either due to a twisting mechanism or a direct blow. Isolated injury to the MCL is also common, especially in football, where the individual is tackled, imparting a valgus stress to the medial aspect of the knee.

   a. **Examination.** Examination will often demonstrate substantial effusion, depending on the length of time from injury to presentation. While several physical diagnostic tests such as Lachman's and anterior drawer are useful maneuvers, this is often difficult in the acutely effused and painful knee, thereby limiting your examination.

      (1) With an **MCL** injury, the patient often presents with pain over the medial aspect of the knee, with considerable tenderness, swelling, and ecchymosis. There is usually no joint effusion unless there is a concomitant medial meniscal injury or an ACL tear. The severity of the MCL tear can be estimated by valgus testing the knee both fully extended and in 15 degrees of flexion.

         (a) **Grade I tears:** Pain and no instability.

         (b) **Grade II:** A partial tear of the ligament, which, on testing, will usually demonstrate less than 1 cm of laxity on valgus stretching.

         (c) **Grade III:** A complete tear, as noted by the joint's instability on valgus testing.

      (2) **PCL** and **LCL** tears are uncommon causes of knee pain unless a direct anterior force to the tibia has occurred. If an athlete complains of the knee having "given way" or "popped out," one should consider patellar dislocation/subluxation. There will often be an effusion as

well as tenderness along the medial superior border of the patella and associated medial quadriceps with apprehension on lateral manipulation of the patella.

When the adolescent or teenager presents with a knee injury, the same concerns apply. Although midsubstance ligamentous tears can occur in these individuals, commonly the tibial attachment of the ACL sustains an avulsion injury off the tibial spine. It is important to recognize this, since surgical fixation is mandatory. If the young athlete presents with a history of anterior knee pain and a sudden worsening of the pain, avulsion of the tibial tubercle should be suspected. Tenderness over the patellar tendon and corresponding tibial tuberosity would be present on physical examination.

- b. **Radiographs.** Radiographs of the knee are particularly important in any serious knee injury to rule out concomitant fractures, especially an avulsion fracture of the tibial spine, capsular avulsions (Segond's), fracture of the tibial plateau, and loose bodies.

- c. **Treatment.** Avoidance of weight bearing, ice, NSAIDs, and immobilization with a knee immobilizer. Prompt reduction of patellar dislocations. All knee injuries should have an orthopaedic follow-up.

- d. **Complications.** When an athlete presenting with a significantly unstable knee on examination and significant injury to three of the four ligamentous structures about the knee is suspected, occult knee dislocation with potential for neurovascular injury must be ruled out. Fortunately, true knee dislocations are a rare event in sports, but they are true orthopaedic emergencies requiring immediate reduction followed by evaluation of neurovascular structures. Chronic instability and disability will often accompany knee injuries with unrecognized significant ligamentous or meniscal tears. Locking, clicking, and giving way after any injury are potential signs of loose bodies or significant missed injuries.

2. **Patellar tendon rupture.** Rupture of the patellar tendon is not a common event. Athletes with a history of patellar tendinitis or Osgood-Schlatter disease often have associated tendon degeneration and may be at greater risk for this condition.

    a. Examination. The patient often complains of acute onset of a snap or tearing sensation in the infrapatellar area with inability to bear weight due to loss of knee extension. On examination, swelling, tenderness, and usually a palpable defect in the infrapatellar area are present.

    b. Radiographs. Radiographs often demonstrate a high-riding patella on lateral view or occasionally a small avulsion of the inferior pole of the patella.

    c. Treatment. Emergency treatment includes RICE principles along with immobilization with a knee immobilizer and close follow-up for surgical repair. Often the high-level athlete never returns to his or her preinjury level of activity.

    d. Complications. In athletes with this condition, use of anabolic steroids should be suspected. In some cases, bilateral ruptures have been reported.

C. Lower leg

  1. Proximal tibiofibular joint. Injury to the proximal tibiofibular joint can occur due to a direct blow during contact sports or a severe pivoting motion at this site.

    a. Examination. The athlete will often complain of pain with associated tenderness over the lateral aspect of the head of the fibula with associated swelling and/or ecchymosis, depending on the extent of the injury. Motion may be appreciated at this joint on vigorous palpation. Subluxation or diastasis can occur.

    b. Radiographs. These are often normal, although oblique fracture at the head of the fibula can occur.

    c. Treatment. Avoidance of weight bearing with ice and NSAIDs.

    d. Complications. An unrecognized injury can lead to chronic clicking, popping, and persistence of pain with some proximal instability of the lower leg.

  2. Stress fractures. Nontraumatic lower leg pain can usually be attributed to tibial or fibular stress fractures or compartment syndromes. Stress fractures are a common source of lower leg pain in individuals involved in running sports.

    a. Examination. The patient often presents with a history of gradually increasing nontraumatic pain in the lower leg. There is pain not only during activity but also occasionally at rest. Common sites are the middle and anterior tibia and the distal fibula. Tenderness is elicited over the involved area with or without associated swelling.

    b. Radiographs. These may be normal, show periosteal reaction, or rarely illustrate a complete fracture. Bone scan and MRI are more sensitive diagnostic tests.

    c. Treatment. Avoidance of weight bearing and RICE.

    d. Complications. Undiagnosed stress fractures can go on to result in complete fracture with displacement.

  3. **Compartment syndrome.** Although an acute compartment syndrome is usually secondary to significant bone and/or soft tissue injury to the lower leg, chronic compartment syndrome or exercise-induced ischemia can be a source of chronic pain in the exercising individual. Symptoms may be confined to the anterior, lateral, or posterior compartment. This often occurs in the athletic individual because of hypertrophy of the muscles of the lower extremity in a fixed space.

    a. Examination. Usually the athletic individual complains of gradually worsening pain with associated paresthesia(s) on increased exercise; these symptoms generally resolve at rest. Physical exam is otherwise often normal. Symptoms can be bilateral in up to 50% of cases.

    b. Radiographs. These are often normal.

    c. Treatment. Conservative treatment initially with rest, ice, and NSAIDs is appropriate. However, with documented elevation of compartment pressures, fasciotomy is often the treatment of choice.

    d. Complications. Chronic compartment syndrome is distinguishable from the more common stress fractures and overuse syndromes of the lower leg, since these often cause pain at rest without associated paresthesias.

D. Ankle

  1. **Sprains.** Ankle sprains are common athletic injuries and some 75% to 80% of sprains are of the inversion type, with injury to the lateral ligaments. However, the majority of significant ankle injuries occur with eversion, affecting the medial aspect and deltoid ligaments of the ankle.

    a. Examination. The position of the foot and ankle and direction of the injury are important historical events. The ability to bear weight after the episode with minimal pain and swelling is consistent with a first-degree injury. Walking with moderate pain and swelling is usually compatible with a second-degree injury. If the individual is unable to bear weight except with assistance or has a significantly altered gait, this suggests a severe second- or third-degree injury. Patients with a significant ankle injury often complain of an audible pop or snap. Often the individual has a history of previous ankle injuries.

b. **Radiographs.** Plain radiographs are indicated when there is significant tenderness, pain, and swelling or when instability is noted on ligament testing of the ankle. Special attention should be paid to the ankle mortise view and the symmetry of the talofibular and talotibial clear space, since any asymmetry of this clear space can be associated with significant ligamentous disruption. Even in the absence of fracture, this can represent significant ankle instability. Displaced malleolar fractures, medial malleolar, posterior malleolar, and bimalleolar fractures should all be considered unstable. Computed tomography (CT) and MRI are useful for evaluating complex fractures or suspected "occult" fractures about the ankle.

c. **Treatment.** RICE principles generally apply. In first- and second-degree injuries, the patient may benefit from an ankle orthosis such as a pneumatic or lace-up ankle splint for support and a rapid return to sport. Severe grade II and III injuries should be fully immobilized for several days and require appropriate follow-up, since they can lead to significant disability if an adequate rehabilitation program is not adhered to.

d. **Complications.** Persistence of pain and swelling 2 to 4 weeks after an "ankle sprain" should alert the physician to the possibility of an underlying osteochondral fracture, diastasis, or talar or subtalar subluxation. Osteochondral fractures typically involve the dome of the talus. CT and MRI are often useful in delineating such injuries.

2. **Achilles tendon rupture.** This is common in running and jumping sports. Athletes with a history of Achilles tendinitis or older individuals with degenerative tendon changes are at increased risk.

a. **Examination.** The athlete often presents with an acute onset of pain accompanied by a palpable pop or tearing sensation in the lower leg. Pain, swelling, and inability to plantarflex the foot are diagnostic. Thompson's test is positive. The patient will often describe feeling as if "I was kicked in the back of the leg."

b. **Radiographs.** Often normal. MRI is the diagnostic test of choice for evaluating the integrity of the Achilles tendon.

    c. **Treatment.** Emergency immobilization in the equinus position (30 degrees of plantarflexion) with avoidance of weight bearing. Surgical repair is usually advocated.

    d. **Complications.** Often the amount of pain and swelling inhibits the physician's ability to examine the Achilles tendon adequately; however, the tendon should be fully palpated so as not to miss this injury.

E. **Foot.** Foot injuries often accompany ankle injuries as the typical ankle sprain often injures the lateral proximal foot at the base of the fifth metatarsal.

    1. **Fifth metatarsal injuries.** Avulsion fractures at the base of the fifth metatarsal should be distinguished from a Jones fracture, which is a transverse fracture through the diaphysis of the fifth metatarsal.

        a. **Examination.** Both present with pain and swelling over the proximal lateral aspect of the foot with difficulty bearing weight.

        b. **Radiographs.** Avulsion fractures are evident as a fracture line through the tuberosity. The Jones fracture shows a horizontal fracture line through the diaphysis.

        c. **Treatment.** Avulsion fractures occur when the peroneal brevis tendon avulses its attachment at the base of the fifth metatarsal. Initial treatment involves the RICE principles along with immobilization with an ankle orthotic device, pneumatic or lace-up splint for 7 to 10 days followed by protected mobilization and rehabilitation. This is in contrast with the treatment of a Jones fracture, which can be treated conservatively with a short leg cast and avoidance of weight bearing for 6 to 8 weeks. In highly competitive athletes, however, surgical repair is the treatment of choice.

        d. **Complications.** A misdiagnosed Jones fracture can often lead to nonunion and chronic pain.

    2. **Stress fractures.** Stress fractures are common in running sports. Although the metatarsals are the most common location, stress fractures of the tarsal bones also occur.

        a. **Examination.** A history of repetitive use with pain and tenderness over the symptomatic area. Swelling or ecchymosis is rarely present.

        b. **Radiographs.** May demonstrate periosteal reaction or an incomplete fracture.

        c. **Treatment.** Avoidance of weight bearing and RICE principles.

        d. **Complications.** Complete fracture with nonunion if unrecognized.

BIBLIOGRAPHY

Brukner R, Khan K. *Clinical sports medicine.* Sydney, Australia: McGraw-Hill, 1993;8–25,337–371.

Mercier L. *Practical orthopaedics.* St Louis: Mosby, 1995:294–326.

Reid DC. *Sports injury and assessment.* New York: Churchill Livingstone, 1992.

Subject Index

Handbook of Orthopaedic Emergencies

Edited by
Raymond G. Hart, M.D., M.P.H., F.A.C.E.P.
Timothy James Rittenberry, M.D., F.A.C.E.P.
Dennis T. Uehara, M.D.

Written by experienced emergency department physicians, **Handbook of Orthopaedic Emergencies** includes 29 chapters covering essential information on orthopaedic principles and procedures and management of specific injuries throughout the musculoskeletal system and spine.

Plus, get specifics on:
- pediatric orthopaedics
- soft tissue injuries
- foreign bodies
- sports medicine
- and much more!

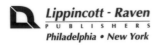
Lippincott · Raven
PUBLISHERS
Philadelphia · New York

ISBN 0-7817-1610-1

9 780781 716109

Orthopaedics